Jam Cornwell

Dr. BOERHAAVE'S

Academical Lectures

Ex Libr ON THE *T. Hussey*

Theory of PHYSIC.

BEING

A Genuine Tranflation of his

INSTITUTES

AND

Explanatory COMMENT,

Collated and adjufted to each other, as they were dictated to his STUDENTS at the Univerfity of *Leyden*.

VOL. I.

Containing the *Hiftory* of PHYSIC, and the Oeconomy of the feveral Parts fubfervient to *Chylification*.

The SECOND EDITION Corrected.

LONDON:

Printed for W. INNYS in *Pater-nofter Row*.

M DCC LI.

Crawford

THE

PREFACE.

Though the deserved Reputation of our learned Author, with the apparent Accuracy and Importance of this Work, may render any Apology for its Publication absolutely unnecessary; yet the Reader may perhaps expect some Reason for its appearing in this manner, collated and translated into English. For this, it is obvious to every one that knows any thing of our Author's Stile, that his great Concifeness, whereby he represents a Multitude of Idea's in a small Compass, is of it self more than sufficient to engage the whole Attention of tolerable Capacities, without any additional Embarassment from a Language, in which the English must be allowed to be less conversant than in their own; infomuch that a late eminent Writer in Physick * laments that the concise Accuracy wherewith our Author has

A 2   wrote

* Dr. Quincy, Lexic. Medic. under the Word *Institution* and *Aphorism*.

The PREFACE.

wrote fhould prevent his being generally read.
*It is therefore with a View of rendering this
Work of general Ufe to thofe who are unhappily
ignorant of the* Latin *Original, as well as to
facilitate it for fuch as are in fome meafure
acquainted therewith, that we have ftript off its
foreign Drefs, and adjufted the Text and Comment, by exhibiting them together; which laft
is an Advantage never yet offer'd to the Public
in any Language. So that the Candidate for
Phyfic is here prefented with the beft Method of
initiating himfelf into fo difficult a Profeffion,
that has ever yet, or will perhaps hereafter appear at any time in the World; containing not
only the whole Learning of the Ancients, but
alfo the immenfe Treafure of all our modern
Difcoveries relating to the Subject; and this
too in a Method and Language the moft eafy,
familiar, and intelligible; that tho' the Student
is now unfortunately deprived of being inftructed
by the Profeffor himfelf in Perfon, yet he may
hereby more leifurely and diftinctly reap the fame
Advantages, without either the Expence or Fa-
tigue of leaving his Country.*

*The Work in itfelf feems to be as well adapted
for the Service of the more Advanced as it is for
Beginners; fince the firft may be fatisfied with
refrefhing their Memories by reading the Text
only, which will to them appear fufficiently evident, without diving into the particular Notes,
that may be often found neceffary to inform the
younger Student; but if the Notes or Comment
fhould*

The PREFACE.

should appear to the former in any Place to be more defective, or less accurate than the Text, there is no Judge so severe, but will readily make some small Allowance, in consideration that the one was an extemporaneous, but the other a studied Discourse. To conclude: If the present Translation of the Text shall appear more correct than others, and the Publication of the Whole as generally useful as intended, it may encourage and hasten the Edition of the Remainder in the same manner with this first Volume.

THE

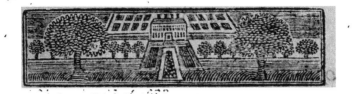

THE
CONTENTS.

Of

CONTENTS.

INTRO-

INTRODUCTION.

Concerning the Origin, Progress, and different States of Physic.

T H E Student that applies himself to Physic, is, from the Nature of the Science, obliged to be acquainted with every Truth that has been advanced in the several Branches of that Faculty, as well by the Ancients as the Moderns ; and when these are once apprehended, he ought carefully to add to 'em his own particular Observations ; registering them in his Mind, in the same Condition as they appear'd to his Senses.—To learn these Truths and Discoveries, he shou'd begin first with the *Institutions* of Physic ; which comprehend the Knowledge of every thing necessary for the Preservation of Health, and the Cure of Diseases. After which, he may proceed to the *Practice* ; which is the putting those Precepts, which he has before learned, in force upon his Pa-

B   tient.

tient.—The Ancients, and ſome of the Moderns, have injudiciouſly excluded every thing from the Inſtitutions of Phyſic, which has not ſome relation to the animal Oeconomy. But a Phyſician, who follows the Practice, ought certainly to be verſed in the medical Idiom or Language uſed by the practical Writers, if he wou'd underſtand what is offer'd to his Attention: and the ſudden Calls for his Aſſiſtance will not then admit of any Delays for Information. Thus the Hiſtory of Inflammation cannot be ſeparately underſtood, without a previous Idea of Obſtruction, joined with the whole Doctrine of the conical Artery, receiving Blood from the Heart. A Phyſician ought therefore to be furniſh'd with a juſt Notion of all Diſeaſes before he ventures upon the Practice; that when he comes to a Patient, he may readily diſcover his known Diſorders by their proper Signs.—But prefatory to theſe Inſtitutions, it ſeems agreeable to add an Introduction concerning the Hiſtory of Phyſic: for it muſt be well worth a Phyſician's Notice, to be acquainted with the Advances by which our Profeſſion has arrived at its preſent State; and no leſs entertaining to take a View of the ſeveral Faces with which Phyſic has appear'd in different Ages.

§. 1. The Perſon who can perform the ſeveral Actions proper to the human Body with Eaſe, Pleaſure, and a certain Conſtancy, is ſaid to be well; and that Condition of the Body is termed Health.

§. 2. But if he either cannot perform thoſe Actions; or if he performs them but with Difficulty, Pain and ſudden Wearineſs; he is
then

then faid to be ill : and that State of the Body is call'd a Difeafe.

The Contents of the two preceding Sections appear. fo fimple and common, that fome may imagine them not at all pertinent to the Art of Phyfic; yet they ought not to be neglected : for it is from the Inability itfelf to perform any of the Actions proper to the human Body, that we arrive at a Knowledge of the immediate Caufe of that Inability. Thus a Pain in breathing denotes a Pleurify ; an Inability to move any Limb at Pleafure, a Palfy, &c.—'Tis a good Cuftom among the *Turks*, that when they have called a Phyfician, they will not follow any of his Directions, till he has firft told the Patient what his Diforder is.

§. 3. Now the Injuries of Weather, with the fudden neceffary and unavoidable Changes in the *Air* [1] ; the Nature of folid and fluid *Aliment* [2] ; Accidents from *Violence* [3] ; the very Actions of *Life* [4] ; and even the *Structures* [5] of the human Body itfelf, muft have fubjected our Species to Diforders ever fince they have lived as *we do* [6].

[1] A Fluid, fo abfolutely neceffary to Life, that we cannot fubfift two Minutes without it ; yet is it fometimes fo deadly and peftiferous, that it often brings Difeafes, and Death itfelf, without any other Caufe.——The Air is a confufed Mixture of all Bodies. The Seeds of all Vegetables float in it. Gold itfelf, tho' fo ponderous, may afcend in it to the Height of fifty Foot ; which is demonftrated by Chemiftry. The Air is fill'd with the va-

rious *Exhalations* which afcend from the Earth,
fome of which arife in the Morning, others at
Noon ; but both very different from thofe which
defcend in the Night.—The *Stars* themfelves produce various Changes in the Air : the *Sun* and
Moon efpecially. have a great Influence on the Atmofphere. The freezing Nights fucceeding fultry
Days in *Mefopotamia*, were trying to the Conftitu-
tions of our Forefathers : tho' nothing cou'd be
more healthy than the temperate Air of *Ægypt* ;
but for *China* and *Eaft-India*, which were inhabited by the other fucceeding Families, the one is unhealthy by its Fogs, and the other by its violent
Heat.—To thefe add, the various Changes made
in the Air by the different Seafons of the Year,
Meteors and Winds, which are very frequent in
the hotteft Countries. The fudden Difference between a hot fultry Air, and a cold, heavy one, fo
much impedes Perfpiration, that it muft neceffarily caufe various Diforders, even fo as to kill nine
out of ten, if we may believe *Sanctorius*. The
nocturnal Air in particular muft have a very confiderable Effect on our Bodies ; becaufe in the
Night, the watery Vapours, raifed from the Earth
by the diurnal Heat, are condenfed and defcend
by their own Weight. I have known Men of *Her-
culean* Strength flung into incurable Rheumatifms
from the cold of one Night, which has been taken
by fleeping in the wet Grafs.—The Winter Air,
is more healthy than the Summer ; becaufe the fro-
zen Surface of the Earth keeps in the Vapors
which would otherwife afcend from it. But the
Earth opening its Pores in the Spring fends forth
its Exhalations, which are very pernicious to Mankind, if it were only by their inducing the fudden
Changes of Heat and Cold.

[a] Our

2 Our firſt Parents were ignorant of the Nature of Eſculent Plants, Fleſh and Garden Fruits; they made tryal upon all, and by woful Experience they learned to diſtinguiſh the deadly from the wholſome: As, in our Times, Sailors in their Voyages to remote Countries, run the Hazard of uſing unknown Aliments. And again, the Aliment which is healthy for a ſtrong Conſtitution in a cold Air, will be inſuparable to a weak Perſon in a warm Air. Nor were the firſt of Mankind ſenſible, till they had experienced, that by the taking of Cold, though pleaſant, Aliments into their Bodies while very hot, and in ſuch a warm Air, there was Danger of cauſing a preſent Pleuriſy and Death.

3 Falls, Strains, unforeſeen Accidents, Stones and Trees blown down by Tempeſts, &c. gave birth to Chirurgical Diſorders. The Want of Mechanical Engines, and the Irregularity of the Ways thro' dangerous Mountains, ſtill increaſed theſe Accidents among the firſt Race of Mankind. Nor was War ever ſilent for any conſiderable Time; ſince we are ſupplied with an Inſtance of it between *Cain* and *Abel*, two of the firſt three Men in the World.

4 The mere Actions of Life will conſume the Body equally with the moſt acute Diſeaſe: Hunger can be bore but for a few Days, and Thirſt but for a few Hours; if Matter is wanting in the Habit to ſupply the bodily Decays: And this Abſtinence kills the ſooner, as the Body is ſtronger and uſed to a more plentiful and ſubſtantial Diet. For the ſtronger the Habit of Body, it is ſo much the more obnoxious to the moſt acute Diſeaſes. A moſt ſevere Peſtilence may be cauſed in a Perſon barely by too much Motion of the Body. I ſaw

a Man

a Man that was order'd to carry Letters in hafte
to *Utrecht*, who, by exceffive running, fo forced
the groffer Parts of his Fluids into the fmaller Veffels, as to render the Obftructions incorrigible by
any Art. Reft and Motion of the Body fhou'd
never exceed proper Degrees, which was a Thing
altogether unknown among the firft Race of Mankind.

⁵ So fmall, thin and tender, are the greater Number of the Veffels in a human Body, that it is more
a Wonder they hold out as they do, then that they
are fo frequently difordered. The largeft Artery, in the Coats of the fmalleft fanguiferous
Artery, is equal to the tenth Part of the Thicknefs of a Spider's Thread : But that fmall Artery
is an *Aorta* with refpect to a fmall Artery in the
cortical Subftance of the Brain. Thro' the narrow
Orifices of thefe fmalleft Veffels the various Fluids
in our Bodies are continually propell'd with a very
great Velocity, by which Means there is a mutual
Attrition produced between the Parts of the circulating Fluids and the Sides of their Veffels, and
fo the Action of Life deftroys itfelf. Thofe Veffels
which we find fo very fmall in an Adult, were fo
much fmaller in the Fœtus as the Adult is larger
than the Fœtus : For in a Conception of but two
Weeks old, there are none of thofe Veffels wanting which will be poffefs'd by it when adult. How
eafily, then, may thefe tender Solids be difordered.

⁶ There is here no Occafion to enter into Doubts
about the State of Innocency, which feems to have
been fhort, and in which the human Body was not
fubject to the prefent Accidents, nor its Structure
the fame ; fince the Powers we now find in it feem
infufficient to preferve it in the State mention'd.

§. 4.

§. 4. The Species were no sooner thus in-fulted with Difeafes, but the Prefence of thofe Difeafes in the Body irritated it to exert a Sort of Mechanical Impulfe, or inconfcious *Automatic* [1] Motion, for their Removal: Which Sort of Automatic Endeavours of the Body to recover itfelf, are found by ftrict Ob-fervation to be exercifed as well in Brutes, as rational Animals; notwithftanding the Caufe of that Motion is undifcoverable by human Reafon, no other being affignable than the Will of the great Author of all Things.

[1] An Automaton is a Machine that performs various Motions without any other Caufe than the Mechanifm of its own Parts within itfelf; which, when once put in Motion, continue fo, from the fame Caufe. Thus a Watch is an Automaton, which, whilft in Order, moves round its Hands by the determinate Motion of its internal Parts. By an automatic Motion, or Impulfe, we there-fore underftand that Motion which refults from the mechanical Structure of the human Body, which we can neither produce nor deftroy by the Influence of the Mind or Will. It is certainly true, that fuch a kind of Motion does exift in our Bodies, how much foever it may be difpleafing to fome Philofophers. The human Body is an Affemblage of fmall elaftick Solids, by whofe conjunct and regular Actions, Life and Health are produced. The Head or firft Spring of Motion, in thefe elaftic Solids is the Heart, which continues its al-ternate Contractions and Dilatations fo long as the Animal lives. But even the fmaller elaftic Solids, which are every where continued throughout the

Body,

Body, have a Power by which they endeavour to
reſiſt and overcome every thing injurious to the
Oeconomy. Suppoſe a human Body, in a great
Heat by violent Motion, to be ſuddenly expoſed to cold: The Blood would certainly be, by
that means, coagulated and its Motion ſtopp'd in
the ſmaller Veſſels, if it were not for the Nature or
inſenſible Action of the Solids ; *viz.* a ſudden Contraction of all the cutaneous Pores, whereby they
exclude the injurious Action of the cold. When
Poiſon has been taken, the Animal muſt inevitably periſh, if its Force gets into the Blood, or its
Action continue long upon the Viſcera ; but provident Nature, or this automatic Motion generally
does, what every expert Phyſician ought firſt to
do, *i. e.* ejects it by Vomit. Nor is the Mind
able to ſuppreſs theſe automatic Endeavours of our
Machines for Self-preſervation. Suppoſe one
Friend tells another, that he is only going to
threaten him with a Blow upon the Eye ; and
therefore bids him endeavour not to ſhut it at the
Offer.: The Mind is at that Time ſecure from
Danger ; but the ſpecious Offer is no ſooner made,
than the Lids of that tender Organ are cloſed, notwithſtanding all the Reaſons and Reluctancy of the
Mind to the contrary. Suppoſe a Piece of Glaſs,
&c. enter thro' the ſkin, if it be not extracted, it
will by its Hardneſs and Acuteneſs always deſtroy
the ſoft Parts in contact ; therefore a Suppuration
follows, that the injurious Body may float in a Cavity full of inſenſible Matter, without offending the
Solids, and be afterwards diſcharged. The conjunct Power of all theſe Actions of the Body for
preſerving its own Health, which ariſes from the
wonderful Structure of its Parts, is what *Hippo-*
crates calls NATURE ; to which he aſcribes ſo many

ny and great Efficacies, and to mention one out of
a Multitude, the Crifes in acute Difeafes. There
is not any one Difeafe but receive Helps from
this automatic Motion, which is exerted throughout the whole Progrefs of a Diforder, tho' it be
inconfcious to the Mind.—Even this fame Principle is no lefs obfervable in Brutes. The Dog de-
vours Grafs to loofen his Inteftines, and expel
their dry and chalky Fæces ; nor will he eat any
kind of Vegetable but his own Sort of Grafs.
Poultry that live upon folid Grain, too compact
to be comminuted barely by the Strength of their
Stomachs, fwallow little Stones, which are rough,
and perform the Office of Teeth in their Stomachs,
upon that folid Aliment : And Poultry that are
fick generally retire into Holes, where they pick
Mortar from the Walls to obtund the offending
Acidity in their Stomachs.—In *Afia* there is a little
Animal in Figure like a Lion, which if it happens to be bit in its Conflict with the Viper, it has re-
courfe to a Plant called Mungos, upon which it
tumbles and revives itfelf ; and then brifkly returns
to the Serpent and overcomes it : Nor were Men
acquainted with the alexipharmic Virtue of this
Plant by any other means.—So *Melampus*, the
moft ancient of the *Greek* Phyficians, of *Argos*,
when he obferved that Sheep who fed on black
Hellebore had a Loofenefs, he transferr'd the Ufe
of that Medicine for the like Purpofe in Men, and
the Plant for many Ages after bore the Name
Melampodes. By thefe Methods Mankind doubt-
lefs acquired a confiderable Notion in Healing.
—In like manner the ufeful Hœmorrhages which
naturally broke out in acute Difeafes, encouraged
Phlebotomy ; a Remedy which muft of itfelf appear otherwife threatning and cruel.—If a little

Sand

Sand falls into the Eye, we find the Eye-lids are quickly and ftrongly contracted, and the Eye by that means thruft further into the Orbit ; whence the large lacrymal Gland being comprefs'd by it, a Stream of Tears follow to wafh out the Sand, and abate the Inflammation caufed by the Friction and Pain in that tender Organ. But what can be more fimple and eafy than to imitate Nature, by injecting fome warm and mild Liquor, to wafh out the foreign Bodies and abate the Inflammation caufed by their Roughnefs.

2 In vain muft a Phyfician endeavour to account for an Appearance in Nature, the Caufes of which he is ignorant ; as we are affured by the different Effects of Medicines. The human Body has a Faculty of rejecting every thing foreign to its Nature, in common with all Animals, Vegetables, and even Metals ; for Gold in its Element, or Mine, will not join itfelf to any thing that will not turn to Gold. The Facts are certain, and obferved by the Refearchers of Nature ; but in vain do we ftrive to explain their Caufes.

§. 5. Another Principle differing from the former, was the uneafy Senfation in the Mind, caufed by the impeded Action itfelf of any Member ; or the Torment of Pain, irritating any diforder'd Part, and oppreffing the Mind with Grief: This excited the Mind alfo to fearch after, and apply Remedies fit to remove thofe Impediments ; which Remedies were hit upon either by natural Inftinct, or by promifcuous Experiments.

Thefe Endeavours of the Mind proceed from its being impatient of Pain, ftriving by all the
Means

Means it can think of to obtain Eaſe : nor is it a
Principle in common with, but quite diſtinct from
that of the automatic Motions of the Body, §. 4.
—Theſe Endeavours of the Mind for Eaſe are reducible to two Claſſes. To the firſt belong *pro-
miſcuous Experiments made without Reaſon or Obſervation :* as by ſtriving to eaſe a Part by variouſly
changing its Situation, applying any thing to a
Wound or Burn that comes firſt to hand, *&c.* —
When any thing falls into the Eye, a Stream of
Tears will flow from the automatic Motion, to
waſh it out ; but the Mind being uneaſy at the
Senſe of Pain, will alſo uſe its Endeavours by various Trials ; as applying the Hand to the Eye,
and rubbing the Eye-lids, *&c.* and ſo forwards
the Actions of the preceding. If a Perſon has a
Pain in his Side, he will diſpoſe himſelf in various
Situations till he acquires the moſt eaſy. And
when any of theſe Trials have proved ſucceſsful,
they will be remember'd and talk'd of by the Patient : and hence aroſe the firſt Rudiments of Phyſic. —The other Claſs of theſe Endeavours of the
Mind for Eaſe, is, when it oppoſes Diſorders with
Remedies to which it is directed by *Reaſon, Obſervation, or the Nature of Things.* Thus the beſt
Remedy for a Man fatigued with great Heat and
violent Exerciſe, is what will dilute the Blood and
mitigate the Acrimony to which its Salts are incli-
ning ; but if we attend to the Appetite, we ſhall
find it deſires for this purpoſe a cool, watery and
acidulated Drink. And as moſt Men die from the
Want of Fluidity and Obſtruction of the Blood ;
it frequently happens, that from this Appetite the
Sick will have a ſtrong Deſire for cold Water before
Death ; the careleſs Phyſician at that time neglect-
ing to take notice of the Appetites, which point to

the

the immediate Cause of the Disease. These Endeavours belong to the Mind; and even in Brutes we cannot attribute them to the Body: for the Body of a Person asleep, or in an Apoplexy, takes no Concern for Aliment, or other Wants. There are many extraordinary Appetites to uncommon Food, in several Disorders, to be attributed to this Principle; which Disorders are by that means frequently brought to a Period. A Person in an acute Fever longs for Grapes, or to be in the Cold; his Friends dissuade him, his Attendants deny them to him: however, he happens to get his long'd-for Dainty, and returns with his languid Fibres braced up, or a loose Belly, discharging the obstructing Viscidities; and thus gets well. A rich Patient of *Amsterdam*, and a liberal Rewarder of the Faculty, longed for pickled Herrings: his Physicians refused them; yet he ventured on 'em, and was cured: the History is extant in *Tulpius*; and there are a hundred Instances of the like Nature, in Dropsies, intermitting Fevers, &c. to be met with in the Writers of Observations. The Girl that has a Chlorosis eats Chalk, Fuller's Earth, or other earthy Substances which obtund Acidities: this Appetite is bad with respect to a healthy Body; but in that present Disorder it directs to a proper Remedy. There are so many Histories of Success in most Disorders from the Gratification of longing Appetites, that I think a Physician ought not inconsiderately to deny them. Nor ought any body to accuse me from hence, with having supposed our Machines to be acted by a sort of fatal Necessity, contrary to a free Agency. I only deduce Consequences from Facts, and assert what I have experienced; being first certain of their Causes and Effects: than which, I know no other way to Knowledge.

§. 6. From

§. 6. From thefe Principles (§. 4, and 5.)
the Art of Phyfic or Healing took its firft
Rife; and in that Senfe (§. 4, and 5.) it was
at all Times and in all Places practifed by
Mankind.

Natural Phyfic, as defcrib'd at §. 4, and 5. was
practifed by Mankind at all Times and in all Places; for the Species were never exempt from Diforders (*per* §. 3.) and Means to remove thofe Diforders were fought after in all Ages (*per* §. 5.)
therefore natural Phyfic was always in Practice;
and no Man was ever deprived of natural Inftinct.
But the Art of Phyfic eftablifh'd by human Knowledge is of a much later Date, for there were not
always People who imitated and improved the
Method of Healing barely founded on Nature.
But human Minds are not limited to the Sphere of
Inftinct, which only confiders prefent Objects, for
that is the State of Brutes; but by comparing paft
Objects with thofe that are prefent, it can attain
to the Knowledge of future Events. From an
Obfervation of the Appearances in the Heavens,
continued feveral Ages, arofe the Art of Aftronomy; till at length they could as certainly foretel
an Eclipfe Ten Years to come, as the daily rifing
and fetting of the Sun. In the fame manner began Phyfic, when a Perfon could diftinguifh Difeafes, and had obferved what good Events had
happen'd in them from Art, Accident, or Nature;
whence he could infer and fafely pronounce, " a
" Hundred have been cured of the Difeafe which
" appears with thefe Signs, by fuch a Medicine;
" and it will be fo in you, my Patient." This
Art of predicting might be greatly favour'd by the
Longævity

Longævity of our Forefathers, by which they were capable of an infinite Number of Experiments, and fo might be furnifh'd with an infinite Number of Cafes by their own Memories, which our fhort-liv'd Generation is obliged to fupply from the ftanding Obfervations of others.

§. 7. From the moft early Accounts of *Hiftory* [1] and Fable, we learn that the Art of Phyfic or Healing was firft cultivated, fo as to prevent future and cure prefent Difeafes, amongft the *Affyrians, Babylonians, Chaldeans* [2], and *Magi*; from thefe it came into *Egypt* [3], *Lybia, Cyreniaca* [4], and *Croto* [5]; and thence it was carried into *Greece* [6], where it principally flourifh'd in the Peninfula of *Cnidos* [7], and the Iflands of *Rhodes* [8], *Cos* [9], and *Epidaurus* [10].

[1] It is no eafy matter to determine the Time when Phyfic firft appeared as an Art, or, which is the fame, when a felect Number of Men took upon them the Care of their Fellow-Citizens Health; yet we ought to diftinguifh or clafs the Times of its Advances according to the Accounts given us. The firft and moft early of which we can only guefs at from the nature of the thing, having no Accounts of thofe Men and their Tranfactions this way. The fecond is fabulous, the Monuments of which we poffefs, but deform'd with Rhetoric, and other arbitrary Ornaments. And the third is hiftorical, taken from the Commentaries of ferious and learned Hiftorians.— It is probable that before and after the Flood there were a few old Sages

more

more particularly curious and delighted with examining their own and others Diforders than the
reft, who from their Curiofity made ftill better
Obfervation of what ufually caufed and cured thofe
Diforders ; that there were fuch, we learn from
Fable, the moft ancient Kind of Hiftory, which
tells us of one *Phœbus* or *Solus* in this Character ;
but this *Phœbus* was *Horus* King of the *Affyrians*,
who, according to *Pliny*, was the Inventor of a
particular Medicine ; and the word *Horo* fignify-
ing Light in the oldeft of Languages, *Hebrew*, does
alfo confirm that he and *Phœbus* were the fame. ——
But it is probable that the Art of Healing took its
firft Rife in *Mefopotamia*, or not far from it, becaufe there was the Birth or firft Seat of Mankind,
and there was fix'd the firft Kingdom that was framed ; in that happy and temperate Region our
long-liv'd Forefathers invented moft Arts. But
from thence Phyfic paffed with Aftronomy and
Languages into *Phœnicia*, and from *Phœnicia* it
might fpread into *Egypt* ; but that *Egypt* did not
produce the firft Cultivators of Arts, may be judg'd
from the Nature of the Country, which was unin-
habitable till they had made it fo by artificial Motes
and Banks. And even many Ages after that, in
Affyria, we find the Art no further advanced than
for one Neighbour to help another in his Illnefs ;
which was the firft Method of practifing Phyfic.

² The *Chaldeans* were the firft Colonies that fet-
tled in *Affyria*, and their Rulers and Judges were
called *Magi*, who formed the Precepts of their
Knowledge into Verfes, being Mafters of every
Science ; fince their very Kings were not permitted to rule unlefs they had been learned of the
Magi, as we are informed by *Pliny*. Among thefe
Magi, *Zoroafter* was one of the moft confiderable,
whom

whom Superſtition has rank'd among the Number of diabolical Sorcerers, thro' the perverted or miſtaken Senſe of the Name *Magi*, or Magicians; much in the ſame manner as the *Romans*, hating the ſeditious and threatning Enquiries of Aſtrologers, expell'd all that bore the Name of Mathematician out of *Italy*. Length of Time has buried from us the Learning of the *Chaldeans* in Oblivion. The vaſt Number of Books which contained the Learning of the Eaſtern Nations, ſhared the Fate of periſhing with their regal Cities, as *Niniva*, *Jeruſalem*, *Babylon*, *Perſepolis*, and *Alexandria*; what now remains to us is but little, and muſt either be taken from *Herodotus*, or deduced from Conjecture. The Writings we poſſeſs of *Sanchoniathon* and *Beroſus* on this Head are imperfect, and for the earlieſt Part of their Hiſtory, we have no Account but in the ſacred Scripture. The oldeſt Hiſtorian is *Moſes*, next to his follows the Book of *Joſhua*, then the Author of the Books of *Kings*, and the *Apocrypha*; and after them come the Writings which remain to us of *Sanchoniathon*, which to our great Trouble are very imperfect. At a long Interval from the preceding came *Herodotus*, who was followed by *Thucydides* and *Xenophon*. That there were Phyſicians in the Eaſtern Parts, is confirmed by the Accounts of *David* (1 *Kings* i. 3, 4, 5.) and *Aſa* (2 *Chron.* xvi. 14.) but that they were not famous in the Time of the *Perſian* King *Darius Hyſtaſpis*, ſeems to follow from his not ſending for his own Country, but *Egyptian* Phyſicians when he had luxated his Foot.

⁵ The *Egyptians* made great Advances in Phyſic; for their Prieſts, who were Interpreters between the Gods and Men, and even their Kings, approved of the opening of dead Bodies, to find

out

out the Caufes of Death ; but that and the reft of their Sciences they kept as hidden Secrets, wrapt up and conceal'd in obfcure Figures or Hierogly-phics. That the Office of Phyfician was very an-cient among the *Egyptians*, may be learn'd from the facred Scripture, where it tells us, that when *Jacob* dy'd in *Egypt* his Body was embalm'd by *Jofeph*'s Phyficians. But that the Number of their Phyficians was very great, will appear from but one fingle Part of the Body being affign'd for the Province of one Phyfician ; fome took upon them the Care of the Eyes, others the Ears, and others different Parts of the Body ; fpending their whole Lives in the Knowledge and Cure of the Diforders of each Part, and being fubjected to Punifhments or Rewards according as they acted : fo that *Egypt* proved another native Country to Phyfic, from whence the great *Plato, Thales, Laertius*, and par-ticularly *Democritus*, and all *Greece*, acquired their Skill, according to their own Confeffions. The *Egyptian* Learning fuffered greatly by the cruel Wars under the *Pharaoh Necho's, Hophra*, and *Pfaminenites*, when *Egypt* was firft fubdued by the *Affyrians*, and afterwards by the *Perfians* ; info-much that the *Egyptian* Phyficians belonging to the Court with Difficulty efcaped the Sword, at the Requeft of *Democedes* of *Croto*, when they had in vain attempted to reduce the luxated Foot of King *Darius*, Son of *Hyftafpes*. But afterwards *Egypt* afpired to its former Glory in this Science, when in following Ages, flourifh'd *Herophilus, Erafiftratus, Ammonius, Diofcorides*, and others, who were fo well fkill'd in all the Parts of Phyfic, that fuch as defired any Knowledge in that Fa-culty, reforted to learn of them from all the Countries around them.

C ⁺ *Cyreniaca*

⁴ *Cyreniaca* was a happy Province amidſt the barren Sands, which produced, among other Philoſophers of celebrated Name, *Ariſtippus*, *Eratoſthenes*, *Callimachus*, and *Carneades*; but no conſiderable profeſs'd Phyſician : tho' after the *Crotonians*, the *Cyrenians* were firſt concern'd in Phyſic there. In that Place alſo grew the famous Plant *Silphium*, which was expreſs'd, as a particular Gift of the Gods, upon the Coin of *Battus*, the *African* King, who built *Cyrene*.

⁵ At *Croto* flouriſhed the *Pythagorean* School, which produced the Phyſician *Democedes* ; who, upon the Slaughter of the Tyrant *Samius Polycrates*, whom he attended, was brought into *Perſia*, where he recovered the luxated Foot of *Darius* by applying Mallows, after it had been made more difficult to cure by the bad Treatment of the *Egyptian* Phyſicians. There he alſo cured an Ulcer in the Breaſt of *Atoſea* ; but being advanc'd with much Wealth and Honour, he affectionately return'd afterwards to his own Country, charged with the Embaſſy of the firſt *Perſian* War. But when the Philoſophers were expell'd from *Croto*, and the *Pythagorean* School burnt thro' Malice, another was erected at *Metapontus*.

⁶ Phyſic ſeems to have paſſed into *Greece* from *Egypt* in the Time of King *Amaſis*, under whom *Egypt* drove a conſiderable Commerce with *Greece*, as we are inform'd by the *Attic* Laws brought out of *Egypt* by *Solon*. The Fame of Phyſic in *Greece* was very inconſiderable at firſt ; the moſt ancient Phyſician that was a Native *Greek*, ſeems to have been *Melampus*, who having found out the Nature of Hellebore by obſerving its Effects on Goats, cured the Daughters of King *Proetus* of an hyſteric Phrenzy, which made them imagine themſelves

changed

changed into Cows, leaving afterwards his own Name to that falutary Plant.

⁷ *Cnidos* was a City in the leffer *Afia*, which feems to have taken the Art of Phyfic from their neighbouring *Affyrians*; in that City flourifhed a celebrated medicinal School, as *Galen* tells us, whofe Methods of Healing are often quoted by *Hippocrates*, who has from thence referved to us many Monuments concerning the ancient State of Phyfic; and this probably may give Rife to that falfe Reflection upon this Father of Phyfic, *viz.* that *Hippocrates* ftole his Obfervations from the *Cnidian* Temple, and afterward fet it on Fire to conceal his Plagiary, by which he appropriated the Wifdom of his medical Anceftors to his own Pen. But the *Cnidian* Phyfic feemed principally to confift in a ftrict Obfervation of the antecedent and confequent Symptoms of Difeafes, without deducing any Indications from them, or referring particular Difeafes to their general Caufes; for which *Hippocrates* defervedly reprehends them.

⁸ *Rhodes* was an Ifland celebrated for the Ingenuity of its Citizens; for their Study in Navigation, and the Healthinefs of its Air, being *Tiberius*'s wifh'd-for Place of Exile; it fome Time enjoy'd a very ancient School of Phyficians, which was fo much decay'd and forgot in the Time of *Hippocrates*, that he does not once mention it.

⁹ *Cos* was the Ifland where the firft School of the *Afclepiads* was fixed; concerning which we fhall be more particular in our Account of *Hippocrates*, §. 13 and 14.

¹⁰ At *Epidaurus* we are told *Æfculapius* was born, where the Worfhip of that God was very ancient and famous, inafmuch as the God himfelf frequently performed Miracles; but when a raging Peftilence came to *Rome*, he fixed his Seat there. In

the Temple of the ſalutary God, the Sick, who
came far and near, uſed to ſleep, and receive their
divine Advice in Dreams.——The State of Phyſic, as we have hitherto traced it, was wholly empirical ; and this Period of it may be conſidered
as its Infancy.

§. 8. The firſt Foundation of Phyſic (as
yet empirical) was therefore raiſed, 1. By
accidental Diſcoveries 1, made without any
Deſign. 2. By natural *Inſtinct* 2. And, 3.
By unexpected or extraordinary *Events* 3.
Which were the firſt Sources of Empiriciſm,
or ſimple Experience.

1 Hereby we intend the Knowledge of unuſual
Effects from ſeveral Cauſes, by ſome Variation,
which the Mind could not diſcern to be ſufficient
in the Agent. Thus Men found that cold Water,
tho' the moſt harmleſs of any Drink, being drank
when the Blood was in a heat, would cauſe a Pleuriſy, and even Death. And ſo the Inhabitants of
Cairo found only by Experience, that when the
Nile overflowed its Banks, on the ſame Day the
Plague would decline and ceaſe.

2 By *Inſtinct* we here underſtand thoſe auxiliary
Means reſulting both from the automatic Motions
of the Body (§. 4.) and the ſpontaneous Endeavours of the Mind (§. 5.): not indeed the Conſequence of human Reaſon, yet ſufficiently conſiderable, and not unworthy to be examin'd into.

3 Theſe *Events* are Effects contrary to the received Opinions of Men ; as if a Perſon in a Fever, who was ſtrictly forbidden all Garden Fruits,
ſhould recover his Health by eating plenty of
Grapes ; or as if the Ancients having experienc'd
the

the cold Air of Service in inflammatory Fevers, should use the same with fatal Consequence in a Pleurisy.

§. 9. The Art thus imperfectly establiſhed, was soon improved and enlarged. 1. By remembering the Succeſs of the Experiments which had been made in it (*per* §. 8.) 2. By regiſtering a Deſcription of the ſeveral Diſeaſes, the Remedies, and their Operations; which were engrav'd upon the Pillars, Tables, and Walls of the *Temples* [1]. And, 3. By expoſing the Sick in the public Markets and High-ways, in order for thoſe who paſſed by to examine them concerning their Diſorders; that if they had known any thing effectual in the like Diſtemper, they might acquaint them with it, and adviſe them the ſame; and hence aroſe Obſervation, deſignedly made to remark the Events of Medicines and Diſeaſes. And thus Empiriciſm, or the Practice of Phyſic by mere Obſervation, became more perfect from each of theſe Principles (§. 8, 9.) tho' as yet the Faculty could only diſtinguiſh the paſt and preſent Events. But the Art was alſo advanced, 4. by *Reaſoning* [2], from comparing the Events obſerved (*per* §. 8, 9.) with the preſent Circumſtances and conſequent Effects which was termed Analogy.

[1] It was a laudable Cuſtom that obtain'd among the Ancients, for any one that eſcaped ſome imminent Danger, to record the Hiſtory of their Preſervation in the Temple dedicated to the Dei-

ty

ty to whom such Preservation was thought owing; thus it was after escaping Shipwrecks, and recovering from Diseases, that a History of the Disease, the Advice, and Means of Cure, might be expressed to future Ages in a Table devoted to that Use. These Tables were the first Books that contained any medical Prescriptions, and Cases, or Histories of Diseases. With Monuments of this kind were filled the Roof and Walls of the Temple at *Epidaurus:* Things certainly of more Use, than the pompous Monuments and flattering Accounts of People which in these Ages make the Ornaments of our religious Buildings.

² When any Body passed by the Bed of a sick Person exposed in some public Place for Advice, they asked what his Disorder was? The Answer might be probably, an acute Fever; the Passenger upon this recalling to mind whether himself or any Acquaintance had been ill, and cured of the like Disease by any Remedy, bleeding, &c. the like Means was then recommended to the Patient on his own Experience; and thus Analogy made another and more perfect kind of Practice in Medicine, which even the Empirics themselves cannot practise without; for notwithstanding they so much condemn Reasoning in Physic, they secretly call in its Assistance.

§. 10. The Art in some measure thus (§. 9.) establish'd, was further improved and perfected, (1.) By appointing certain Persons as *Physicians* ¹ for the Cure of only one or a whole Class of Diseases. (2.) By those Physicians taking exact Accounts or *Histories of* the several *Cases* ² or Disorders which came under their Care. And, (3.) By their accurately observing and

and defcribing the feveral *Remedies* 3 applied,
with their Operations and Ufes.——Phyfic being thus hereditary in but a few Families, and
engroffed 4 by a fmall Number of Hands, efpecially among the Priefts, it brought them
much Honour and Wealth, tho' the Art itfelf
was by that means extremely cramp'd in its
Advancement.

¹ Certain Priefts were appointed by the common Laws among the *Egyptians* for the Practice
of Phyfic, who had an Income for their Service
at the Public Expence, and were confined in their
Practice under particular Reftrictions. As, (1.)
That no one prefume to practife beyond the Bounds
of the particular Difeafe or Clafs which had been
made his Province, but that each profefs and act
only for the Cure of fuch Diforders as had been
cuftomary for his Family. That (2.) every Phyfician practife agreeable to the Books of *Hermes*,
and not to act otherwife at his Peril; but to be
under certain Penalties for male Practice. That
(3.) no Phyfician prefume to excite Evacuations
till the fourth Day of a Difeafe. That none but
Glyfters and gentle Remedies be ufed before the
third Day in Fevers, ftrictly refraining from Vomits and Purges. That (4.) none but Phyficians
prefume to practife Medicine.—Thus Phyfic muft
have evidently received confiderable Advances a-
mong this wife, rich, and flourifhing People, who
fo ftudioufly endeavour'd to cultivate it.

² Great was the Accuracy and Induftry of the
Ancients in their medical Obfervations, or Accounts of Difeafes; they patiently and carefully remark'd not only the paft and prefent Condition of
the Difeafe, but alfo the Patient's Age, Sex, Habit,

bit, Strength, and Diet; yet fo little were they addicted to Hypothefes, precarious Reafonings, and
drawing Conclufions from their Obfervations, that
Hippocrates reprehends them for Timidity in thofe
Refpects.

3 The Medicines of that Age were taken chiefly
from Plants; in the gathering and preparing of
which the Ancients were extremely induftrious, as
we may judge from the *Cratonic* Epiftle of *Hippocrates*, where he very minutely points out the native Soil, Time of gathering, and Method of keeping Hellebore.

4 The Priefts, being covetous of Wealth and
Reverence from the People, and in order to increafe the Refpect and Number of their Patients,
concealed the Art under the Pomp of Superftition
and Fable; by thefe Means depriving the Public
of its Benefits, they referv'd the Art as a Secret to
themfelves and Families.——Thus when *Iphiclus*
afk'd the Advice of *Melampus* for Impotency, after
the fpecious Apparatus of Sacrifices and Augury,
he ordered him the Ruft of a Knife that had been
ftuck into an Oak; by this formidable, but vain
Shew of Religion, he endeavour'd to conceal that
fimple Preparation of Steel, which had been flowly
diffolved by the acid Juice of the Tree, and was
certainly a moft excellent corroborating Medicine.
A military Captain, who had a fpitting of Blood,
befought *Æfculapius* for a Remedy; the Priefts,
who were verfed in Phyfic, anfwer'd, inftead of the
God, " that he muft take the Kernels of Pine-
" Apples mixed with Honey," a very proper
Medicine; by which he was cured.——Even *Hippocrates* himfelf bound his Pupils by an Oath not to
divulge the Myfteries of their Profeffion to the
profane Commonality. But throughout the whole
Univerfe Phyfic was originally practifed by hardly
                                                    any

any but the Priefts ; thus it was among the *Jews*
and *Egyptians* ; in the Ifland *Lemnos*, where the
Priefts of *Vulcan* practifed Phyfic ; among the
Indians, whofe Priefts were diftinguifhed by the
ancient Name of *Brachmans* ; and laftly, among
the *French* and *Germans*, where they were called
Druids.

§. 11. Add to thefe (§. 9, 10.) that (1.) the
Infpections of Carcafes by Priefts in their daily *Sacrifices* [1], (2.) the Cuftom of *embalming* [2]
and opening the Dead, (3.) the Infpection of
Wounds, happening in all Ages, and (4.)
laftly, the dreffing of Carcafes by the *Butcher* [3],
each afforded fome Knowledge of the anatomical Structure of found Bodies as alfo of the
immediate and abftrufe Caufes of Health,
Sicknefs, and Death.

[1] Sacrificing was a religious Rite among the
firft of Mankind, as we learn from our Accounts
of *Abel* and *Noah* in the facred Hiftory ; and from
the very ancient, though fabulous Account, of the
golden Age. But as no Sacrifice would make
Atonement, or pleafe the Deity, but fuch as were
made of Victims perfectly found, therefore the
Priefts were obliged to be follicitous in their En-
quiry after the Signs of their perfect Health, and
to learn what States of the Vifcera imported that
the Animal was unfound, being to anfwer for the
Succefs or Mifcarriage of his Oblation from the
morbid or healthy Appearance of their Fibres.

[2] The Cuftom of *Embalming* is very ancient,
even before the Time of *Jofeph* ; in order to which
they were obliged to open the Body, take out the
Vifcera, and fill up their Spaces with a Compofition

tion of Spices; but all this could hardly be done for many Ages together, without frequently detecting the latent Caufes of the moft fevere Difeafes, as well as the Structure and Situation of the Parts; and hence the firft Foundation of *practical Anatomy.*

^s The Butcher diffecting brute Animals, could not avoid feeing the natural State, Situation, Number, Figure, &c. of their Vifcera, and various Humours; but frequent and deftructive War afforded Opportunities of difcovering many of the Mufcles and larger Veffels, with the Articulations of Bones, to the naked Eye in the yet living Subject; infomuch that fome have attempted to extract a Syftem of Anatomy from *Homer*, who has in reality writ Hiftories of Wounds fkilfully and anatomically ftated.

§. 12. And laftly, the Art feems to have been in a manner compleated, (1.) By the Diffection of *living Animals* [1] made with a philofophical View, and an accurate Infpection of human Bodies after they had been kill'd by fome Difeafe. (2.) By taking a more exact Acccount of the Caufes of Diftempers, diftinguifhing their Stages into Beginning, Increafe, Height, and Decreafe, Terminations, Variations, and different Symptoms. (3.) By a more perfect Knowledge of Medicines, artfully chufing, preparing, and applying them; having firft obferv'd their Strength and Operations.

[1] *Democritus*, being fkill'd in the Learning of the *Egyptians* and *Phœnicians*, fpent a long Life in Experiments, particularly in the Diffection of

Brutes,

Brutes, to difcover the Caufes and Seats of Difeafes. The living Diffection of brute Animals alone
afforded always the greateft Advances to Phyfic;
without this neither would *Herophilus* have difcovered the lacteal Veffels in Kids, *Euftachius* and
Pecquet their *Receptaculum Chyli*, and thoracic
Duct in the Horfe and Dog; nor *Harvey* his celebrated Circulation of the Blood. But thefe Diffe-
ctions were made with a double View, one merely
in the way of common Butchery; the other with
a View to Philofophy and Phyfic, *Democritus*
feems alfo to have joined Mathematics with his
phyfical Experiments, having wrote of Gravity, a
Vacuum, and the Elements.

§. 13. At length *Hippocrates* [1], in the fame
Age with *Democritus*, being well fkill'd in all
thefe (§. 7, to 13.) Particulars, and furnifh'd
with numerous wife Obfervations of his own
as well as of others, form'd the beft of them
into a *Greek* Syftem of Phyfic; and was the
firft that truly deferved the title of Phyfician:
for being of incomparable Reafon and ample
Experience, fupported by a found Philofophy,
he laid a juft and rational Foundation of Phyfic for future Ages.

[1] *Hippocrates* was a Man of happy Genius and
great Learning, verfed in the Philofophy of *Democritus*, which was the pureft of any Syftem, being founded on three Principles, Atoms, Gravity,
and a Vacuum; which have been in our Age again
reftored by the moft folid Reafonings of Sir *Ifaac
Newton*. Being defcended from the great *Æfculapius*, the medical Knowledge of his Anceftors in a
manner glow'd and improv'd in his Blood from the
very

very Birth; he imbib'd the Learning of the School at *Cnidos* and of the *Egyptians* in his Travels; so wealthy, that he is said to have sent his Son *Thessalus* with a Ship armed and freighted with Medicines as a Gift, to attend the *Athenian* Fleet in their Voyage to *Sicily*. He had under him a Class of young Physicians, who were employ'd in making Experiments; which, when communicated to *Hippocrates*, he shew'd the Use of them to Physic. In his Practice he succeeded beyond any Mortal, being requited with divine Honours for his Service in the Plague at *Athens* and *Thessalia*. He was no inconsiderable Anatomist, tho' he did not publish his Writings on that Subject; for he learn'd the Structure of human Bodies from a careful Dissection of their Parts, and observed that the *Intestinum jejunum* was almost empty of Aliment. He was so well skill'd in Surgery, that the Merit of no one comes up to him. He seems to have been a Lover of the Mathematics, from the Letter to his Son *Thessalus*. When he asserts Philosophy to be useless with regard to Physic, he speaks of moral Philosophy, upon which alone the *Pythagorean* School was then employ'd. He made himself well acquainted with the Opinions of his preceding and contemporary Physicians, and was the first that by just Reasoning joined the Theory to Practice in Physic. He has given us such Histories of Diseases from his own Practice and Observation, illustrated with the Experiments of his Pupils, as may vie with the best of our Moderns; and especially in acute Diseases, as the Pleurisy, Phrensy, Quinsy, &c. he has been so ample, that his Successors to this Day can add but little; to be satisfied in this, any body may, like *Duretus*, compile an Index of the Particulars relating to one Disease interspersed thro' the Writings of *Hippocrates*,

crates, and afterwards let them be compared with what is given us on the like Difeafe by other Authors. His Works have been revifed by *Aretæus*, but more perfectly by *Galen*. ⁝⁝⁝ ⁝ ⁝⁝⁝ ⁝⁝

§. 14. This Work of *Hippocrates* continued improving among the *Afclepiads* [1], and was afterwards digefted into a more regular Method by *Aretæus* [2]; and being ftill further improved at various Times by feveral Artifts in different Countries, it was brought into the School of *Alexandria*, and came at laft into the Hands of *Galen*.

[1] The Defcendants of *Æfculapius* preferved the Doctrines of *Hippocrates* entire to the Time of *Tiberius* and *Galen*. The whole Family being thus blefs'd with the rich Treafure of Obfervations that had been made and left them by their Anceftors, and being alfo furnifh'd each with their own Knowledge and Experiments, were by thofe Means informed how to moderate Nature; to excite her Forces when languifhing, and to reftrain her Powers when too violent. They learn'd the Virtues of Medicines not from fuperftitious Writings, but from the real Facts and Experiments of many Ages. —— Their Method of Practice was like what follows: they knew by Experience that a Pleurify, accompany'd with particular Appearances in the Spittle, Refpiration, Heat and Pain, ufually ended in a fatal Mortification within the Space of three Days; but they found it had been alfo obferv'd by one of their Anceftors, that a Patient in the fame Cafe recover'd by profufe bleeding from a Wound till he fainted, whereas others in the like Difeafe perifh'd at the fame time; therefore imitating the

Advice

Advice of Nature, they bled plentifully, and exhibited lenient, watery, and diluent Medicines; which Method they found to fucceed the beft in all acute or inflammatory Cafes. But they alfo learned by the Obfervations of their Anceftors, that a Pleurify attended with a free Refpiration, a thick Spittle, with little Particles of Blood, and other Circumftances of Heat and Pain, imported that the Difeafe would terminate the firft Day; in which Cafe they therefore left the Difeafe to Nature; for they had found bleeding under thefe Circumftances to fupprefs the fpitting, prolong the Difeafe, and render it more dangerous.

² Before *Aretæus* we ought to have given *Herophilus* and *Erafiftratus* their due Praife, as two fkilful Improvers of Anatomy. *Herophilus* is even faid to have diffected three hundred human Bodies, many of which, being Criminals, were opened alive: No wonder then he fhould perceive white Veins (*i. e.* the Lacteals) in the Mefentery; which, by the way, is an Argument that the Anatomy of the *Greeks* was not fo fuperficial as many have imagined. *Erafiftratus* wifely obferved, that an Inflammation happen'd whenever the Blood paffed out of its proper Veffels into thofe which only convey Spirits, meaning the Lymphatics. But thefe curious Writings perifh'd in the Conflagration of the *Ptolemæan* Library, which happen'd in the time of (the firft or) *Julius Cæfar*. The Library was founded by King *Ptolemeus Philadelphus*, and was fupported by the fucceeding Kings in *Alexandria*, to which City the moft fkilful Men in all Arts were folicited at the public Charge. *Alexandria* was frequented by the Learned of every Nation, for the Promotion of Learning, and particularly Phyfic. From hence came *Galen*: And here *Attalus* King of *Pergamus* founded a Library, and made phyfical Experiments

periments of Poisons on Criminals. But *Aretæus* of *Cappadocia* was the first, who being skill'd in the Writings of *Hippocrates*, and other *Greek* Phyficians, reduced Physic into a more regular System, and added what had been left upon the same Subject by other most eminent Physicians. After him, *Asclepiades* of *Bithynia*, in order to advance his Fame, boasted he had secret Medicines, by which he preferv'd his Health, kept off Difeases, and wou'd prolong Life: He also gloried in having reftored a dead Woman to Life, who seems to have been in an hysteric Fit. Nor was the Notion of *Theffalus* more vain, who contracted the Study of Physic to the Space of but six Months: Omitting the whole Physiology, he wou'd have the whole Care of a Physician consist in knowing whether the Parts of the Body were too ftrict or lax; to tighten them when too lax, and to relax them when too tenfe. But then the first of the *Latin* Physicians, *Celfus*, deliver'd the Doctrine of *Hippocrates* in his own Language with the greatest Purity, and interfperfed many excellent Opinions of the other ancient Physicians. It is uncertain whether he, coming of a noble Family, learnt Physic only by reading; or whether he was employ'd in the Practice: tho' the latter seems most probable; at leaft this is certain, that he was a Man of very great Learning, and has wrote of Physic with the greatest Perfpicuity, and digefted things into the most regular Method.

§. 15. *Galen* [1] made a Collection of their refpective Writings, digefted what was confufed, and took a great deal of Pains to explain every thing *into the Clouds* [2], according to the Peripatetic Philofophy; doing almoft as much *harm to Phyfic* by the one, *as he did it good* [3] by the other:

other : for by loading the Art with tedious Explications of every thing by the four Elements, the Cardinal Qualities, their several Degrees, and the four Humours, he has shewn much more Wit *than Truth in his Theory* 4.

Galen was a most expert Logician, extremely well versed in the peripatetic and natural Philosophy, as he also was in the several Opinions of the Ancients : à Man of acute and fertile Genius, writing in a pure and elegant Stile ; and in every respect truly a great Man. He lived about a hundred and ninety Years after the Birth of Christ, when *Severus* was Emperor.

He confused every thing by striving to make the genuine Observations of *Hippocrates* correspond to the false System of the Peripatetics ; and whenever he enquired after the Cause of any Appearance, he obscured the Truths of the Divine old Man by his mistaken Conjectures. He built upon the following System : " That Bodies are made up of " rude Matter, extended in threefold Dimensions, " and endued with a substantial Form, which de- " termines and distinguishes the Body to be of this " or that Kind. That, among the sensible Affe- " ctions of Bodies, there are four radical or pri- " mary *Qualities :* Heat, Cold, Humidity and " Dryness ; by which the Action of all Bodies is " to be explain'd, and from whence arise the pri- " mitive *Elements* ; viz. Fire or hot and dry, Air " or hot and moist, Water or cold and moist, and " Earth or cold and dry. Which Qualities deter- " mine the Nature of all Bodies in which these " Elements exist. But that in the human Body " there are four primitive *Humours* ; viz. Bile, an- " swering to fire, or hot and dry ; Blood, cor- " responding to air, or hot and moist ; Phlegm,
" akin

" akin to water, or cold and moist ; and Melan-
" choly or Atrabilis, related to earth, or cold and
" dry. That out of thefe Humours, intermix'd,
" and retaining their elementary Qualities, arife
" *Temperaments* of People. That alfo thefe Qua-
" lities have different Degrees, not varying their
" Nature, but only differing as to more or lefs,
" intenfe or remifs. Thus in Heat there are four
" *Degrees :* The firft, which nourifhes the natural
" Heat of the Body ; the fecond, which caufes
" Fever ; the third, which excites Inflammation ;
" and the fourth, which caufes Burning and Mor-
" tification. That this fame Theory holds good
" with refpect to the Virtues of Medicines, which
" have not only the fame cardinal Qualities, but
" alfo a like Number of Degrees in each. Thus
" Medicines, which are potentially hot, if they
" are fo in the firft Degree, they reftore the vital
" Heat of the human Body ; if hot in the fecond,
" they caufe a Fever ; if in the third, an Inflam-
" mation ; and in the fourth, a Mortification.
" Therefore the chief Bufinefs of Phyfic confifts in
" our having a juft Notion of the Qualities and
" their Degrees in Difeafes and Medicines. For
" when it was once found by us that the Cold in
" a quartan Fever afcended to almoft the fourth
" Degree, the natural Heat was then reduced to
" near one Degree and a third, and the Difeafe
" only wanted a Degree and a half of the greateft
" Cold, by which means the cold Phlegm over-
" came the fiery Bile ; it was therefore neceffary
" here to give Medicines of a Degree and a third
" hot, in order to reftore the healthy Tempera-
" ture, as Theriaca, &c. And thus in Prefcrip-
" tions, Opium, which is almoft of the greateft
" Cold, fhou'd be corrected with Euphorbium,
" which has the greateft Heat."——Admirable

D　　　　　　　Skill,

Skill, thus eafily to eftimate and proportion the
Nature of Difeafes and Medicines, if it were not
founded upon fo weak a Bafis as a fubtle but falfe
Imagination.

It muft be acknowledged that Phyfic was made
much more perfect on the Account of *Galen*, for
as he was furnifh'd with almoft all the Learning of
the Ancients, he has referved to us many things of
Confequence which are no where elfe to be found :
He was excellently fkill'd in the Writings of *Hippocrates, Herophilus, Erafiftratus, Afclepias*, with
thofe of the methodic and empirical Sects : His
Merit appears from having accurately defcribed
Difeafes, Pulfes, and feveral uncommon Diforders,
from an occular Infpection and a very ample Practice ; befides, he digefted and reduced whatever
Obfervations related to one Difeafe, and were interfperfed thro' a great Number of Books, to their
general Heads, under one general Title ; and by
that means left us a very methodical Syftem of
Phyfic in all its Branches, containing almoft every
thing that had been difcovered in that Age.

The Theory of *Galen* was built entirely upon
the Schemes of a fertile Imagination, and metaphyfical Subtilties, by which he and his Followers endeavour'd to account for the Appearances of Nature, who in a manner flipt thro' their Hands, in
the fearch, while they loft themfelves in the Cloud.
The Powers of Bodies which he aims to eftablifh
are not in the leaft fufficient. Aqua-fortis acts not
by heat, cold, or any other galenic Faculty, but
merely by the Salts with which it is faturated. Alfo
Mercury cures the Pox by Properties very remote
from any comprized in the Claffes of the galenic
Scheme. His Degrees in Difeafes and Medicines
are taken not from unerring Nature, but a precipitate and frantic Imagination ; by which, in fhort,

he

he did Phyſic more damage than all his Skill in the Ancients, many Years Practice, and Knowledge in the *Materia Medica,* cou'd ever repair.

§. 16. Learning after the ſixth Century being almoſt aboliſh'd in *Europe,* by its being over-run with barbarous Nations from the North (the *Goths*) who were quite rude in their Genius, Language and Manners, ſo as to *efface the Arts* [1] and almoſt the Memory of them ; *from the ninth to the thirteenth Century* [2], Phyſic was nicely cultivated by the *Arabians* in *Aſia,* *Africa* and *Spain*; whereby Surgery in particular, with the *Materia Medica* and its Preparations grew more complete and correct : but then the falſe *Galenic* Theory (§. 15. N. 2.) ſpread and peſter'd the Art more than ever; but this not without the Approbation of moſt of the ſucceeding Profeſſors : about that time they began to be inquiſitive after the Sciences in *Spain,* eſpecially in thoſe Parts next the *Saracens,* who expell'd the *Goths*; and there the firſt Reſtorers of Learning were ignorantly call'd *Magi* or Magicians, in the worſt Senſe of the Word. Here they began to expound the Writings of the *Arabian* Phyſicians, in public Academies; being as yet ignorant of, or at leaſt not accuſtom'd to, thoſe of the *Greeks.*—— Even from the Time of *Galen* to the Beginning of the ſixteenth Century Phyſic receiv'd ſcarce any Advancement; for almoſt the whole Buſineſs of his ſucceeding Phyſicians, by which they were deſirous of Praiſe, was either to en-

large

large the Works of *Galen* with Commentaries,
or contract them into Compendiums.

Arts and Sciences have always fhared equal
Fate with the Deftruction of Empires. The Learning of the eaftern Nations had been long before
abolifh'd in like Manner. In *Egypt* the Arts and
Sciences, particularly Phyfic, flourifh'd under the
firft *Ptolemies* ; but fuffering by the Conflagration
of a great Library (of 700,000 Volumes in *Alexandria* ; fix Hundred only of which were fpared at
the Requeft and Clemency of *Areus* and *Auguftus*)
they languifh'd to nothing, and their chief Profeffors went over to *Rome* ; by which means the Arts
and Sciences were extinguifh'd with the Strength of
the Empire. But in the fifth Century after the
Birth of Chrift, a northern Storm of *Barbarians*
fpread thro' the more polite Part of the World ;
who extinguifhed the fmall Light of Learning that
then remained. For being a furious People, and
averfe to Science, of which they were ignorant,
they burnt up the Libraries, together with the U-
niverfities and Cities : unhappy Age ; when Men
being only folicitous of animal Life, neglected the
diftinguifhing Ornaments of Wifdom. The *Roman* Language was firft ruined by the *Longobards*
that fubdued *Italy* ; and by intermixing and cement-
ing it with foreign Words, they fpread a Sea of
Barbarifm throughout *Europe*. At length, in the
feventh Century, *Mahomet*, an Enemy to polite
Arts, eftablifh'd a new Religion upon his own
Principles : in a little time he confirmed his Doctrines, both in *Paleftine*, *Arabia*, *Egypt* and *Affyria*,
preferring his own *Arabic* Language before the Sa-
cred and Learned, and tranflating every thing into
that Language, began to revive the Arts and Learning of the *Greeks*. His Caliphs or Chief Priefts
travelled

travell'd with Money and Authority over *Europe*, *Afia* and *Africa*, in order to deftroy the Language of others and eftablifh their own.

In the ninth Century, *Spain*, where the Arts had taken Refuge, was fubdued by the *Saracens* of *Africa* ; who laying afide their Victories for a comfortable Peace, and being a People naturally of fome Genius, began by Degrees to fearch in the learned Books of the *Greeks* : they then clothed in *Arabic* the Writings of *Hippocrates*, *Ariftotle* and *Galen*; in fhort, the whole Nation was fo enamoured with the Beauty of Learning about the End of the tenth Century, that they erected a confiderable Academy in *Morocco*, for the Education of Students at the public Charge : they alfo collected a Library with fo much Affiduity, that the King himfelf and the Chief Prieft thought it not beneath them to lend a hand, and be prefent at their Exercifes. At that time the *Arabians*, who were otherwife cunning and thoughtful People, fo nicely drefs'd up the *Galenic* Syftem, that it prevail'd much upon the Minds of Men who were employ'd about mere Ideas, and fatisfied with abftract Notions. All Truth was fought for in *Ariftotle*, and fometimes in *Galen :* when any Author had fhewn that his Opinions were agreeable to the Sentiment of either of thefe Fathers, they were allow'd to be true by univerfal Confent.—They not at all meddled with Anatomy, nor made any great Progrefs in the Practice of Phyfic ; they were indeed a little more curious in Botany and Surgery : but Chemiftry, they either firft brought into *Europe*, or, at leaft, greatly improved it. They alfo added the Preparation of Medicines to Phyfic, infomuch that the generality of Compofitions ftill retain their *Arabic* Names, Syrup from *Surep*, Juice ; Julep from *Juleb*, Rofewater, *&c.* The Principal *Arabian* Phyficians were

D 3 *Rhafes,*

Rhases, Avenzaor, Avicenna, Averhoes, and, in Pharmacy, *Mesue.* The Fame of the *Arabians* thus promoting Physic at *Toledo* and *Corduba,* excited the Learned in most Parts of *Europe* to travel to that Part of *Spain* which was possessed by the *Moors,* to learn the Arts, and especially Physic. These *Arabians* bringing their Books into *Italy,* when there were hardly any other to be found there ; the ignorant Populace every where vainly reckon'd them to be Magicians, as seeming to be learned beyond the Bounds of human Capacity.

§. 17. *At length* [1] they were confuted and corrected in their prejudiced and vain Notions by two Expedients ; *viz.* by the Hippocratic Doctrine being restored and prevailing in *France* on the one hand, and by anatomical and chemical Experiments on the other. About the Year 1453 several *Greek* Manuscripts were brought out of *Bysantia,* and translated (by *Chrysoloras* [2], *Gaza, Agyropulus, Lascaris, Chalcondulas, Trapezuntius, Mysurus,* and others) at *Venice,* and elsewhere ; by which means the *Greek* Language and Authors were again restored to use. About the same time *Aldus* happily publish'd the *Greek* Physicians together by printing, which was then lately discovered. Also *chemical Experiments* [3] were soon after introduced, by *Arnoldus Villanovanus, Lully, Basil Valentine* and *Paracelsus;* who applied Chemistry to Physic and Philosophy : and then Anatomy revived ; which was first closely prosecuted by the industry of *Jacobus Carpus* [4] in *Italy.*

About

[1] About thefe Times the Spani/h Phyficians, whofe Nation by degrees recovered their own Country, correfponded and communicated in their Learning with the Italians; they began publickly to expound theWritings of the Arabian Phyficians in an Academy at Padua; and in the beginning of the 13th Century they tranflated Galen into Latin.

Thus by degrees Barbarifm began to be extinguifh'd, but flowly; almoft every Body being blinded and prejudic'd in favour of the Peripatetic Doctrine.

[2] During the whole fifteenth Century the unfortunate Greeks flying from their ruined Country into Italy, brought thither their Language, Books, and ancient Monuments, as their chief Treafure, and the Springs of true Learning; and in the 16th Century the Works of Hippocrates came into a general Efteem, being in a manner a new Book, fince Galen only had been in ufe with the Arabians, and commented upon in France, where they had alfo tranflated Avicen. About the fame time Galen arofe more pure and entire, out of the vaft Volumes of the Arabian Phyficians, fo as to be publifhed by himfelf; then alfo the Latin Tongue began to recover its former Purity, and at the fame time a new Defire infpired the Minds of Men after true and ufeful Knowledge; they now began to perceive that Galen was preferable to the Arabians, and Hippocrates ftill better than Galen; in the former of whofe Writings Fernelius and Duretus were well verfed, and being improv'd alfo by their own Experience, they diffipated the Efteem that had prevailed for the Arabians; and in this manner the rational or Hippocratic Practice of Phyfic was renew'd, and the falutary Art in a great meafure reftored to its priftine Splendor.

D 4

[3] The

[3] The firſt Chemiſtry appeared chiefly in the Monaſteries, where there were ſome idle People, Smatterers in Learning, who began to contrive in what manner they could make Gold. *Baſil Valentine* firſt applied Chemiſtry to Phyſic in the 14th Century; then flouriſhed *Paracelſus* at *Baſil*, who was a *Helvetian*, born in the Year 1494, about the Time of *Veſalius:* he being ignorant of the learned Writings of *Galen* and the *Arabian* Phyſicians, to which he had an utter Averſion, founded a new Sect of his own, which gained ſo much Authority in a few Years, that the Princes of *Germany* would hardly admit any to be their Phyſicians who were not Chemiſts. This Man raiſed his Fame chiefly by the Uſe of Mercury, in which Age only he and *Carpus* durſt venture upon the Exhibition of it, particularly in the Venereal Diſeaſe, which at that time raged exceſſively; ſo that as the Eſteem for the *Arabians* was overturned by the Doctrines of *Hippocrates* prevailing in *France*, in *Germany* the ſame *Arabian* Phyſicians were expunged by the Arms of *Paracelſus*. But in the beginning of the 17th Century there happened yet a greater Diviſion in the Schools and *Galenic* Doctrines than before. *Helmont* at that time, who was a Man of ſome Experience, of an acute and daring Genius, alſo verſed in the Opinions of *Galen* and the Philoſophers, as well as the Anatomy of *Veſalius*, quickly perceived that neither the Syſtem of *Paracelſus*, who was ignorant of Anatomy and Phyſic, nor the Verboſities and Controverſies of the Schools, would either of them direct to the Truth. But the Remedy which he applied was in effect worſe than the Diſeaſe, for he ſo founded Phyſic upon Chemiſtry, that he would have no other certain Way either to its Theory or Practice. After *Helmont, Sylvius de la Boe* firſt introduced Chemiſtry

in

in the Univerſity at *Leyden*, and perſuaded the
Stewards to build a publick Elaboratory for it.
Chemiſtry is certainly a good Servant to Phyſic,
but it makes as bad a Maſter.

⁴ *Carpus* ſoon began to eſtabliſh Anatomy in
Italy after his Return from Exile. The firſt that
publiſh'd any thing upon Anatomy was *Mundinus*,
in the Year 1450; after him *Jacobus Berengarius
Carpenſis*, who firſt uſed Mercury in the Venereal
Diſeaſe, by which he acquired much Wealth and
Eſteem; he made a great Number of accurate Diſſections of Men and Brutes, publiſhing a Commentary upon *Mundinus*, and afterwards his own Anatomy, which being very ſcarce, I lately received
from *Italy*, and peruſed with much Pleaſure in the
Year 1731. But in the Year 1539 *Veſalius*, the
great Reſtorer of Anatomy, began to write upon
this Subject.

§. 18. At length the immortal *Harvey* ¹, by
the Diſcoveries which he demonſtrated, overturned the whole Theory of the Ancients, and
founded Phyſic upon a new and more certain
Baſis, upon which it at preſent reſts.

¹ He overturn'd the monſtrous and vain Hypotheſes which then prevailed in Phyſic, by publiſhing his incomparable Writings upon the Circulation of the Blood, and Generation of Animals;
wherein " he demonſtrates the human Body to be
" an Engine, all whoſe Offices depend upon the
" Circulation of the Blood, which alone being
" ſtopt, the whole muſt periſh;" from which
Theſis alone the whole Theory of the *Galeniſts* and
Chemiſts was overturn'd, and all the Learning of
the Ancients; that only ſubſiſted which was founded
and approved by Experiment; ſo that the whole
                                          Progreſs

Progress of Physic may be commodiously divided
into the ancient before *Harvey*, and the modern
after his Time ; for he so happily managed his
Discoveries and Opinions, that he seems to have
gained the Consent of almost all the Physicians before his Death ; for *Hippocrates*, who was a careful
Observer of Nature, being certain of the Causes,
has alone left us the truest Accounts of her Appearances ; nor is the Doctrine of *Harvey* contrary
to that of *Hippocrates*, but rather an Explanation
of it.

§. 19. Since his Time it has been variously
improved, without *adhering to any* [1] particular
Sect [2], not only by new and certain Discoveries in *Anatomy* [3], *Botany* [4], and *Chemistry* [5],
but also by *physical* [6] and *mechanical* [7] *Experiments*, in Conjunction with the real Facts
which have occurred in the Practice of Physic
itself. From hence it appears that the Art of
Physic was ancienily established (1.) by a faith-
ful Collection of Facts observed, whose Effects
were (2.) afterwards explained, and their *Causes* [8]
assigned by the Assistance of Reason ; the *first* [9]
carries Conviction along with it, and is indi-
sputable ; nothing being more certain than Demonstration from Experience, but the *latter* [10]
is more dubious and uncertain ; since every Sect
may explain the Causes of particular Effects
upon different Hypotheses. Tho' it is certain
that Physic may be as well supported by just
Reasoning, as by Observation and Experience.

[1] At present Physick may be learned without
adhering to any particular Sect, by rejecting every
thing

thing that is offered without Demonſtration, and by collecting and retaining only what has been offered and approved to be real Truth both by the Ancients and Moderns. *Hippocrates* adhered to no particular Sect, he propoſed nothing but what muſt neceſſarily be admitted by every one. An *Italian* Phyſician ſent me a little Book which he had, entitled, *Piccola de Arte Medica* ; in this ſhort Compendium was compriſed whatever Propoſitions could be admitted for Axioms, or undoubted Facts by Phyſicians ; I would advife you my Hearers, as much as póffible, to the ſame Study ; for you will find no other certain way of advancing in the Science.

² By this Term we underſtand a probable Opinion which has been receiv'd by many People, but yet is not ſo evident as to compel every reaſonable Perſon, ſkill'd in his Profeſſion, to allow it for true ; but it is of the utmoſt Conſequence to diſtinguiſh what relates to the Sect or Opinion from Obſervation, or Matter of Fact. Towards the Height of an inflammatory Fever a burning Heat is felt throughout the Body ; this is evident, and obſerved by every one ; but *Galen* and his Followers tell us, that this Heat ariſes from Exceſs of Bile ; the Chemiſts, from a Redundancy of Sulphur in the Blood ; *Helmont*, from the Fury of an *Archeus* ; all theſe Opinions are uncertain, and belong to each Sect ; we ought therefore to reject them, to preſerve the Art ſecure and uncorrupted with falſe Conjectures, retaining only what reſults from Obſervation, or what follows of conſequence from the Facts or Obſervations, ſo evidently, that no ſkilful and unprejudic'd Perſon can refuſe their Aſſent. We have undoubted Experiments in Phyſics, Mechanics, Anatomy, Botany, Chemiſtry, and the Practice of Phyſic ; all which we ought to

admit

admit for true, fo far as they are Experiments;
nor are we to add any Suppofitions or Confequences, but what are deducible from them by fevere
and juft Reafoning. All the Facts and Experiments which the Anatomift perceives in the Diffection of Bodies muft be admitted for true; thefe
are true in the Works of *Galen*, and will remain
fo in the Works of all fucceeding Anatomifts; but
when we proceed to explain the Ufes of thofe
Parts, there is great room to err, as we frequently
do. Chemiftry teaches us the Changes which Bodies fuffer of themfelves, and when applied to
Fire; for Experiments themfelves teach no Falacy:
but when we apply the Phænomena of one Body
to account for the Appearances of another, and
then draw Conclufions in refpect to the human
Body, we are frequently deceived. Thus if any
fhould fay, that the fixed Salt of *Tachenius* is proper in the beginning of a Dropfy, his Affertion
will be juftified by Experience; but if he proceeds
to explain the Manner in which it operates, it is
very poffible he may be altogether deceiv'd. And
thus in Botany, the Kinds and true Characteriftics
which have been imprinted on Plants from their
Origin by the Creator, never fuffer any Changes;
but in their Virtues and arbitrary Characteriftics
given them by Men, they frequently vary and
deceive us. Phyfics, which faithfully recounts to
us the Appearances of Nature, juftly deferves our
Refpect and Attention; but in explaining their
Caufes it often ftumbles; and being blinded by
Hypothefes, falls into the firft Error which is neareft: but mechanic Laws are eternally the fame, and
muft remain perpetually true; tho' in our Application of them to Bodies not fufficiently known,
we are frequently deceiv'd. For Example in the
Loadftone, we know all Bodies gravitate or tend

to each other, this Law is univerfally true, nor is
the Magnet excepted from it; but if one fhould
proceed to explain the Nature and Action of the
Magnet by the Laws of Gravity, he will be altogether deceived, becaufe it poffeffes Properties diftinct from any which refult from Gravity ; for if
one Magnet be placed near another, and the low-
ermoft at free liberty to fall in the Direction of the
oppofite Poles, it will not anfwer Expectation.
The practical Phyfician affures us, that the Treatment of Difeafes which have the fame Appearance
with thofe obferved in the Time of *Hippocrates*,
fhould not differ from that ufed by him ; but if the
fame Treatment fhould be ufed in another Difeafe,
differing or miftaken by its Signs, or wrong Name,
or ufed in an improper Stage of it, we can hardly
expect to fucceed ; fo that in this refpect we feem
to be more happy than our Anceftors, in that not
being feduced to Errors by any Authority, we only
admit Facts, to which we are compell'd by the
Force of Truth and free Confent, or embrace fuch
things only as are evinced by Experiments, or are
fo apparent from them, that we cannot confute
their Evidence.

Literary Commerce has conduced much to the
Improvement of Phyfic, when that was facilitated
by the Inftitution of public Pofts, or Conveyances
of Letters ; but much more by real Experiments,
made by the Invention of various Machines, to lay
the Truths of Nature more open to us ; and laftly,
by the Inftitution of learned Societies, for the Improvement of Philofophy, natural Hiftory, the
Arts, and Phyfic, at *London* and *Paris*.

³ There is no room to doubt in Anatomy, fo
far as it regards the Structure, Situation, and Connexion, &*c*. of the feveral Parts ; but when a Phyfician adds to it the Ufes of thofe Parts, the motion
of

of their Fluids, &c. and endeavours to explain them upon too narrow Principles, he is in the utmoſt Danger of Error.

4. Botany has added much to the Perfection of Phyſic, it teaches us the characteriſtic Signs by which we are to diſtinguiſh one Plant from another; and has been ſo much improved within the two laſt Centuries, that if it was purſued with the ſame Vigour, there would be great room to hope for its arriving to Perfection in a ſhort time. *Micheley* and *Vaillant* have done Wonders in this Branch.

5. Chemiſtry is the Obſervation of thoſe Changes which ariſe in different Bodies from the Application of certain degrees of Fire; ſo far as it exhibits Experiments, it may be certainly relied upon; but our Reaſonings in it are often fallacious; an Ounce of Antimony taken inwardly gently purges the Bowels, but when prepared by Fire, it occaſions the moſt violent Vomiting; the ſimple Appearance of theſe Effects is moſt certain, but the Explanation of them various and arbitrary. If any one remarks the Principles which are obtained from Blood applied to a certain degree of Fire, he will find there firſt aſcends Water, then Salt, and in the Retort remains an Earth (*per* §. 227.) Of theſe Facts one cannot be deceived; but if you ſhou'd by haſty Reaſon conclude from this Experiment, that the Blood therefore contains ſuch Salts and Oils as you thus obtain, it wou'd be an Error with a witneſs; if a Chemiſt takes upon him to account for the Appearances of Bodies, he forgets his own Character, and acts the Part of a Philoſopher, or too often, of a Rhetorician.

6. One Part of Phyſics is experimental, declaring only the Appearance of Bodies obſerved by our Senſes; *v. g.* that Gold is the moſt heavy of
Metals,

Metals, nineteen times heavier than Water, diffolvable in Mercury, &c. and this Part of it cannot deceive a Perfon. The other Part of Phyfics
is rational or theoretical, which by Reafon accounts
for the Properties of fome Bodies by the Affections
of others, which are capable of being made the
Subject of our Senfes and Experiments; and in this
latter one may be frequently and eafily deceived.
Nitre and Sulphur expofed to the Fire, go off
with a confiderable Explofion, this we are certain
of; but that the Explofion which happens in
Thunder proceeds from the fame Caufe, we are
not affured of, even we are fatisfied to the contrary.

. 7. Nothing is more evident than the general
Rules which are deduced from mechanical Experiments; but nothing is more uncertain than what
Mechanicians affert from thofe general Rules concerning the human Body; they make phyfical and
mechanical Experiments upon Bodies with a View
to deduce general Rules from them, which Rules
are fuppofed to be true in all Bodies fubject to the
fame Experiments. Thus we are told, that a Body
falling from a given Height will acquire a certain
Velocity; that the *Momentum* of the falling Body
will be proportionable to the Quantity of Matter
and Velocity, hence concluding that the Impetus
of a folid Body falling upon another from a certain
Height can admit of no Error in its Effects; but
great Care fhould be taken never to apply thofe
Rules to Bodies upon which the like Experiments
have never been tried; a Rule of this kind may
hold good in a thoufand Bodies, and yet be fubject
to an Exception in the next: this hafty Prefumpti-
on has been the Caufe of many Errors among many
Mathematicians, who have applied their geometri-
cal Propofitions taken from Bodies of particula-

Difpo-

Difpofitions to the human Body ; for what is afferted concerning Veffels of an indeterminate Refiftance,
and of incompreffible Fluids, which are not vifcid,
is not equally true with regard to the flexible and
elaftic Veffels, as alfo the compreffible and vifcid
Humours in the human Body ; therefore they who
think that all phyfical Appearances are to be explained mechanically, are in my Opinion mifled.
I am even far from being of Opinion, that thofe
general Laws which are infufficient to explain the
Appearances of fimple Bodies, fhou'd be capable of
accounting for 'em in that which is of all the moft
compound, *viz.* the human Body.

[8] The moft confiderable Genius's have been generally fubject to this Fault, that they endeavour
to obtain a Knowledge of all Things, *by detecting
their Caufes* ; hence it happens, that being mifled
by Experiments, they form general Conclufions,
which are not practicable, or elfe inconfiderately
conclude, that Propofitions deduced from a few Experiments will hold true throughout Bodies in general.

[9] What is demonftrated to us by our Senfes cannot be difproved in any Age, nor oppofed by any
Authority, unlefs by that of the Scepticks. The
Circulation of the Blood will be equally true and
undeniable a thoufand Years hence, as at the prefent
Time. Such is the Advancement of Phyfic in our
Days, that if we continue our Diligence, its Copi-
oufnefs and Certainty muft be indifputable. There
are indeed fome who affirm Phyfic to be wholly
conjectural, which is falfe ; it has this in common
with all other Arts, that it is imperfect, but that
Imperfection is the Default of the Artift ; which is
generally greater in the Profeffors of this, than of
other Arts. Befides, the Uncertainty of fome
things in Phyfic, do not diminifh the Evidence of
other

other Propositions, of whofe Certainty we are fatisfied. *Hippocrates* tells us, that the Knowledge
which is changeable is no Knowledge ; we may be
certain as to the Effects of Things ; all the Difficulty lies in their Caufes, in which we fhall commit no Error, if we firft confider their Effects attentively, fo as to deduce the Caufe from them
with Evidence.

¹⁰ The Confequences which we deduce upon the
trueft Principles, often deceive us, and become fubject to many Exceptions under different Circumftances. It may feem ftrange indeed to fome, that
the divine Reafon of Mankind fhould be fo weak
in real Facts, which are fo obvious to our bare
Senfes ; but our Errors in that refpect proceed not
fo much from the Weaknefs of our Reafon as from
our want of Thought, and too precipitate Judgment ; the Ideas we obtain from Things are certainly true in themfelves, but we affign Caufes from
Effects too haftily, before we have fufficiently examined them. For Example, in Heat, the Ancients obferved that a healthy human Body was always fome degrees hotter than the temper of the
ambient Air ; that this Heat was continued from
the very Birth, and then found that the Heart was
the firft Organ that acquired this Heat moft, and
the laft that grew cold or retained it longeft ; it
therefore feemed reafonable to them, that the Caufe
of this Heat muft refide more immediately and conftantly in the Heart ; and that therefore the Heart
muft be as it were the Spring of all Heat in the
human Body. All this they experienced to be
true ; but they fucceeded very lamely in their At-
tempts to detect the Caufes by thefe Facts ; when
neither the Nature of Heat nor the Action of the
Heart were as yet difcovered. They ought therefore to have poftponed their Judgment till the ne-

E   ceffary

cessary Data were assigned for this Affair, as we
find it was in the Time of *Harvey*: they might
then have learned, that in every Second of Time
the Heart ejected two Ounces of Blood, with a
brisk Force into the *Aorta* ; and also, that it again
received equal Quantities of Blood in the like Space
of Time. But an Hour contains 3600 of those
small Spaces of Time, and the natural Heat of a
Man continues through all the Parts of his Body so
long as the Heart continues to propel that Quantity
of Blood into the *Aorta* in that Space of Time ; if
it abates the Number of its Contractions in the given Time, the Man must begin to grow cooler,
and when it wholly ceases, his Body must become
as cold as the Air. If they had considered these
Circumstances, they would have assigned the Cause
and Seat of the Blood's Heat not to the Heart itself, but to the determinate Velocity with which
the Blood moves through the Heart. But who
would have suspended their Judgment on this Affair, from the Time of *Hippocrates*, down to our
Day ; the Space of 2200 Years ? that would have
been declaring himself ignorant in one of the most
considerable Articles of his Profession ; yet is it
what ought to have been done ; and with such
Patience only can Physic be purged from its Errors, and established upon the most true and certain Principles. Therefore when a Difficulty of
this Nature offers itself, not accountable for but
upon Hypotheses, we should restrain our Judgment, and leave the Doubt to be solved by our
Posterity, when they shall have attained Light
enough from Experiments which have escaped us.
It therefore behoves us to defer our Opinions about
the Use of the Spleen, and some other Parts in A-
natomy, with the Virtues of many Plants, the
Causes of contagious Diseases from Poisons, *&c.*
till

till Time fhall bring the Truth to Light. By this means Phyfic, 'tis true, will be reduced to a fmall Compafs ; but then it will be true, certain, and always the fame. But while, from the imperfect Ideas of many Experiments, we attempt to deduce Theorems, and eftablifh Opinions, it is impoffible that Phyfic fhould be free from Falacy and Errors : Such Speculations are fitter for the Lucubrations and Entertainment of the Learned, than to direct the Practice of a Phyfician, who being mifled by fome fuch fpecious but falfe Theory in a City, might turn out to be of the moft fatal Confequence to its Inhabitants.

Of the Parts and Principles [1]
of PHYSIC.

§. 20. FROM the fecond Head (§. 19. (2.) Phyfic has been loaded with many *ufelefs* [2] and *fallacious* [3] *Hypothefes*; to *expel* [4] *which*, we are to confider that the whole De-fign of the Art is to keep off and remove Pain, Sicknefs and Death, and therefore, to preferve prefent and reftore loft Health ; fo that every thing neceffary to be known by a Phyfician, is reducible to one of thefe two Heads.

[1] By *Principles* we here underftand, not the conftituent Parts or Elements of Bodies, but the Means of Demonftration, or Truths ; not depending upon others, but by which others are to be eftablifhed.

2 Among the *ufelefs* Hypothefes, we may reckon that of the *Pythagoreans*, explaining the Nature of Bodies by Numbers ; the fubtil Matter of the *Cartefians* ; a fubtil and rambling *Æther* ; the *Fuga Vacui*, &c. But the Ingenuity of Mankind has been generally unwilling to take up with fuch Principles as are the moft obvious to our Senfes, and ufeful to our Intereft ; they think we cannot underftand Nutrition, unlefs we are firft acquainted with the Nature of Wheat, nor can we underftand the Nature of that, unlefs we are acquainted with the Nature of the conftituent Principles. But their Search does even not terminate in the conftituent Principles or Elements, but they muft endeavour to find out by Conjecture in what manner the univerfal Matter of all Things does by a fubftantial Form put on the Texture and Difpofition of Wheat. But if thefe Things were poffible to be known, as they certainly are not, they would have no manner of Ufe with regard to the Affairs of human Life.

3 Such is the Nature of *fallacious* Hypothefes, that when the Principles which are laid down for the Bafis are only imaginary, the whole Train of Confequences which are thence deduced, muft be evidently falfe, and amount to nothing. *Cartefius*, who contrived a philofophical, but imaginary Hypothefis, concerning the Structure of the World, founded upon the Laws of Motion, and a fubtil Matter filling all Spaces, whirling about certain Axes, made the Parts of his Scheme correfpond fo well with each other, that it was fubject to little or no Objection, except the Falfity of its Principles. If in like manner fome Geometrician fhould attribute the Properties of a right-angled Triangle to an oblique angled one, like the Theorem of *Pythagoras*, he might thence deduce a new Syftem of Geometry, hanging very well together, but in reality no more

than

than a Dream; which, upon the removal of its Principles, muft vanifh into nothing.

4 Every thing which does not conduce to the Prefervation of Health, and to the Cure of Difeafes, may be purpofely omitted in Phyfic, notwithftanding they may be both true and curious: becaufe a Phyfician may perform his Office without their Affiftance. See my Oration relating to this Subject, *de repurganda Medicina.*

§. 21. The *Object*[1] therefore of Phyfic in the *Human Body*[2], is Life, Health, Difeafe, and *Death*[3], with the Caufes from whence they arife, and the Means by which they are to be regulated, reftored, or prevented.

[1] By the *Object* of Phyfic we here underftand every thing which is abfolutely neceffary to be known or done by a Phyfician; which, fo far as it confifts in Contemplation of the Mind, is Theory; but fo far as it relates to Action, it is, from the thing itfelf, called Practice.

[2] In the *human Body*, not as a metaphyfical Entity, not as a Mind, but as a living and animated Machine; for the Confideration of the two firft do not at all come under the Province of the Phyfician.

[3] Death deferves to be confidered by the Phyfician, both to avoid it, and to prefage it when unavoidable: it is prognofticated to be at hand from the Symptoms obferved in dying People; but the great Danger of a Perfon's Dying, can be only judged of from a previous Confideration of the Nature of the fatal Accident. Suppofe a large inacceffible Artery to be punctured, though the Wound feems to be ever fo flight and fmall, yet it may be fatal, as we find by Experience, becaufe all the

Blood

Blood may be let out thereby till the Nerves of the Heart become paralytic. Fatal Events of this kind ought to be remarked, that we may be capable of judging in what Cases our Affiftance may be neceffary, as in this to ftop the Hæmorrhage.

§. 22. Phyfic is therefore the *Science* [1] or Knowledge of *thofe things* [2], by whofe Application and Effects Health may be preferved when prefent, and reftored when loft, by the Cure of Difeafes.

[1] It has been much controverted among Phyficians, whether Phyfic ought to be termed an Art or a Science. The Matter feems to be thus: Cogitation confifts of two Parts, Underftanding and Will. Underftanding or Senfe is by the Ancients diftinguifhed into five Degrees; the I. Firft is fimple Perception by our Senfes, thus we know Light and Sound exift, becaufe we hear and fee. The II. Second is Science, or the Knowledge of Things by their Caufes; as if one fhould affirm it as a Rule, that hard Bodies upon Friction grow hot, and that therefore he may in this place affert that Heat will arife from the Friction of two hard Bodies together at this time, as they have done before. The III. Third is habitual Action or Art which produces thofe things into Being, which were before formed by Science. Suppofe, for Example, a Statuary, whofe Mind is furnifhed with a requifite Knowledge for the Formation of fome Image: he retains in his Mind the Idea, we may fuppofe, of *Hercules*, to which the Block of Marble is to be carved, he knows what Parts are to be removed to difcover the included *Hercules*, and he alfo knows how to ufe the Inftruments by which the fuperfluous Stone is to be feparated; this is the Science of a

Statuary;

Statuary; but when the Sculptor himfelf comes, he examines the Piece of Marble, divides it into the Head, Trunk, and Limbs, and makes Cavities, which are to ferve afterwards for the Throat, Eyes, &c. till at length by continually removing fmall Parts of the Stone in this manner; the naked *Hercules* at length appears; all this is the Work of the Statuary, his Art or his Science put in practice. In like manner the theoretical Part of Phyfic may be termed a Science, but the Practice of it is to be ranked among the Arts. But there are other Reafons why it fhould be rather called a Science; firft, *becaufe its Theory is put in Practice not by fimple Imitation*, but by the Knowledge of Caufes. Phyficians not only know by Experience that warm thin Liquors abate Fevers, but they alfo underftand that it does fo, by relaxing the Fibres and diluting the vifcid Blood. But the Dyer is ignorant of the Reafon why he adds Allum, Tin, or Gums, in his Art; as he is alfo of their Action. Secondly, becaufe Phyfic is a previous *Knowledge of Things to come.* We do not preferve prefent Health, nor remove prefent Difeafes, that is not in the Power of Man; we only place Health again in the room of that which was juft loft, or in the room of the Difeafe which at prefent exifts. I cannot be faid to cure a Pleurify on the third Day, nor is it in my Power; I only prevent the Difeafe from being conftantly prefent, fo as to turn to an *Empyema*, or Death. Nor can I be faid to preferve prefent Health, but only to caufe a Perfon to be in Health the next Day. IV. *Fourthly, Prudence*, or the Direction of Art with regard to future Events, which chiefly relates to Things belonging to human Life. V. Fifthly, *Wifdom*, which comprehends the four other Degrees,

E 4   In

² In like manner, as a Statuary ought to know the Inftruments, and Methods of ufing them, to effect his Defign, and then to judge what Parts of the Stone are to be removed to expofe the Image to View ; fo a Phyfician ought not only to be acquainted with every kind of Remedy, and the Method of ufing the fame, but he ought alfo to underftand the Nature of Health and Difeafes, that he may judge what is to be removed of the Difeafe, that the loft Health may be recovered.

§. 23. Therefore the Neceffity, *Ufefulnefs* ¹ and *Dignity* ² of Phyfic, are hence fufficiently apparent.

¹ The Service of Phyfic is evident from the Effects we daily find from the Practice of it ; without it a great Part of Mankind would not live out their Days ; and ftill a larger Number of great Men being opprefs'd with Pain and Difeafes, would fpend their Lives ufelefs to the Public. Some have indeed objected, that every Man may be his own Phyfician ; but it will readily appear, that a Man employed in other Affairs, cannot be fo perfectly acquainted with the neceffary Doctrine of Phyfic, as thofe who have made it the entire Bufinefs of their whole Life ; nor is it poffible they fhould have the like Opportunities of learning Anatomy, Pharmacy, &c. And as for thofe Reflections which are caft with Contempt upon Phyfic by the Illiterate, they have arofe from the Ignorance of fome unfkilful Practitioners, and not from the deferving Art itfelf.

² The Ufefulnefs of Phyfic in a Republick is both well known and efteem'd, efpecially as it is fo extenfive as to touch the Life and Health of every individual Member ; the Efteem for it has
always

always been fo great, that People afflicted with
Difeafes had rather apply themfelves to any ignorant Perfon than be without Phyfic; but it is very
evident, that thofe who know any thing of Phyfic
will not inconfiderately commit themfelves to the
Rafhnefs of Pretenders. The moft ancient He-
roes, and even the bold *Achilles*, were not altogether unfkill'd in Phyfic; nor did they think it beneath them to practife it with their own Hands.
Our Saviour is a remarkable Inftance in this refpect, who being invefted with divine Power, alfo
made it his particular Care to relieve the bodily
Diforders of Mankind.

§. 24. There are two Methods which may
be relied upon as certain for the Attainment
of our Profeffion, which may be efteemed its
folid Foundations; the *Firft* is an accurate
Obfervation[1] of all the Appearances offered to
our Senfes in the human Body, whether in
Health[2], *Difeafes*[3], *Dying*[4], or already *Dead*[5];
whether they proceed from internal Caufes refiding in the Animal, or from the Action of
external Bodies, Accidents, or the Art itfelf.
The *Second* is a ftrict Confideration and Difcovery of the feveral latent Caufes, concealed
from our naked *Senfes*[6] in human Bodies, by
a juft *Reafoning*[7]; which is really neceffary,
to prevent future ill Accidents, and fecure the
good Events. Phyfic thus eftablifhed upon
Judgment and Obfervation, can be only attained by a juft Reafoning from the feveral Facts,
(1.) which have before been *thoroughly confidered*[8] in every refpect; from comparing thofe
Reafonings

Reasonings with Nature or Experience, and
with each other; and from diligently remark-
ing which of them appear agreeable or disagreeable to Truth; that from the whole we may
be enabled to draw just Conclusions in regard
to present and future Events; which Conclusions may then be *relied upon* 9 with Certainty
as Matter of Fact.

1 Observation here is the Attention of the Mind
to such Changes as happen in human Bodies, all
which Changes proceed from Motion, which Motion is produced originally in the Body, as a Machine; some of these Changes are obvious to the
Senses, others are not so; the Motion of our Fluids
thro' their Vessels does naturally escape the Notice of all our naked Senses; therefore a Physician
ought to be acquainted as well with the Objects
which do not fall immediately under our Senses,
as with those that do; for the Knowledge of the
first is equally necessary to Physic with the last,
tho' it be only attainable by Analogy, from comparing the Parts less known, with those which are
wholly obvious to our Senses.

2 The State of the Pulse, and Respiration, the
Colour, Heat, Tension, and Moisture of the Skin,
the Brightness of the Eyes, &c. as they appear in
healthy Bodies, in order to distinguish the morbid
Changes in the same Appearances; from a due
Consideration of all these Signs, may be deduc'd
an Estimate of the Danger, or the Probability of
Recovery, and State of the Powers of Life, or of
the Disease; all which were largely consider'd by
the Ancients, but have undeservedly been treated
with much Neglect in the present Age.

By

³ By enquiring into all the prefent Circumftances of the Patient's Cafe, and by afking him and his Attendants after every thing, which will not fall under his Cognizance without.

⁴ *Hippocrates* was extremely well verfed in the Symptoms of dying People, and accurately remark'd the prefaging Signs of Death ; but the fucceeding Phyficians have been very negligent herein. We indeed fay a Man is dying when the Difeafe prevails and tends to Death; thus in a *Phrenitis*, which will prove fatal on the fourth Day, the Patient begins to die in the middle of the third Day, and the whole Syftem of the Body, efpecially the Brain, is gradually deftroy'd.

⁵ To fearch out by practical Anatomy the latent Caufes of Difeafes, of which we are often fo greatly ignorant, and to remark all the Changes which have been made by Death throughout the whole Body, and all its Vifcera. Surprizing is the difference even in the external Appearance of the dead from the living Body; the engaging Livelinefs of the Eyes, and Purple Tincture of the Cheeks, which fo allured our Fellow-Creatures but a few Days ago, do in this State vanifh, and leave a ftill, pale, and horrid Spectacle. But no lefs are alfo the Changes made by Death within the Body, infomuch that *Ruyfch* taking the Hint from hence, has filled the Veffels of dead Bodies by Injection, and reftored again the lively Appearance which Death had deftroy'd.

⁶ An Inftance of this we have in the *Sanctorian* Perfpiration, a Difcovery of the utmoft Confequence in Phyfic, which that Author obferved in his own Perfon, and has done more Service to Phyfic than all the fubtil imaginary Schemes and Interpretations of *Galen*, which were made during the whole 13th Century. This Method of improving
ving

ving Phyſic by ſenſible Obſervation, was follow'd
by the *Cnidian* Phyſicians, who are on this account
praiſed by *Hippocrates*, by whoſe own diligent Obſervations the Art of Phyſic in that Day was greatly perfected; he carefully remark'd every thing
which happen'd in the diſeas'd human Body, whether from external or internal Cauſes; whether
from the eating of *Wolfs-Bane*, the Bite of a Viper,
too large a Doſe of *Scammony*, ſudden Cold, and
the like, *&c.* which have undeſervedly been much
neglected by the Moderns.   We ought to make it
our chief Study to collect all the Obſervations and
Experiments we poſſibly can, and diſpoſe them
under their proper Heads; but an Experiment or
Fact is with regard to the thing itſelf, an Appearance obvious to the Senſes of the Enquirer;
our Mind adds nothing to the Appearance, but
barely the Perception of it.

⁷ We are ſaid to reaſon when we compare the
Ideas we have before experienc'd with each other,
that we may be diſtinctly informed of every Property appertaining to each Idea, and thence form
a Judgment of the Agreement or Difference between each; nor is there any thing more required
to Knowledge, than this Compariſon diſtinctly and
patiently proſecuted.   But the Phyſician above all
ſtands in need of juſt Reaſoning, to aſſiſt him in
the Diſcovery in many things of the human Body,
particularly the great Claſs of Diſeaſes which lie
concealed from the Obſervation of naked Senſe;
God has alſo given reaſonable Faculties to our
Minds to make new Diſcoveries of Truth and Invention; we cannot expect ſuch Diſcoveries from
careleſs Obſervation, and accidental Experiment,
but from thoſe which are deſignedly made with a
ſtrict Attention of Mind, to convert them to ſome
Uſe.   Obſervation or Experience alone will not
make

make a Phyfician; for any two Difeafes are never
fo much alike, but a fmall degree of Reafoning
may diftinguifh the difference.

⁸ All the Obfervations which we have made
upon any Head ought to be committed to Paper,
examined with the ftricteft Attention, and applied
to the prefent Circumftances of our Patient's Cafe,
that by confidering every Particular, we may by a
flow and folid Judgment determine the latent Caufes of Difeafes. Take an Example of this ; in the
Method of detecting the latent Caufes of Difeafes
by external Appearances: we obferve that in the
living human Body there is a conftant Refpiration,
in which the Air is alternately preffed into, and
expelled out of the Lungs ; we alfo obferve, that
the infpired Air is colder and dryer than the ex-
pired, which is warmer, and more humid ; alfo
that in Infpiration the Air is forced through the
Mouth and Nofe to the narrow Opening of the
Glottis, thence into the wider Cavity of the *Larynx,*
and from that into the round *Trachea* and conical
Bronchia ; and at laft, from the Branches of the
Bronchia into the fmall Air Veficles of *Malpighius.*
In Infpiration we know the *Diaphragm* becomes
flat, and draws down the Ribs, by which means
the *Thorax* is dilated, and the *Abdomen* compreffed.
In Expiration fucceeds the Reverfe of all thefe ;
the Ribs return clofer to each other, and the
Diaphragm returns into the *Thorax,* of a concave
Figure. In Infpiration the Veficles of the Lungs
are dilated, the fmall Veffels fpread upon them,
varioufly agitated, opened, and the Blood more
freely admitted into them ; in Expiration the fame
Veffels are compreffed together, and their contained Blood ftrongly propelled thro' them ; for the
Blood is forced from the Heart into the Lungs
thro' a conical elaftic Artery ; but in a conical converging

verging Veffel, every part of the contained Fluid
ftrikes againft its fides, which muft therefore be
dilated in proportion to the Force of the arterial
Fluid; fo that the Blood being expofed to the
Action of the Air in the Lungs, is forced into the
larger Veffels by the Contraction of the Heart, but
into and thro' the fmaller Veffels by the compreffing Force of the diftended Veficles, which is returned upon them; the Blood is therefore in the
Lungs intimately mixed, greatly attenuated, and
fo fitted for circulating thro' the fmalleft Veffels.
This Doctrine of Refpiration we ought to apply to
the difeafed Patient, and compare it with the feveral Appearances or Symptoms prefent in the Body.
Another Example of phyfical Reafoning, extended
beyond the ordinary Obfervation of our Senfes, may
be given in the Pulfe, which is a latent Action,
concealed from the Eye; yet notwithftanding we
may obtain a diftinct and full Idea of it; *viz.* that
the Artery is always full of Blood, and the Heart
drives it forward with a confiderable Force, are
both demonftrable from the Diffection of living
Brutes; but every Liquor, when it cannot proceed
in its Courfe, refifts; therefore in the Arteries,
which are full, their interior Portion of Blood cannot return back, becaufe of the fucceeding Blood,
which ftrikes againft that which went before;
therefore the preceding Blood not moving forward
with the fame Velocity with which the latter was
propelled by the Heart, it muft confequently expand the conical Artery, fo as to form the Pulfe;
all which is equally certain with what is daily offered to our common Senfes.

    If Phyficians were to unite their Endeavours,
and form a Society for the collecting of every thing
true and ufeful from the Writings we now poffefs,
and afterwards digeft them into Aphorifms under

proper

proper Heads, it must certainly form a System of
Physic capable of solving any Difficulty in the Art
with as equal Certainty as the Problems in any
other Science.

§. 25. In order to discover Truth in this
Manner by Observation and Reason, it is re-
quisite we should fix on some Principles whose
Certainty and Effects are *demonstrable* [1] to our
Senses, which may serve to explain the *Phænomena* [2] of natural Bodies, and account for the
Accidents that arise in them; such only are
those which are purely material in the human
Body, with *mechanical* [3] and physical Experiments; for we are not sensible of any other
way of attaining to a true Knowledge of the
universal and particular Affections of Bodies.

[1] Demonstration is an evident Proof of some
dubious Proposition, so that no Body who admits
the general Principles, can deny their Assent; these
are purest in the Mathematics, tho' there are many Demonstrations no less evident in Physic, especially those which are taken from Anatomy. But
there is no necessity for the Principles of any Art
to be proved in that Art, it is sufficient if their
Certainty is by any means demonstrated in other
Arts.
[2] These ought to be first adjusted with Distinction, Clearness, and Certainty; with Distinction,
which points out one Being from any other; as if
one was to define a Circle to be a right Line continued upon a Point till one End meets again with
the other; with Clearness, which consists of simple
Notions or Ideas easily conceived by any Man in
his Senses, as that two and two joined make four;
with

with Certainty, which cannot be denied by any reasonable Person, or which must always appear true upon Examination.

 [3] The universal Laws of Nature, or Affections of all Bodies, depend on mechanical and physical Principles, upon which alone their Actions are explicable; the same Laws are also true in the human Body, for its Matter appears to be universally the same with that of all other Bodies; so that what may be said to be true of all Bodies, may be also affirm'd true in our own. Thus, if one should affirm, that by the Friction of two Bodies would arise Heat, the same will also be true upon the Friction of solid Parts in the human Body. But then there are other Principles not to be explained by these universal Laws, but by some particular Disposition in the certain Body; these Properties are called physical. But a Physician ought to consider both the Affections of Bodies in general, as well as those only proper to the human Body, that from a judicious Comparison and just Reasoning, he may never subject the human Body to those Laws only, to which the generality, but not all Bodies, are liable.

§. 26. But as there are in the human Body many other *Appearances* [1] not intelligible upon those Principles, they therefore are not to be demonstrated and explained by such Principles; if we would avoid Error, we must take a very different Course for that Purpose; this will readily appear to any one who considers and admits for true the following Propositions, which are elsewhere demonstrated.

 [1] Such as Memory, Understanding, Reason, and the Knowledge of past and future Appearances; which

which are peculiar to the Mind, a Being without Figure or Extension, and conscious of Pleasure and Pain.

§. 27. We are to consider, (1.) That Man is composed of a *Body*,[1] and *Mind*,[2] *united*[3] to each other; (2.) that the *Nature*[4] of these are very different, and that therefore, (3.) each has a *Life*,[5] *Actions*[6] and Affections differing from the other; yet (4.) that there is such a reciprocal Connection and Consent between the particular Thoughts and Affections of the Mind and the Body, that a Change in one always produces a Change in the other, and the reverse; also, (5.) that the Mind performs some Actions by mere Thought, without any Effect upon the Body; and that it has other Thoughts, which arise barely from some Change in the Condition of the Body; on the other hand also, (6.) that there are some Actions performed by the Body without the Attention, Knowledge, or Desire of the Mind, which is neither concerned therein as the Cause or Effect of those Actions; that there are also some Ideas formed in the Mind of a Person in Health by its past Actions; and lastly, that there are other Ideas compounded both of the past and present. That, (7.) whatever we observe to arise from Thought in the human Body, is to be only ascribed to the Mind as the Cause. But, (8.) that every Appearance which has Solidity, Figure, or Motion, is to be ascribed to the Body and its Motion for a Principle, and ought to be demonstrated and explained by their Properties.

F

perties. That, (9.) we cannot underſtand or explain the Manner in which the Body and Mind reciprocally *act upon each other*[7] from any conſideration of their Nature ſeparate; we can only (10.) remark by Obſervation their Effects upon each other, without explaining them; and when any Difficulty or Appearance has been traced ſo far, that it only remains to explain the manner of their reciprocal Action, we are to ſuppoſe ſuch account *Satisfactory* [8], both becauſe it may be ſufficient for all the Purpoſes of the Phyſician, and as it is impoſſible for him to ſearch any further.

[1] By the Body we underſtand that Part of us which is extended in three Dimenſions, has a Form, and is fitted for Motion or Reſt, &c.

[2] By the Mind we underſtand that Being which thinks, and perceives itſelf thinking, and the thing thought of.

[3] The Union of the Body and Mind is ſuch, that the Mind cannot reſiſt forming to itſelf the Ideas of Pleaſure and Pain, when the Body is in a particular manner affected; nor can the healthy Body refuſe to obey the Action of the Mind under particular Circumſtances.

[4] By the Nature of the Body or Mind, we underſtand every thing which we are ſatisfied belong to each. The eſſential Nature of the Mind is to be conſcious, or to think; but to think of this and that particular thing, is accidental to it. The eſſential Nature of the Body is Extenſion and Reſiſtance. Theſe Attributes have nothing in common to each other, nor ought one to conclude from Similitude, that two Beings are reducible to one general Claſs. When I think of Extenſion, it

does

does not infer any thing of Thought; and when I reflect upon Thought, I can perceive no Connexion of it with Extension; therefore the Idea of the Body has nothing in common with that of the Mind, and the reverse. In the same manner, there is no Connexion between the common Ideas of Time, Sound, Gravity, Light, &c. *Socrates* made a proper Answer to *Crito*, when he was ask'd in what Place he should chuse to be buried? *viz.* " You will not find *Socrates* when you prepare my " Tomb, nor shall I be sensible of what you then " do for me." Nor are there Reasons wanting to prove from the present Condition of the Mind, that it may live hereafter without any Commerce with its Body. The incomparable Mathematician *Vietus*, who first restored Algebra to us, received the Enemies Letters from his King, to expound their mystical Signs; while he was studying to explain their Meaning, he was taken up with the most profound Meditation for three whole Days and Nights, insomuch that he was not the least sensible of what had been transacted without his Knowledge, taking no more Concern for his Body, than if it had been long deserted as an Enemy by his Mind. In like manner, we find *Archimedes* in a Consternation when he first was ordered to answer King *Hieronus* concerning the mix'd Gold in the Crown, till at last lighting upon the Experiment, *i. e.* going into the Bath, he cry'd out Victory. And in the same manner a *Roman*, who was in a deep Consternation or Extasy, being not at all terrified at the formidable Advances of the *Syracutians* in Battle, made a great Conquest without once breaking his Lines.

The Life of the Body is, 1. To generate Motion under particular Circumstances, as the Loadstone approaches to Iron. 2. For its constituent

Parts

Parts to attract each other; from whence proceeds that Refiftance to the Force of external Bodies, or *Vis inertia.* 3. To gravitate, or tend towards the Center of its Planet. And then, 4. comes the Affeftions proper to particular Bodies. The Life of the Mind is, 1. To perceive the Appearances of all external Objects, by the Changes they make in the Organs of Senfation. 2. To judge or compare the nature of two Ideas with each other, and then to deduce fome Confequence, as that they are of the fame Kind, or different; as we conclude from our Notions of a Circle and Triangle, that a Triangle is not a Circle. 3. To will any thing. In a word, the Life of the Mind is, to be confcious. Thefe are all the Functions of the Mind; for paft Actions are uncertain, and they may be all referr'd to the fingle Act of its Confcioufnefs..

⁶ The Action of the Body is to communicate Motion to other Bodies; the Paffion of it is to receive fome Change in itfelf from another Body or a Mind. The Action of the Mind is Volition, which every Body is acquainted with, but no one can explain. The Paffions of the Mind' are the Changes it receives from external Objects by the Senfes. Suppofe the Mind to be thinking of a Circle, and in the interim a Cannon to go off, it will lofe the Idea of a Circle, and acquire that of Sound; this is the Sufferance of the Mind, becaufe it can neither retain the Idea of a Circle, nor refift that of a Sound. There are alfo fome Affections in the Mind different from the preceding, fuch as violent Paffions, or involuntary Commotions, which the Mind cannot refift, and the Faculty by which it moves and determines the feveral Parts of a human Body, agreeable to its Inclination.

We

⁷ We cannot underſtand why two Principles, which have no Agreement in Power, ſhould thus concur in the ſame Functions, tho' there have been three Hypotheſes framed to explain the Intercourſe of the Body and Mind; the firſt is, by the *phyſical Influx*, which ſuppoſes the Thing thought of, and the Thought itſelf, to be one and the ſame; which we ſhall hereafter demonſtrate to be abſurd, in as much as our Mind is ignorant of its own Nature. The ſecond is the Syſtem of *occaſional Cauſes*; and the third ſuppoſes a Harmony eſtabliſh'd by God, taking it for an infallible Rule, that determinate Actions of the Mind muſt be neceſſarily attended with correſponding Motions in the Body, and the contrary; and this laſt ſeems to be the trueſt Opinion, but it leaves us equally in the Dark with the other.

ᴮ If any Action is to be explain'd which is compounded both of the Faculties of the Mind as well as of the Body, ſuch as Walking, Pain, voluntary Reſpiration, &c. a juſt Account ought to be firſt given how far, and in what manner, the Body is concerned in the Action, and then alſo of the Mind; if this can be done, it is enough, without diving into the manner of Connexion between the different Actions; the Explication of the corporeal Actions appertains to the Phyſician, and thoſe of the Mind to the Philoſopher; but their Connexion can be explained by no Man. Heat may be conceiv'd to ariſe in Bodies without any relation to a thinking Mind, as Mill-ſtones grow hot in their grinding; but Motion is not explicable from the Affections of the Body, nor even from the Properties of the Mind, therefore Heat and Motion are not accountable from the Mind; and if you ſhould ſay that the voluntary Motions of the Muſcles proceed from the Act of Volition in the Mind,

you

you explain the thing not in the leaft, becaufe there is nothing in the Idea of Motion which is alfo to be found in any Affection of the Mind. We call an Explanation of a thing the Demonftration of Agreement or Relation between its own Properties and the fame in another; but this is here not only impoffible, but alfo quite ufelefs to a Phyfician; for the great Bufinefs of a Phyfician is to be acquainted with the Means of reftoring loft Health, and no Cure can be effected by him, but through fome Change made in the human Body by the Application of others ; therefore this Search after the Connexion between the Body and Mind not appertaining to a Phyfician, is to be rejected, among thofe (§. 20.) which are ufelefs to the Art. The Phyfician, who cures Difeafes of the Body, is not follicitous about thofe of the Mind; for when the firft is fet to rights, the latter will quickly return to its Office. Thus when the Eye is blinded with a Cataract, the Mind cannot perceive fenfible Objects by it, the Aid of Phyfic is therefore call'd in to couch the Cataract, or deprefs the opake cryftalline *Lens*; after which the Rays of Light finding a free Admiffion to the *Retina*, the Mind will be fenfible of vifible Objects by it; and thus the Bufinefs of Phyfic will be done without the Affiftance of Optics. When a Perfon is in a *Delirium*, or Swoon, the Phyfician cannot recall the Mind, which has no relation to his Bufinefs; but by applying Vinegar, or other Volatiles to the Nofe, he can reftore the fick Machine to its former Motions, and then the Mind will alfo exhibit its former Actions, and this full as well as if he underftood the manner of Connexion between the Actions of the Body and thofe of the confcious Mind.

§. 28. We

§. 28. We may alſo affirm, that the *prima-ry phyſical Cauſes*[1], in what manner, and the ultimate *metaphyſical Cauſes*[2], for what End, the moſt general Appearances are in a deter-minate manner affected, are neither poſſible, uſeful, or neceſſary to be inveſtigated by a Phyſician; ſuch as the Origin of primitive and *ſeminal Forms*[3], of *Motion*[4], the *Ele-ments*[5], &c.

[1] *Primary Cauſes* are thoſe productive of ſecon-dary ones; but we always meet with God in our Search after theſe, and this puts a Stop to our fur-ther Knowledge; for God is an infinite Being, and if we compare the whole Univerſe with him, it will be found almoſt nothing.—In our Search after *phyſical Cauſes*, we ſhould not be over ſollicitous to determine every thing in which Experiment will not aſſiſt us; for we never can be certain of the Truth of ſuch Diſcoveries, and if we were, it would be of little or no Uſe to Mankind; we are thus wholly ignorant of the Origin and Communication of Motion in Bodies; for Motion is no more eſ-ſential to the Idea of Body, than a Circle is to that of the Mind. Let thoſe Philoſophers appear, who hold that an Aſſembly of Gods joined toge-ther to form the Univerſe, and explain by one ſimple and univerſal Experiment, why any Body in motion communicates part of its motion to the next which it touches; an ingenious Perſon would anſwer, God made it ſo. We ought therefore to reſt upon Experiment, and lay aſide uſeleſs At-tempts to explain the moſt general Laws and Prin-ciples obſerved in Nature; taking Example by the wiſe Ignorance of the Chemiſts, who barely rela-ting the Appearances offer'd to them, are not con-

cerned

cerned about the firft Caufe. *Barthol. Schwartz*
having difcovered the furprifing Experiment of
producing Thunder and Lightning, by the Application of Fire to a Powder made of Nitre, Sulphur, and Wood-coals, mix'd in a certain Proportion, never enquired into the Caufe of that Phæ-
nomenon by which almoft the whole Face of the
habitable World has been chang'd. The Moderns
have found, that two Grains of Gold diffolved in
three times as much *Aqua regia*, and precipitated
with half that Quantity of Oil of Tartar *per deliquium*, forms a Powder, which applied to a certain
degree of Fire, will blow up a hundred Weight.
The Chemift ftops at the bare Appearance ; but
the Philofopher taking a Courfe very different
from the Experiments of the Chemift, ftudies the
Formation of a mechanical Engine, by which two
Grains will raife a Weight of a hundred Pounds;
and thus each of them obtain their Ends by different Means.

2 By metaphyfical Caufes, are meant thofe general Attributes of Beings which are abftractedly
effential to them as Beings; which are therefore
very univerfal, and remote from Action.

3 An Element is the Matter of which a Body is
originally compofed, and into which it may be
ultimately refolved. Great has been the Controverfy in all Ages about the Elements. Some con-
tend for Water only, others for Air, and others
again for Water and Fire; but the greater Number
are for the four Peripatetic Elements; tho' the
Chemifts alfo build upon their Salt, Sulphur, and
Mercury ; but neither of thefe can be properly an
Element, for it is effential to an Element to have
its Part abfolutely fimple and homogeneous ; but
then how can Matter thus homongeneous form the
great Variety of Bodies we meet with ? If you re-

treat

treat to the *Monades*, or Atoms of *Pythagoras*, and universal Matter, you do not take our Eyes with you to convince us ; nor can we be certain whether there are fuch or no, fince you tell us of things from which the Mind can never receive any real Ideas.

⁴ Some of the Chemifts acknowledge befides Matter, Form and Vacuum, a feminal Principle ; which fo determines the Structure of vegetable Bodies in their Growth, that they can appear in fuch a particular Form, and no other. If an Anifeed be fowed in a pure Earth, moiftened with Rain-water, and forwarded with a Heat equal to that of a fetting Hen, it will produce the Plant Anife, whofe Smell, Tafte, and Structure, differs from all other Plants in the Univerfe ; and in the Vegetation of the Plant there is alfo a new Production of Seeds, each of which is capable, under proper Circumftances, of producing the like Plant ; if thefe Seeds were wanting, the whole united Power of Nature together could never produce the fame Plant ; therefore, according to the Opinion of the Chemifts, this Seed muft contain a Principle, which from Earth and Water always produces that particular Plant, which no other Seed can produce. In like manner they fuppofe Metals to be formed of a feminal Subftance, which grows or vegetates in the Bowels of the Earth with a fubterraneous Heat, by means of a particular Juice ; which Opinion is confirmed by philofophical Experiments, and fupported by many Reafons.

⁵ The Origin of Motion is to be look'd for in God ; if we fubftitute any other primary Caufe, we do him Injuftice. I may fay that it becomes a true Philofopher to confefs his Ignorance of firft Caufes, which he is never likely to attain to ; but notwithftanding fecondary Caufes may be ufed to as

good

good Purposes as if we were acquainted with their
first. If I learn by Experiment the Virtues of any
Plant for the Cure of Diseases, I may do as much
Service with it in Physic as if I had created the
Plant. If every thing useless to the Art was to be
in this manner expunged, as we in this Section ad-
vise, Physic would lose nine Parts out of ten, and
be by that means purged of its Drofs, and restored
to its native Simplicity.

§. 29. But a Physician may, and ought to
furnish himself with, and reason from, such
Things as are demonstrated to be true in *Anatomy* [1], *Chemistry* [2] and *Mechanics* [3], with natural and experimental *Philosophy* [4], provided
he confines his Reasoning within the Bounds
of Truth and simple Experiment, *per* §. 25.

[1] He that desires to learn Truth, should teach
himself by Facts and Experiments; by which
means he will know more in a Year, than by ab-
stract Reasoning in an Age. Proper Experiments
have always Truth to defend them; also Reasoning join'd with Mathematical Evidence, and founded upon Experiment, will hold equally true; but
should it be true, without those Supports it must
be altogether useless. Nature distributes the Faculty of Reason to all Men equally alike, but he will
excel in Reasoning who has made the best Use of
Experiments, having consider'd the Structure, Situation, Figure, Size, and other Peculiarities, obvious to our Senses in the several Parts of the human Body.

[2] Chemestry acquaints us with those Changes
which arise in Bodies from Mixture, and the Application of them to Fire. Suppose one Substance

of

of a particular kind to be mix'd with another, and applied to a determinate degree of Fire, the Confequence will be a Production of new Appearances, which is the Bufinefs of the Chemift to remark; nor does ever Chemiftry deceive us, if it proceeds no farther than real Experiments, and their Effects; upon the Addition of the beft Oil of Cloves to rectified Oil of Vitriol, they run into a violent Commotion, and exhale Cloulds as thick as Pitch, which quickly turn into Flames.

Mechanics teach us to apply the general Laws of Motion to all Kinds of Bodies. Every Body is extended, refifts Motion, is moveable, capable of Form, &c. The Effects of all thefe general Qualities, and the moving Powers thence arifing, are applicable to every particular Body; nor can we be deceived therein, if the Body to which they are applied be diftinctly and carefully confidered in all thofe Refpects. Mechanics therefore fuppofes a previous Knowledge of the Structure of all the Parts in the human Body, to which we would apply mechanical Laws; and in this Senfe Phyfic is no more than the Knowledge of fuch Things as are tranfacted in the human Body, either by the common Affections of Bodies, or by the determinate and particular Structure of the Parts in the human Body. It therefore appears that Mechanicians, ignorant of the Structure of the Parts whofe Actions they would exprefs by Numbers, muft run into the Exceffes of Error; which Defect has been charged upon ourfelves, for what has been formerly advanced in an Oration *de ufu Mechanices in Medicina*; tho' there are fome, Enemies to the very Name of Mechanics, who affert, that our Bodies are not fubject to the fame Laws with all others.

§. 30. It

§. 30. It is neceſſary for the Phyſician, in furniſhing himſelf with theſe Principles and Experiments, to begin firſt with ſuch as are moſt ſimple, certain and eaſy to be under-ſtood; after which he may proceed to thoſe which are more compounded, and ſo by de-grees to the moſt complex, obſcure, and dif-ficult.

§. 31. He that would learn by Experiments, ought to proceed from Particulars to Generals; but the Method of inſtructing academically, proceeds from Generals to Particulars; which is the Method we ſhall obſerve.

A Profeſſor ſkill'd in the Science which he teach-es, firſt lays down general Rules, by which the Nature of each particular Subject is to be defined; but an Inventor of Diſcoveries ought to learn the Properties of every particular Body by proper Ex-periments, that he may afterwards reduce them into Claſſes, according to their Affinity: The firſt Me-thod is in the Schools termed Analytical, the other Synthatical. The Inventor, *Ariſtotle*, when he ob-ſerved that Oxen, who had Horns, wanted fore Teeth in the upper Jaw, and finding they were alſo wanting in Stags, Goats, Sheep, and other Ani-mals with which he was acquainted, took occaſion to affirm, that all Animals that had Horns wanted upper Teeth. But *Ray*, teaching the Nature of Animals, lays this down for an Axiom; from which he infers, that neither the Ox, Stag, nor Range Deer, have Teeth in their upper Jaw becauſe they are horned.

§. 32. From theſe Conſiderations appears the Order of our Doctrine; for in the firſt Place

we

we are to confider ¹ *Life*; then Health, afterwards Difeafes; and laftly their feveral Remedies.

¹ Life is the Sum or Aggregate of all the Actions
refulting from the Structure of the feveral Parts in
the human Body; when all thofe Actions are performed with Eafe and Perfection, it is called
Health.

§. 33. Hence the firft general Branch of
Phyfic in our Inftitutions is termed PHYSIOLO-
GY, or the Animal Oeconomy; demonftra-
ting the feveral Parts of the human Body, with
their Mechanifm and Actions; together with
the Doctrine of Life, Health, and their feveral Effects, which refult from the Mechanifm
and Actions of the Parts. The Objects of this
Branch have been ufually denominated *Res
naturales*, Things natural or according to Nature.

§. 34. The fecond Branch of Phyfic is called
PATHOLOGY, treating of Difeafes, their Differences, Caufes and Effects; or Symptoms;
by which the human Body is known to vary
from its healthy State. This Branch is diftinguifhed into (1.) *Diagnoftic* Pathology, fo far
as it defcribes the Difeafes of the Body; (2.)
Ætiologic, when it treats of their Caufes; (3.)
Diatritic, when it confiders their Differences
and future Events; and laftly, (4.) the *Symp-
tomatologic* Part of Pathology, is that which
explains the various Effects or Symptoms of
Difeafes.—The Objects hereof are termed *res*

contra naturam, Things preter-natural, or contrary to Nature.

§. 35. The third Part of Phyfic is termed SEMIÓTICA, which fhews the *Signs* diftinguifhing between Sicknefs and Health, Difeafes, and their Caufes in the human Body; it alfo imports the State and Degrees of Health and Difeafes, and prefages their future Events. The Objects of this Branch are the *Non-naturals* as well as the *Naturals* (§. 33.) and *Preter-naturals* (§. 34.)

§. 36. The fourth general Branch of Phyfic is termed HYGIENE, or *Prophylaxis*; which teaches us what Remedies are proper, and how they are to be ufed; to preferve Life and prefent Health; and, as much as poffible, to prevent Diftempers. The chief Object hereof is the *Non-naturals*, or *Res non-naturalis*.

§. 37. The fifth, and laft Part of Phyfic, is called THERAPEUTICA; which inftructs us in the Nature, Preparation, and Ufes of the *Materia Medica*; and the Methods of applying the fame, in order to cure Difeafes and reftore loft Health. This Branch is called *Methodus Medendi*, fo far as it points out the Means and Cure; which are comprized under three Heads: (1.) *Pharmacy* [1], or the Preparation and internal Ufe of Medicines; (2.) *Dietetics* [2], or Regimen, refpecting a Regulation of the Diet, Air, &c. And (3.) *Surgery* [3], comprehending manual Operation with Inftruments, and topical Remedies.

By

¹ By the *Materia Medica* we here intend all Remedies, taken as well from Diet as Pharmacy; in which ample Signification *Diascorides* has described the *Materia Medica.*

² Natural Remedies, as they come first to our Hands, are very often unfit for the Stomach, too strong in their Action, nauseous to a Patient, or else not sufficiently exalted in their Virtues. Physicians have therefore industriously contrived to render them more innocent, grateful, and efficacious, by subjecting them to various Preparations, Compositions, and Changes; and this is the Business of Pharmacy, whether Galenical or Chemical.

³ The *Methodus Medendi* points out to us the curative Indications, with the Time and Method of applying Remedies, being the immediate Foundation of the extemperaneous Prescription of Medicines, and of the general Rules to be given by the Physicians for the Patient's Recovery.

§. 38. Having thus distributed Physic under its proper Heads, agreeable to the Nature of the Art itself, as well as the most convenient Method of teaching and learning the same, which is also approved by the established Custom of the Professors through many Ages past; we shall next proceed to treat of the several Branches separately in that Order.

P H Y-

PHYSIOLOGY.

§. 39. **T**HE human Body, we find by
Anatomy, is composed of *solid*
and *fluid Parts*.

Fluids are those Bodies which consist of insensible Parts, have so small a Degree of Cohesion, that they easily separate from each other, and give way to a smaller Force than will remove the whole Body ; we say, consisting of insensible Parts, to distinguish them from a Heap of Sand, which might otherwise claim this Definition of a Fluid.

Solids are those Bodies whose Parts cohere together so strongly, that the whole is sooner removed by any Force from its Place, than its Parts separated from each other. There are various degrees of this Firmness or Solidity ; those Animals Solids are the most firm which resist Separation with the greatest Force ; such as Tendons, some of which cannot be pulled asunder by the Force of two thousand Weight ; those Parts are the least solid which have so weak a Cohesion, that they may be separated by a Force not much greater than what they sustain in the healthy living Animal ; such as the cortical Part of the Brain. Those Parts of the Animal are the most fluid which are separated from each other with the least Force, and are the most easily put in Motion ; such as the perspirable Matter of *Sanctorius* ; but those are the least fluid which are the most viscid and ropy, such as the *Mucus* of the Nose, &c.

§. 40. The

§. 40. The ſolid Parts of the human Body are either membranous Pipes, or Veſſels including the Fluids, or elſe *Inſtruments* [1] made up of theſe, and more ſolid Fibres, ſo formed and connected, that each of them is capable of performing a particular Action by the Structure, whenever they ſhall be put in Motion ; we find ſome of them reſemble *Pillars* [2], *Props* [3], *Croſs-Beams* [4], *Fences* [5], *Coverings* [6], ſome like *Axes* [7], *Wedges* [8], *Leavers* [9], and *Pullies* [10]; others like *Cords* [11], *Preſſes* [12], or *Bellows* [13]; and others again like *Sieves* [14], *Strainers* [15], *Pipes* [16], *Conduits* [17], and *Receivers* [18]; and the Faculty of performing various Motions by theſe Inſtruments, is called their *Functions* [19]; which are all performed by *mechanical Laws* [20], and by them only are intelligible.

[1] *Inſtruments* are compound Bodies, which by the Size, Figure, Connection and Diſpoſition of their Parts are capable of performing determinate Actions for particular Uſes. Thus the *Dentes Molares* are compoſed of the moſt compact and boney Matter, fit for dividing the more ſolid Aliments ; Their Surface is rough and unequal, fit for holding faſt and grinding the Food ; Their Articulation in the Sockets of the Jaws is the moſt firm, that they may not be looſened or pulled out in the Action ; Their Size too is determinate, ſo as to be proportionable to their Office, and the Jaw in particular, as well as the human Body in general ; all which Circumſtances concur to this effect ; to wit, the Diviſion of hard, tough, and ſolid Aliments, by the rough Surfaces of thoſe Teeth. Several of theſe ſimple Inſtruments are uſually joined together into

one

one Organ, or compound Inftrument, as Mufcles and Bones make up the Hand, &c.

² *Pillars* are perpendicular Supports, fixed upright under the Body which they fuftain.

³ *Props*, are every thing which fuftains the whole, or fome Parts of the Body, from receding out of their proper Places. Thus the Feet are the general Supports to the whole Body, the Veffels to their contained Fluids, &c.

⁴ *Crofs-Beams*, are Supports, whofe Direction is parallel to the Horizon, or otherwife inclined, as the Ribs, Clavicles, and the digaftrick Mufcles, with refpect to the Tongue, &c.

⁵ *Fences*, are hard and refifting Parts, which keep off external Violence from the more tender Parts, which they defend : thus the *Cranium* is a Helmet to the Brain, the *Sternum* a Shield to the Heart and Lungs, &c.

⁶ *Coverings*, are flat and flexible Fences, being tough as Leather, defending all the external Parts of the Body ; fo tough and hard is the Skin fometimes found, that there are feveral Inftances of Bones being broke by external Violence, without any Injury fuftained by that Part.

⁷ *Axes*, are fixed Points, upon which Leavers turn to raife fome Weights, fuch as the *Trochanter major* to the *Glutæi* Mufcles ; the *Patella* to the extending Mufcles of the Leg, &c.

⁸ *Wedges*, are fharp edged or pointed Bodies, having feveral Sides, and a larger Bafis, fitted for cleaving and cutting hard Bodies afunder ; like the *Dentes Canini*, and *Incifores*.

⁹ A *Leaver* is an inflexible right Line, moving upon a fixed Point, to which it is faftned ; fuch as all the long Bones.

¹⁰ *Pullies*, are either moveable or immoveable Points, over which a Cord defcends in an angular

Direction

Direction to raiſe ſome Weight ; as in the Tendons of the digaſtrick Muſcles of the lower Jaw, and the *Trochleares* of the Eye.

11 *Cords*, are flexible Lines whereby Powers raiſe Weights to which they are faſtned ; ſuch are the Tendons, Nerves, Muſcles, &c.

12 *Preſſes*, are inflexible Plains which approaching each other by imcumbent Weights or Powers, preſs upon the intervenient Body ; ſuch as the Heart, Stomach, &c.

13 *Bellows*, are Machines which take Fluids into a large Cavity, and expel them through a narrow Aperture ; ſuch are the *Thorax* and Windpipe.

14 *Sieves*, are Plains perforated with many ſmall Holes, which only tranſmit ſuch Parts of Bodies as are leſs than the Diameter of thoſe Perforations, retaining and ſeparating thoſe Parts which are groſſer ; ſuch as the ſmalleſt Blood Veſſels, with their lateral Lymphaticks, which exclude the red Part of the Blood with the other Glands.

15 *Strainers*, or rather *Filters*, are Plains perforated with the moſt minute, but oblique Apertures, which tranſmit the thinneſt Part of Fluids, and keep back the more groſs ; ſuch as the lacteal Veſſels in the Inteſtines.

16 *Pipes*, or Veſſels, are the Tubes diſtributed through every Part of the human Body, in which are contained their proper Fluids in Motion. There are three Kinds of theſe Veſſels, which keep their contained Fluids in a continual progreſſive Motion ; Arteries, Veins, and the intermediate Veſſels which connect them ; the two firſt being conical, and the laſt cylindrical.

17 *Conduits* are another kind of Veſſels, through which Liquors are conveyed, but not conſtantly, they being ſometimes empty, at other times full : ſuch as the Auricles and Ventricles of the Heart, &c.

the-

the Figure of them is various, neither conical nor cylindrical.

[18] A *Receptacle* is a hollow Body, which receives some Fluid, in which it continues for a certain time; the Bladder for Urine; Bile and *Semen* are confiderable Receptacles; the *Folliculi Adipofi*, are expanfions of the Extremities of the Arteries; the Pituitary *Sinus*, the fimple Glands, and *Mucus Receptacles* of *Vaterus* in the *Uterus*, &c. whence it appears that there are many Fluids in the human Body which are not kept in a continual Circulation.

[19] A *Function*, or Office, is the Power of acting, which depends upon the Structure of the Organ; but the Function put in Practice by Motion is the Action of the Organ.

[20] If the feveral Parts of the human Body agree thus with the Structure of mechanical Inftruments which we have juft now enumerated, they muft alfo neceffarily act by the fame Laws; for the Force of every one of thofe Parts confifts in the Motion which they produce; and by whatever Means that Motion is effected in the human Body, it is always performed agreeable to the general Laws of Mechanicks. There are indeed fome who think that thefe Actions ought not to be explained by mechanick Laws, fince the mechanical Caufes of them are unknown to us; but in faying this, they fhew very little Confideration; for we are not treating of the Caufes, but the Effects fubject to mechanical Laws. There are many, and confiderable Motions performed in Nature, of whofe Caufes we are ignorant; but the Motions themfelves are always fubject to thofe univerfal Laws which appear to be true in all fenfible Bodies; even the Loadftone, the Caufe of whofe Action is moft concealed from us, performs its Motions by certain and known Laws; which once obferved, never fails to be true when applied

to future Experiments. The human Body performs various Motions, the Caufes of which are abfolutely concealed from us ; but the Effects of thofe Motions are the Elevation of Weights by fixed Cords, the Propulfion of Fluids through their feveral Veffels, &c. which Effects being fimilar to thofe which are produced by mechanical Caufes, are not governed by any other Laws.

§. 41. The fluid Parts of the human Body are included in their refpective *Solids* [1], or Veffels, by which they are kept in a conftant and *determinate Motion* [2] or Circulation ; being often *feparated* [3] from each other, *mixed* [4] together again, and varioufly *changed* [5] in different Parts of the Body, whofe Veffels and continuous Parts are *moved* [6] by them ; the Sides of the Veffels are *wore away* [7], changed in their Figure, and again renewed by them ; all which Actions are performed agreeable to the *Laws* [8] or Principles of *Hygroftatics* [9], *Hygraulics* [10], and *Mechanics* [11] ; by which they ought therefore to be explained, yet fo as to have a ftrict regard to the *particular Nature* [12] or Texture of each Fluid ; and upon thefe Principles alone depend entirely the Actions of each Part, fo far as we are capable of knowing by all Kinds of Experiments.

[1] All the great Difcoveries and Knowledge in thefe Parts which we now poffefs, is owing to the Induftry of the Moderns ; for the Ancients, tho' they were not ignorant that our Fluids had a Motion, yet they did not look for the Caufe of that Motion in their Veffels ; nor were they at all curi-

ous in determining their Nature, Elasticity, and conical Figure ; but we are now sensible that the Fluids of the human Body exert no less Force to dilate their Vessels, than their containing Vessels do by their Contractions exert in order to drive them forwards.

² There is nothing in the arterial Blood itself which should determine it to flow to Parts remote from the Heart, nor to make it return to the Heart in a contrary Direction ; the Determination of that Motion is from the Heart.

³ A Separation is again made of the different Liquors, which before apparently formed one similar Fluid flowing thro' one Canal ; after which Separation, those different Liquors continue their Course apart thro' different Vessels of their own ; all this is perform'd in the Arteries : thus the *Aorta* receives the Blood, which was before intimately mix'd, from the pulmonary Vein, and distributes in such a manner thro' the Body, that the sanguiferous Arteries contain the red Blood, the Lymphatics its pellucid Part, the Vessels of the salival Glands draw off their Fluid, the semeniferous Tubes the *Semen* ; and so in the *Pancreas*, and other Parts, particular Fluids are convey'd off distinct from the Blood.

⁴ The Fluids are so intimately mix'd again with each other, that there is no Part of one but may be found to contain some Part of the other ; this Intermixture is performed chiefly in the larger Conveyances, as in the *Vena cava*, near the Heart, where all the Lymph, Chyle and Blood, returning from the several Parts of the Body, are pour'd into one Mass ; as also in the Sinus of the pulmonary Vein, the Sinus's of the Brain, and other venous Receptacles.

What

⁵ What a Power the Veſſels exert in changing the Condition of their included Fluids, is apparent in the Bile, which may be formed merely from Bread and Water; but how very different is the Nature of Bread from that of the Bile? and yet the Bread and Water ſuffer no other Action to convert them into Bile, but that of Mixture with the other Fluids already in the human Body, in Conjunction with the determinate Action of the Veſſels in each Part.

⁶ All the Motions in the human Body proceed primarily from the Fluids; the Bones are moved by the Muſcles, the Muſcles by their Nerves, and other Veſſels, and theſe again by their contained Fluids.

⁷ The Attrition ſuffer'd by the Sides of the Veſſels from their Fluids, is in proportion to the Velocity of their motion; if the Blood in the Arteries is impell'd againſt their Sides with a double Velocity, they will be alſo repell'd again by them with a double Force. The Arteries in the cortical Part of the Brain, tho' ſo many times ſmaller than the Hairs on one's Head, do ſuffer an almoſt infinite Number of Shocks from the Force of Pulſation; they muſt of neceſſity be therefore continually ground away and impaired, and muſt conſequently require continual Reparation by new Particles.

⁸ Fluids are in general ſubject, I. To the ſame Laws and Affections which are demonſtrated to obtain thro' all Bodies whatever. II. To thoſe which hold true with reſpect to the Particles of ſolid Bodies; for the component Parts of Fluids are no other than ſolid Corpuſcles. And, III. To thoſe proper to themſelves as Fluids.

⁹ By *hygroſtatic* Laws we mean thoſe Affections of Fluids uſually denominated hydroſtatical, with-

out refpect to any particular Qualities in Water, as the latter Term would feem to import. *Archimedes* going to treat of the Laws of Gravitation in Fluids, firft of all propofes four general Axioms. As,

I. That the whole Aggregate of the Fluid is perceptible by our Senfes.

II. But that no fingle Particle of it is fo to the naked Eye.

III. That the Particles and whole Aggregate of the Fluid gravitate.

IV. That their compotent Parts may be feparated by the leaft Force.

From whence he deduces the general Laws, to which are fubjected all the Fluids hitherto known, refpecting barely their Fluidity, without regard to the determinating Properties of particular Fluids, or the Nature and Form of their containing Veffels. Therefore as thofe general Laws hold true of all Fluids, they may be alfo as juftly applied to the Fluids of the human Body.

[19] *Hygraulics* is alfo rather ufed by us here than the received Name *Hydraulics*, becaufe we would not be underftood to regard Water in particular, which does not include the feveral Properties of the Fluids in the human Body. Hygraulic Laws or Principles exhibit the Phænomena of Fluids moving thro' particular Veffels or Tubes; but the Veffels in the human Body are fome of them *cylindrical*, giving no Refiftance or Change by their Figure to the motion of the Fluid; as in thofe *Tubuli* which form the *Anaftomofes* of the evanefcent Arteries with the incipient Veins; and others of them are *converging* and conical, where the Section or Diameter of the Tube is always leffening, and the Refiftance of it continually increafing, by which means alfo the Impulfe and Friction of the Fluid

against

againſt the Sides of the Veſſel are perpetually augmented; while other Veſſels are *diverging*, where
the Sections of the Tubes are continually enlarging,
ſo as to diminiſh their Reſiſtances. The cylindric
Veſſels in the human Body, are thoſe between the
Arteries and Veins, the Perſpiracles of the Skin, *&c.*
The conical converging Veſſels, are all the Arteries, and the *Vena Portæ*, after its Entrance in the
Liver; and the diverging Veſſels are all the Veins
and excretory Ducts.

¹¹ That Fluids are alſo to be conſider'd mecha-
nically, is apparent from their component Parti-
cles being Solids; therefore when the Parts of a
Fluid perform any Action, they do it by the ſame
Laws by which Solids act; and the Effects or
Action of a Fluid is no more than the Sums of the
Actions of their component ſolid Particles.

¹² Were the Fluids of the human Body poſſeſs'd
of no other Properties but ſuch as are in common
to pure Water; and were its Veſſels metalline Tubes
infinitely reſiſting, the forementioned Principles
would then be of themſelves ſufficient to explain
their Actions; but many of our Fluids contain
elaſtic Globules, and all of them are compounded
of Oil, Salt, Earth and Water, variouſly attracting and repelling each other; their containing
Veſſels are alſo made up of elaſtic Fibres, admitting reciprocal Elongations and Contractions;
therefore the Fluids in the human Body do not
ſtrictly follow either hygraulic or hygroſtatic Laws,
but they ſtray from thoſe Principles in proportion
to the difference which obtains between them and
common Water; nor are our Veſſels ſubject to the
Laws laid down by *Herones* for Tubes infinitely
reſiſting Fluids in motion; the Particles of the
Blood are continually attracting each other, and
run into Coheſions proportionable to their Con-
tacts;

tacts; which is an Affection not common to all Fluids, but only peculiar to the Blood, and some others. In an intermitting Tertian the Patient becomes chill'd, and shakes or trembles with a continual Anguish or heavy Pain; in a while after he grows hot and feverish, and the Fit leaves him with a Sweat, and a lateritious Sediment in his Urine. In the same manner it will return again in 36 Hours time, and probably continue thus for seven Fits successively, the Disease growing still worse and worse at each Fit till the fourth, and from thence gradually diminishing to the seventh. The manifest Cause of all this Disorder is apparently an Obstruction in the smallest Vessels; but no Mortal will ever explain all these Appearances by the Principles of Hygraulics and Hygrostatics, because they arise from a Change made in the constituent Particles of the Blood.

§. 42. By human *Life*[1] I would be here understood to mean, in the common Sense of the Word, that Condition of the several fluid and solid Parts of the Body, which is absolutely necessary to maintain, the mutual Commerce between that and the Mind to a *certain Degree*[2]; so as to be not perfectly removed beyond the Power of being restored again. It would be inconsistent with my Design here, to give as yet a more ample Definition of Life; nor can I give a more clear Idea of Health, before we enter upon its Principles, than that at §. 1.

[1] Life cannot be defined well till its Physiology, or Nature and Principles of Action, have been first considered; for it is the Sum or Aggregate of all the

the Actions performed in the human Body ; to give a particular Deſcription of which is the Buſineſs of Phyſiology.

2 It is ſometimes no ſmall Difficulty for us to diſtinguiſh between a dead and living Body, as in People almoſt drown'd, in Syncopes, &c. where the moſt apparent Signs of Life are abſent. A young Nobleman, the only Son of a great Family in *Brabant*, being taken out of the Waters for drown'd, without any apparent Signs of Life, was thus cold and lifeleſs convey'd Home ; in which manner he continued, as every Body imagined and reported, to be dead ; but a Perſon ſkill'd in Nature had the apparently dead Body rolled upon a Caſk, and ordered Air to be blown up the *Anus* with a Pair of Bellows, continuing as it were to torture the Body till it had recovered an evident degree of Reſpiration and Senſe, and afterwards all the Faculties of Life, ſurviving the (otherwiſe) certain Death for many Years.——The youngeſt Daughter of a *Dutchman* living in the Colonies of *America*, dy'd of an epidemical Fever ; hereupon a Slave of *Angola* runs to the crying Mother, and promiſes he would quickly reſtore the dear Soul to life ; then gather'd ſome very ſtrong Plants, which after chewing he ſpit up the Noſe of the Body, and opened its Mouth ; and after repeating the Experiment ten times, the Patient recovered her Life ; what Remains there could be of Life in that State is difficult to determine, tho' the Motion of the Heart, Blood, and Reſpiration, had all ceaſed, and according to the receiv'd Definition the Patient was really dead ; but the *African* Slave thus vellicating the tender Nerves in the Noſe (of the Body not yet touch'd with Putrifaction) by the moſt ſtimulating vegetable Juices, ſo far agitated that which moves the Nerves, as to excite them to Mo-

tion,

tion, make the Heart contract, and propel forwards its Blood. The Condition of the Girl now mentioned seems to be in a sort of Medium between Life and Death. If by Life we mean a circular Motion of the Fluids thro' the Heart, Lungs, and *Cerebellum*; and If by Death we understand such a Dissolution of the vital Organs, that they are quite irrecoverable, the mean State of these two will be a Stagnation, or absolute Rest of the Fluids, yet capable of being put in Motion.

§. 43. But in order to obtain a just Knowledge of what is necessary to make (these, §. 42.) Life and Health present in the Body, we ought, (1.) to make an accurate Survey and Collection of the several Appearances to be met with in them both, (2.) to enquire into the *Subjects* [1] in which those Appearances are seated, (3.) to investigate the *Causes* [2] from whence they arise, (4.) the *Instrumants* [3] by which they are performed, and, (5.) the Effects which they thus produce.

[1] For the Life of the Heart is very different from that of the Hair and Nails, nor can we understand Life as an Aggregate or Whole, till we have accurately surveyed what it is in every single Part of which the Body is composed.

[2] A *Cause* of any thing is a Being whose Existence gives Being to some Effect or other, and upon whose Non-existence that Being or Effect must also cease to be; so long as the Heart continues its Motion, so long does Life remain; but whenever that Organ ceases to move, Life itself also ceases to be; the Motion of the Heart is therefore the Cause of Life.

[3] *Instruments*

₃ *Instruments* are immediate Caufes, by which the firft Caufe produces its ultimate Effect. Suppofe I have a mind to drive a Nail into the Wall with a Hammer, the firft material Caufe is a Motion excited in the Body by the Influence of the Mind or Will, and the next is an increafed Velocity or Influx of the nervous Fluid into the Mufcles, which firft elevate, and then deprefs the Arm; the third Caufe is the Hammer, of a determinate Figure, ftriking the Nail; the ultimate Effect will therefore be Motion in the Nail, by which it will penetrate into the Wall; the firft Caufe then is Motion in the *Senforium*, or Origin of the Nerves; the Inftruments are the intermediate or fecondary Caufes between that and the ultimate, *viz.* the Nerves, Mufcles, and Hammer.

§. 44. But as thefe Particulars (§. 43.) to be obferved are almoft infinite in Number and Variety, in order to learn or teach them methodically, we ought to range them under proper Heads and Claffes, and then treat of each by itfelf in order.

§. 45. And firft we ought to begin with thofe Actions which are corporeal (*per* §. 30): but thefe are either, (1.) thofe in common to both Sexes, or, (2.) proper to but one of them; the former of thefe are therefore to be confidered firft.

§. 46. The corporeal Actions in common to both Sexes may be next diftinguifhed into, (1.) thofe performed by Adults, or, (2). by the Fœtus and *incipient* ₁ Animals; but of thefe again, the firft is to be confidered before the laft; (*per* §. 30.)

The

The Order of Nature would direct us to begin our History of the human Body where the Body itself begins to be formed ; but that is repugnant to the Rule, which commands us to begin first with those things which are the most obvious and easy to be known. The Mechanism and Nature of the first Rudiments of the human Body are entirely conceal'd from us ; even the Knowledge we have of the Mechanism and Action of the several Vessels and Viscera in a *Fœtus*, is first taken from a Comparison with those of Adults ; and where the Adult will reflect no Light by Analogy to the Nature of some Parts in the *Fœtus*, we are in a manner left in the Dark.

§. 47. But all these Particulars (§. 43, 44, 45, 46.) are linked together in such a manner, that by mutually performing the Office of Causes and Effects to each other, they seem to make a continued Circle without Beginning or End ; which make it an almost insuperable Difficulty to consider them in a *just Order* [1], without any Disagreement to the Rules of good Method.

[1] An Enquirer after Truth should adhere to the Rule of laying down nothing but what he has before demonstrated in some preceding Proposition ; but whenever one begins to explain the Actions of the human Body, we shall always find there are some things necessary to be premised which are not as yet demonstrated. The Heart is by every one acknowledged for the primary Machine, from whence the Motion of the Blood and Life arise ; but the Action of the Heart cannot be understood before the Nature and Action of a Muscle has been explained,

explained, together with the Blood and the nervous Fluid from the Brain and *Cerebellum*; but these Spirits again arise from the Blood, propell'd to the Brain by the Force of the Heart, whose Action we are investigating; and thus our Enquiries may run in a Circle, without finding any beginning, where it will not be necessary to call in the Ideas of other Parts, in order to explain those we first treat of. It is beautifully observed by *Hippocrates*, that "every thing in the human Body "is so disposed in manner of a Circle, that you "will find the End where you would look for "the Beginning, and the Beginning where one "might expect the End." And *Pitcairn* affirms for a Truth, that one Part of the Body is not formed before the other, but that all the Viscera were created and made at one and the same time; for all their Effects prove in the End to be the Causes of those very Effects.

§. 48. Tho' of all Methods that seems to be the best, which beginning with the *Aliments* [1] at their first Assumption into the Body, proceeds to consider the successive Changes which they undergo in the same; not leaving them till formed into the solid and fluid Parts of the Body itself, and producing their several Actions: For as the whole Body is made up of those Aliments, which we are capable of strictly examining by our Senses, and as its various Actions are also performed by their repeated ingestion, this must be apparently the most easy and certain Method of attaining to a Knowledge of the human Body.

If

ɪ If the Law of Order or Method directs us to make our Beginning at the firſt Rudiments of the human Body, it even then ſeems moſt juſt to begin firſt with the Aliments; for what we receive primarily from our Parents, is ſo ſmall a Particle as to be imperceptible to us; whereas every Grain by which we exceed that Particle, ſo as to be enlarged to this ſenſible Bulk, is taken from the Aliments.

§. 49. The Aliments then, are either Solid or *Fluid* ɪ; and therefore capable of being eat or drank. The Subſtances uſed for theſe Offices, were, in the firſt Ages of Mankind, only *Water* 2, and the natural Products of the *Earth*3; as we learn from ſacred and prophane Hiſtory, as well as from the ancient Poets and the Nature of Things; but ſoon after, Men began to feed upon ſome of the *Fluid* 4 and ſolid Parts of Animals, with thoſe of Fruits and eſculent Vegetables, variouſly prepared by Art.

ɪ Something of *fluid* Aliment is often taken in from the ambient Air, abſorbed by the *Venæ inhalentiæ* of the Skin. *Paracelſus* even aſſerts that he ſaw a Man nouriſhed by means of Plaſters, which were applied to the *Hypochondria*.

2 *Water* is the Principle from whence *Thales*, *Paracelſus*, *Helmont* and *Boyle* deduce the Origin of all Bodies, whether animal or vegetable; and *Moſes* by divine Inſpiration aſſerts, that Fiſh and Fowl, which make a very great Part of the Animal Creation, were produced from this Element. We find the Uſe of Water as a Drink to be extremely ancient, both by the Conſent of profane as well as ſacred Hiſtory, and other Monuments

of

of Antiquity. By facred Hiftory we alfo learn, that
Noah, and by the profane that *Bacchus*, were the
firft that introduced the drinking of Wine, both
of them living a long time after the Creation of
the World ; but before their Times we may juftly
conclude that every Man was well contented with
pure Water for his Drink, which makes the fluid
Vehicle for nourifhing and fupporting the whole
animal as well as vegetable Claffes of the World.
The drinking of Ale, whofe Invention is by Antiquity afcribed to *Ofiris*, was not cuftomary for
many Ages after *Noah* ; and even in our own prefent Times, all the Drink we ufe is in a ftrict Senfe
nothing but Water ; for if that Fluid receives any
Addition by Art, it is rather to render it more
agreeable to drink, than to make it a better Menftruum to allay our Thirft, and diffolve the more
folid Aliments.

Before the Ufe of the Plough was invented,
our Species liv'd entirely upon the Fruits of the
Earth ; and when that was contrived, they feem
to have liv'd many Ages after without hunting the
Cattle for Food, fince they had no Weapons for
that Purpofe. The Creator favour'd our firft Parents with eating of Garden Fruits only, but he
afterwards indulged *Noah* with Flefh of all Kinds ;
which Account is alfo agreeable to that of the
golden Age, given us by the Poets ; and *Pythagoras* alledges the Authorities of the moft ancient
Times, when he fo ftrictly commands Men to abftain from Flefh.

Among the fluid Parts, we may reckon Milk
and Eggs for the chief ; the Ufe of which was
even granted Men by *Pythagoras*, in Imitation of
Nature, who had appointed Milk for the firft
Suftenence of the new-born Infant, for which innocent Aliment fhe has therefore given it a natural

Appetite

Appetite by Inftinct; for the firft Action learned and practifed by the new-born Infant is that of fucking, and if the Nipple is denied it, the Finger is commonly put into the Mouth and fuck'd inftead of it.

§. 50. Even fince thofe early Times, *many People* [1] have been fupported all their Lives with nothing but *Vegetables* [2] and Water; and what is more, whole Nations have been contented to live in that manner; a Man was formerly fhow'd about for a Spectacle in thefe Parts, who lived upon nothing but Grafs and *Hay* [3]; while others have lived almoft wholly upon *Fifh* [4]; others barely upon *Flefh* [5] and Milk; whilft the Moderns fpread their Tables with almoft *every Kind* [6] of Vegetable, Fifh, Fowl, and Quadruped; which Luxury of the Appetite is ftill farther heightened by the various Artifices of Cookery, as the like Extravagance was formerly fatirized among the *Romans*.

[1] The *Brachmans*, or moft ancient Philofophers, which were from their Habit called by the *Greeks Gymnofophifts*, and who were particularly efteemed in the Time of *Herodotus* for their Antiquity and ftrict Morality, never admitted any thing but Vegetables, and fome of the fuperfluous Humours of Animals (as Milk, Eggs, Honey, &c.) to be their Food; but their Healths were not any ways impaired by that Courfe, their Lives were rather of the greateft Extent, and their Minds fitted for Meditation, and the Culture of every thing curious and learned; even fome of them, *Zoroafter* and *Pythagoras*,

Pythagoras, are in a manner faid to be the firft Starters of philofophical Knowledge; and even the moft devout Chriftians of later Times, retreating into the fandy Defarts from the public Tyranny, have fupported a long and healthy Life only by vegetable Roots, and other natural Products of the Earth, with fimple Water, which they met with in their Walks.

² Many of the firft Colonies of the ancient *Greeks* fed only upon Beech, or the efculent Oak, which is alfo now brought over to furnifh the Tables of the Great in *Spain* and *Holland*. A very ingenious Gentleman accuftomed to a very regular way of living in *Holland*, began to live wholly upon Grafs, but was obliged to defift from it becaufe of a confequent Diarrhæa, which yet was without any Danger, and is cuftomary to the Cattle in Springtime. And in this manner the *Perfian* Army, being fed only upon Herbs, fuffered a very great Lofs of their Soldiers by violent Diarrhæas. All the maritime Ports of *Afia*, from *Balfora* to the *Ganges*, for the Space of a Thoufand Miles in Length, were fed only upon Plants. The Religion of the *Bramines* was alfo received among thofe Inhabitants. The very robuft Natives of *Brafil*, who before the Approach of the *Europeans* often grew to the Height of feven Foot, and were no more decrepid at a Hundred than the *Europeans* at Seventy, lived upon nothing but the Grain *Mayz*, Sugar and Oranges; but now they are feduced both with the Cuftoms and Difeafes of the Chriftians.

³ A Child being left in a Defart by his Mother, was educated among the Sheep and Goats, by which Means he learned to eat Grafs; and when he was taken, he would pick out thofe from the feveral Plants brought him which were ufually

   chofe

chofe by one Sheep; his Voice was like that of
the bleating Cattle, being made a Shew to the
common People in *Holland*. A noted Ruler in
the States of *Holland*, famous thro' moft Parts of
Europe, took it into his Head to try upon how
little a Man might live; he fed for feveral Months
upon nothing but Peafe, without any apparent
Detriment from fo unaccuftomed a Diet, while the
Table of his Family was all the time fpread with
regal Plenty.

⁴ Such were the Countries of the *Iɛthyophagi*, or
Fifh-eaters, mentioned by *Herodotus*, and the People who inhabited upon the Borders of *Æthiopia*;
and in our Time the *Laplanders*, and other Inhabitants of the more northern Parts, make the Fifh
they have lately taken, ferve them for Flefh; and
thofe which have been dry'd, for Bread.

⁵ The *Æthiopian* Nation defpifing Grain, liv'd
wholly upon Flefh and Milk, acquiring the Name
of Long-livers, it being as cuftomary for them to
attain the Age of a Hundred and Twenty, as Seventy Years among us. The *Abyfinians*, their Po-
fterity, even to this Day live almoft in the fame
manner; to whom *Lewis* XIV. fent an Embaffy,
which was treacheroufly flaughter'd by the Multitude; along with the Embaffy perifh'd *du Roule*,
and *Auguftus Lippius*, the latter of whom was a celebrated Botanift. God permitted our Species to
eat the Flefh of Animals foon after the Flood, but
with this Reftriction, that they fhould not eat their
Blood, in which was the Spirit of Life. It was
formerly judged that the Soul of Brutes refided in
their Blood; for which reafon it was not lawful to
eat Blood; but God rather feems to have been unwilling that our Species fhould eat the recent Parts
and Juices of living Animals, that they might not
become more fierce and perfidious by fuch a Diet,

as

as now obtains among the People called *Anthropo-phagi*, or Man-eaters, whose Society and Manners are the most brutal and inhuman. And much in the same manner we find that Brutes who feed upon the Flesh of other Animals alive, are the most fierce, mischievous, and untractable.

[6] We *Europeans* daily make our Aliments of Water, Milk, and all Sorts of fermented Liquors; with every Kind of Fowl, Fish, and Quadruped, and an infinite Number of Vegetables and Pulse, variously mixed and prepared by Preserving and Cooking, with Salt, Vinegar, Oil, &c. and yet Life is tolerably healthy, and long enough by a sober Use of them; even the Learned *Bacon*, as well as *Celsus* before him, condemn a too severe and simple Diet, preferring a sober and licentious Variation in our Food.

§. 51. So that by a proper Use of the several mentioned Aliments (§. 49, 50.) whether simple, *mixed together* [1], *crude* [2], or variously prepared, we find that the Life, Growth, *Nutrition* [3], and Procreation of Mankind, is principally supported and carried on. Nor does the different Nature of the Food make any *great Alteration* [4], in the *Substance* [5], or various Actions of the Body; the Parts and Organs of a human Body in Health have therefore the *Faculty* [6] of converting the various Aliments into a Matter similar to their own, and fit for *augmenting or restoring* [7] such Parts of the Body as are decay'd or consumed.

[1] The Great Man which we lately mentioned (§. 50. N. 3.) to have lived only upon Pease, after he had acquired his Health by that means,

quickly returned to his accuftomed Varieties, and that without any Impairment to his Health.

² A Gentleman of Learning delighted with the Profpect of a ftrong Camp in *France*, began to take a drawing of it, for which he was taken up as a Spy, confined in a fubterraneous Prifon, and lived for feveral Months upon nothing but Horfe-beans and Water. He found for the firft few Days, that this unaccuftomed Diet difagreed with him very much; but it became at length fo natural to him, that he has often declared in Company, after he was fet at Liberty, that he hardly ever enjoy'd better Health and Spirits than when he lived under Confinement upon that Diet. It is alfo a common thing for People to live many Years upon nothing but a Milk-diet, for fear of the Gout. And even I myfelf have lived a confiderable Time upon the pooreft Whey and Bifcuit, without the leaft Prejudice to the Strength and Action of my digeftive Organs.

³ From fo foft and fluid a Subftance as Milk only, arifes Bodies even fo compact as the Bones, tough as the Tendons, and ftrong as the Ligaments.

⁴ It is a mere Fable, that the Drinkers of Wine lofe the Strength of their mental Faculties, by abftaining from that Liquor; for I have known a wife Man, who was much addicted to Anger, live upon Whey only for the Space of fix Months by my Directions. The Counfels which he gave during that thin Diet, were not the leaft inferior to his others. *Calanus*, the Gymnofophift, who lived only upon Wheat and Water, was inferior to none of the *Greeks*, either in Quicknefs of Underftanding, or Sharpnefs of Wit.

⁵ The Blood of a Man, who feeds upon almoft every Kind of Aliment, and that of the Ox, who feeds upon Grafs only, is found to be almoft directly

ly the fame; and upon a chemical Analyfis, there
is no fenfible difference to be perceived ; but by
feeding too long upon Fifh, the Blood of Animals
has been known to contract an Odour like that of
very ftale Fifh. Nor is this to be at all wondered
at, fince the vital Juices of Animals and thofe of
Vegetables, differ only one degree from each other ;
nor is there any greater difference between our Juices
and thofe of other Animals ; even Plants themfelves
are thus known to convert their Aliment into a Nature very different from its crude State ; the Aloe
makes its bitter Juices from the fame Earth and
Water as furnifh the moft fweet and aromatic Juices;
and in this one fingle Botanic Garden at *Leyden* are
nourifhed many thoufands of Plants by the Juice
of one common Soil, which is afterwards converted
into as many different Kinds of Liquors as there are
Plants.

⁶ There is an entire Renovation of all the Nails
from their Roots in about fix Weeks time, in fuch
People as cut them every Week for neatnefs. A
broken Bone will be more ftrongly united than before in lefs than the Space of two Months ; and the
Hair of the Head is wholly renewed in about four
Months, as may appear from computing the Weight
of Hair taken off at each time, infomuch that the
whole human Body is almoft entirely changed in
about fix Months ; and yet all thefe Maffes of our
Body, fo often changed in our Life, are renewed
and made out of our Aliments. But tho' thefe *ex-
uviæ* differ in different Climates and Habits of Body,
as do alfo the Aliments, yet the fame Hair, Nails,
Cuticle, and other Parts of the Body, are again made
from the Aliment, notwithftanding their different
Nature, when the Organs exert their due Force,
by which they affimilate the Aliments into a Subftance like their own ; but when that Force is ab-

H 4   fent

sent in them, the Aliment acquires a foreign Nature, and causes a Disease. *Hippocrates* observes, that the former Races of Mankind, who fed upon the crude Grain, were subject to, many Diseases, which are now avoided by preparing the Aliments.

⁷ Suppose all the Parts of the Body to be in their healthy State, deprive them of Aliment, and the whole will shortly perish; but allow them no more than the brownest Bread and clean Water; and the several Parts of the Body will be as perfectly nourished and renewed, as from eating the richest Varieties. There is therefore a certain Power in the human Body, which can change the Nature of Bread and Water into that animal Substance of the Body, from which it before so widely differed; which Power does also produce the several Fluids in the human Body, differing from Water, from the very same Aliments, in Conjunction with that universal Basis of all Liquors. Nor could all the Powers in Nature by any means conspire to make Blood, with the other, fluid and solid Parts of the human Body, from these Aliments; if this Power, resulting from the Texture and Actions of the Parts, was once absent. The conjunct Action of all the Bodies in the World could never so much as form one human Tooth, from any or all of our Aliments, without that Power in the human Body itself, which converts the Substance of the several Aliments into that of the Teeth, and each other Part. This Power is often call'd *Nature*; being the aggregate Sum of all the Functions proper to the several Parts concerned in the Assimilation of the Aliment, or Conversion, of them into the Nature and Substance of the several component Organs of the human Body.

§. 52. But

§. 52. But daily Obfervation and Experience informs us, that this Affimilation of the Aliment, may be performed with more or lefs Eafe in the human Body; (1.) according to the different Nature of the folid and fluid Aliments in their crude State, and, (2.) according to the different artificial Preparation and Changes which they undergo, in order to facilitate that Affimilation of them afterwards in the Body.

§. 53. Therefore all Sorts of *ripe* [1] Corn or Bread Pulfe *(Cerealia* [2]) after they have been dried, *cleanfed* [3], and *ground* [4], are firft mix'd up with *Water* [5], then well *fermented* [6], and afterwards varioufly *cook'd* [7] by Fire; by which means they are much better fitted for continuing the feveral Actions, and renovating the feveral Parts, of the healthy human Body. But the Parts of Animals we find by Experience are better fitted for the fame Purpofes, by varioufly *cleanfing* [8] and preparing their Parts by *beating* [9], expofing to the *Air* [10], *pickling* [11], and drying, *boiling* [12], potting, *roafting* [13], baking, or *frying* [14], &c.

[1] For before they are ripe they are very watery, flatulent, and afford but very little Nourifhment.

[2] By this Name we comprehend all thofe Plants which bear apetalous Flowers and farinaceous Seeds upon knotty and brittle Stalks, of which the principal are, Wheat, Barley, Spelt, Rye, Oats, Millet, Rice, Maiz, &c. Before Wheat was cultivated Men ufed Acorns in their ftead. Among the feveral Sorts of Corn, Oats and Barley turn the
fooneft

foonest fowre, which therefore afford the beft Aliment in putrid Diforders.

3 Threfh'd and winnow'd from their Chaff, or common Integuments that defend the Grain from being injur'd by Infects, which being hard and indigeftible, ought not to be drels'd with the Meal; but tho' we juftly feparate the Grain from its ufelefs Chaff, we might as properly retain the Bran, or inmoft Coat of the Grain, which would render the Bread more wholfome.

4 That is, ground into coarfe Meal, or finer Flour; but even then it requires futher Preparation to render it digeftible. Horfes fed with the crude Pafte of Meal do indeed grow fat, but then they become weak and unactive.

5 Water converts Meal into a moft vifcid and ropy Pafte, which would of itfelf produce a *Leucophlegmatia*, or pituitary Swelling, Palenefs and Weaknefs throughout the whole human Body; it is even fcarce diffolvable in Water, for Lads ufe Pafte as a Bait for their Hooks, to catch Fifh with; it very quickly fattens Poultry, and other Cattle; but that Obefity is morbofe, and often fuffocates fuch Fowls as have been thus cramm'd.

6 Meal may be kept many Ages uncorrupted, if it be defended from Infects, and the Moifture of the Air; yet it is no fooner mix'd with Water into an uniform and ductile Pafte, and furrounded with a warm Air, but the whole begins to fwell, and acquire an inteftine Motion in its Parts; the Surface appears full of Eyes, or fmall Holes, and exhales a ftrong or fowerifh Odour; it alfo taftes fharp and acid, *&c.* and fuch a State of it is call'd *Fermentation*; the Meal by that Operation lofes its glutinous Quality, becomes fryable, and more eafily mifcible with Water. But Experience affures us, thofe things digeft the moft eafily which dif-

folve

folve the moft readily in Water, and thofe the moft difficultly which are leaft apt to mix with that Fluid; hence fat Subftances of all Kinds are very difficultly digefted and affimilated. But as fuch an acid Smell and Tafte is both unhealthy to the Body and unpleafant to the Palate, the Fermentation ought therefore to be ftopt before it arrives at that degree; and this is done with Fire, by baking the Dough into Bread.

[7] Baking frees the Dough from a great Part of its fuperfluous Moifture, and at the fame time difcharges the acido-aereal Fumes of the Fermentation, which thereupon ceafes; thus by degrees the Fire makes a hard Cruft upon the Surface, raifes the Bread, and renders it more dry, firm, and eatable. If it be bak'd a fecond time in the like Heat, it is then call'd Bifcuit; which, if kept free from Infects, will keep found for Years in the very hot and moift Air under the Equator, where it corrodes Iron. Bread thus prepared eafily diffolves in Water, notwithftanding its Hardnefs, without becoming glutinous, and is of all Breads by much the moft wholfome.

[8] Cleanfed from their Impurities and Hairs, that the fame might not happen in us as does to the wild Goats, who fwallowing Hairs into their Stomachs, have them ftuck together by glutinous Vifcidities, fo as to form a hard Ball, being the Caufe of many confequent Diforders, and even Death; alfo freeing them from their Blood, according to the Direction of *Mofes*; which is a moft neceffary Cuftom in the hotter Countries, becaufe the Flefh of thofe Animals who retain their Blood, quickly putrifies.

[9] Beating of Flefh always renders it the more tender, lufcious, and eafy of Digeftion; for the Juices are extravafated out of the broken Veffels,

and

and diftributed between the flefhy Fibres. The
fame Effect has alfo hunting or chafing the Animal with Dogs before it is kill'd ; fo that the Game
which are this way taken, are generally much pre-
ferr'd to home-fed and kill'd Animals of the fame
Species, as being of a much higher Relifh.

 10 Keeping of Flefh a moderate time in the Air
alfo renders it the more tender, grateful to the Palate, and eafy of Digeftion ; infomuch that a Perfon may eat double the Quantity, without any Prejudice to his Stomach, that he could of frefh-kill'd
Meat ; for when the Juices of the Flefh begin to
ferment, and incline towards a Putrifaction, the
Parts of the Humours become more volatile, their
Salts more pungent, and the folid Fibres more
tender ; but the fame Air, if it be cold, and agitated with ftrong Winds, prohibits Putrifaction,
and more efpecially fo when full of Smoke, which
is replete with the volatile acid Salt of burning
Wood, an utter Enemy to Putrifaction.

11 Meat is pickled with a Defign either to preferve it from Putrifraction, to give it a more agreeable Tafte, or to render it of more eafy Digeftion
in the Stomach ; the firft Intention is anfwered by
rubbing in common Salt, Nitre, Wine, Vinegar,
and drying in the Wind or a Stove ; the two latter
Intentions are anfwered with Salts, Acids, Sweets,
and Spices.

12 Flefh boiled in Water communicates almoft
all its Virtue to the Broth, infomuch that by changing the Water, and repeating the boiling, every
thing which is agreeable to the Palate and nourifhing to the Body may be extracted, fo as to
leave an infipid and ufelefs Skeleton. If this Broth
be infpiffated it poffeffes all the Virtue of the Flefh,
and being diftilled with an intenfe Fire, affords a
larger Quantity of volatile Salt than the Flefh, being

ing itfelf more fapid, and fubject to putrify in a
fhorter time ; for the Flefh may be kept in a temperate Air about three Days, but ftrong Broths,
and Gravy or Soops, begin to corrupt after they
have ftood but twelve Hours.

14 By roafting we underftand the dreffing of
Meat either by a naked Fire, or in a clofe Veffel,
without any Addition of Water. Roafting at a
naked Fire forms a hard and brown Cruft upon
the Surface of the Flefh, which keeps in the Juices
ftrongly agitated by the Fire, and by that means
more ftrongly tending to an alkaline State ; the
Fat becomes yellower, and more bitter, and the
whole Joint of Meat is render'd more lufcious,
dry, and eafy of Digeftion ; the open Fire thus
performs that Change upon the Salts and Juices of
the Meat in a fmall time, which a moderate Heat
does in many Days ; but the fuliginous Vapours
of the Fire which adhere to roaft and boil'd Meats,
not only renders them difagreeably black, but alfo
in conjunction with the Change they make in the
Meat, they very often produce inflammatory Fevers, efpecially when eat in too great Quahtities.

14 Frying is the dreffing of Meat in a Pan over
an open Fire with Butter or Oil ; by this Method
the Meat becomes of a very bad Digeftion to a weak
Stomach, where it quickly turns rancid and alkaline ; hence Meats thus drefs'd are as bad as Poifon to febrile Patients, and ought to make the
leaft Part of a falutary Diet ; for the Flefh this
way drefs'd fuffers a much more violent Heat than
that which is boil'd, fince Oil requires fix hundred
Degrees of Heat, by the Thermometer, to make
it boil ; whereas Water will boil with two hundred
and twelve Degrees ; fo that the faline and oily
Parts of the Meat are render'd fo much more acrimonious by the intenfer Heat.

§. 54. The

§. 54. The Materials for *Sauces* [1] and Pickling, are chiefly *Salt* [2], *Vinegar* [3], *Oils* [4] and *Spices* [5].

[1] It now remains for us to speak of those Substances used for Sauces, to excite the Appetite, and promote Digestion, as well as to render our Aliments more agreeable to the Taste. For these Purposes come in use Salts of all Kinds, of which some are acid, as Wine, Vinegar, Juice of Citrons, Lemons, *Sevile* Oranges, &c. These being mild Acids, give an Appetite to weak Stomachs, and prevent that Rankness and Sickness which otherwise so frequently happens from oily and Flesh Aliments; nor do they excite an Appetite by augmenting any Ferment of the Stomach; they rather promote Digestion, by preserving the Aliment in a found State during its Division in the Stomach. The Salts of a muriatic Kind, like the common, are both Enemies to Putrifaction, and Increasers of the *Saliva* in the Mouth; being of such considerable Use, that there are but few Nations who can do without them. Vinegar too is a volatile acid Salt, generated by a repeated Fermentation; its Acidity is both mild and grateful, not coagulating any of the animal Fluids (except Milk) whatever may be reported of it by the ignorant Populacy; but it dilutes and attenuates the Fluids, corrects and prevents Putrifaction in them, and in some degree strengthens and constringes the solid Fibres. Spices and Aromatics, are such vegetable Substances as exceed the rest in the Strength and Agreeableness of their Smell and Taste, joined with a pungent Warmness upon the Tongue; some of which are indigenous to *Europe*, notwithstanding the generality of them are brought from the *Indies*. Thus our *Angelica* Root, *Acorus*, *Southern-wood*, &c.

deserve

deferve as much the Name of Aromatics as Pepper
and Ginger. Thefe Aromatics abound with a fubtil Oil, in which is conceal'd the volatile Strength
of the Vegetable as a Spice, termed by Chemifts
their *Spiritus rector.* By that Principle they wonderfully agitate the Nerves, and ftimulate all the
folid Parts to more large and frequent Vibrations
or Contractions ; for which reafon they are faid to
be hot ; for by increafing the Motion of the Solids,
and their contained Fluids, they alfo produce Heat.
If a Thermometer is inferted into a Heap of Pepper, it fhows not the leaft Heat by any Afcent ;
and if Pepper be applied to a dead Body, it does
not in the leaft make it warmer than before : But
when taken into the living Body, by ftimulating
the folid Fibres, and augmenting the Contractions
of the Veffels, they increafe the Motion of the Blood,
which produces Heat.———To thefe we may add
every kind of Pickles, which through the Luxury
of our Appetites are every Year increafing ; and
may all of them be reduced to fome of the fore-
mentioned Claffes, fuch as the choice *Garum* of the
Romans, a Pickle made of the ftrongeft Salt and
the Liver of the Fifh *Scombrus,* intimately diffolved
together ; the *Ruffian Caviaro,* made from the fe-
miputrid Ovary of the Fifh *Accipenfer* ; the *French
Botargue, Anchovies,* &c. the Strength of all which
depends principally upon the Sea-falt.

² The Flefh which would putrify in three Days
time if left to itfelf, may be preferved found for
many Years, if it be frequently rubb'd with dry
Bay-falt, or immerged in a ftrong Brine made of
the fame Salt. Common Salt will alfo have the
fame Effect, as will alfo *Sal Gem, Sal Ammoniacum,*
Salt-petre and Allum, except that the Allum communicates a difagreeable Relifh to the Meat.

³ Vinegar,

3. Vinegar, diluted with Water, made a very wholsome Drink amongst the *Roman* Soldiers; they gave this to our Saviour at his Expiration, not out of Derision, but as being the first Drink at hand. Wine and Vinegar prevent the Putrifaction of Flesh by their Acid; thus Brawn is preferved in Wine.

4. Oil or Butter preferve Flesh, by covering it, and excluding the Air and Insects, fo that it may be conveyed from *Britain* to the *Indies*, according to Mr. *Boyle*.

5. Flesh which is frequently rubb'd with Pepper and Ginger will not putrify, becaufe thofe Spices keep out Infects, and dry up the Moisture.

§. 55. Garden *Fruits* 1 are indeed of fo foft a Texture when full ripe, that they require little or no Preparation to render them digeftible in the Stomach.

1 Garden Fruits, which are reftrained to their particular Seafons of the Year, are all of them of a foft, pulpy Texture, and inclined to acid. When they are full ripe (which may be generally known by the Tafte of each, being the moft perfect in their Kind, and in the Apple-kind, by the Blacknefs of their Seeds or Kernels) they are then of very eafy Digeftion; but they are all in general apt to breed Wind in the Bowels, which may however be much prevented by dreffing them with Fire, or fcooping fuch as may be that way eaten, as Apples and Turnips in particular. An Apple which was placed in *Boyle*'s exhaufted Receiver, difcharg'd twenty times its Quantity of elaftic Air in the Space of twenty-four Hours; which Air is fometimes found to be twice more heavy than that of our Atmofphere. Therefore Garden Fruits muft be un-
wholfome

wholfome to fome by their Acidity and Flaculency, as they put on a State of Fermentation in the Sto-mach, efpecially when eaten crude, and in very warm Weather. If the Elaftic Air which they thus generate in Fermentation finds a free Exit either up-wards or downwards, it is forwarded by no ill Con-fequences ; but if it is confined in the Stomach by a Stricture of its two Orifices, or even in the Bow-els, it has been known to occafion great Diftention, excruciating Pain, violent Inflammation, and even Death. Nor are we without Inflances of the fatal Effects of the fuffocating Air arifing from the Juices of Garden Fruits in their Fermentation, and burft-ing through the fmall Crevices of their including Cafks. But when Fruits have once paffed the Acti-on of the Fire, which extricates the Air, they are then quite inoffenfive to the digeftive Organs.

§. 56. As for Drink, the beft is *pure run-ning Water* [1], which may be drank *crude* [2] ; but if it contains Infects, their Eggs or other foreign Bodies, it may be better fitted for Ser-vice, by philtrating through a Pumix or other porous Stone ; alfo by gently *boiling* [3], and let-ting it ftand to fettle a while. But as to Drinks made by a *Decoction* [4] of Fruits or any Sort of Grain in Water, the Nature and Ufe of them may be eafily underftood ; nor is the Compo-fition and Ufe of Malt Liquors lefs known, particularly *Ale* [5], made by fweating and dry-ing the Corn in the Mow, cleanfing it from its Chaff, macerating in Water till it begins to vegetate, then by drying in a Kiln, grinding, and infufing in fcalding Water, then boiling, fermenting, and clarifying. The Formation

I   and

and Ufe of *Wines* 6 are alfo as equally intelligible; made by preffing out the Juice of ripe
Grapes, fermenting and refining the fame.

1 *Water* is the common Drink of all vegetating
Bodies, the *Vinum Catholicum* of the Alchemifts,
without which they affirm nothing can grow and
increafe, whether it be animal, vegetable, or mineral. The pureft Water is alfo found to be always the lighteft, becaufe every foreign Body mixed with Water, as Sand, Earth, Minerals, &c.
is heavier than the Water itfelf; upon which account the *Æthiopians* are faid to be long-liv'd,
whofe very light Waters would not fuftain a Piece
of Wood. Rain-water is the pureft, or moft fimple; not that which falls down in Showers through
the Air, and becomes a Lixivium, by diffolving
all the volatile Salts, and other Bodies floating
therein; but that which defcends from the Clouds
by the Attraction of the higheft ftony Mountains,
thro' which the Water is ftrained, and freed from
every thing foreign, and then runs down in pure
Streams thro' fandy Currents towards the Foot of
the Mountain.

2 Pure Water is beft drank crude; fo that *Nero*
did not act wifely, when being fick of every Sort of
Wine, and exhaufted with the Fatigues of Luxury, at laft drank Water, but after it had been firft
boiled in golden Veffels.

3 The Rain-water which defcends thro' the Air
in Showers, and is retained in Veffels, is found to
be replete with the invifible Eggs of Infects and
Seeds of Plants; infomuch that by letting it ftand
expofed to the warm Air in a Glafs Veffel, you
will quickly perceive it generate many Kinds of
fmall Weeds and minute Kinds of Animals; the
fame will alfo happen if you keep it ever fo clean
in

in Glaffes; but when once the Water has fuffer'd
boiling, then all the vegetating or prolific Power
in the minute Ova of the Plants and Animals is
deftroy'd; yet more boiling than once will be pre-
judicial to the Water, the Water having fome part
of its Subftance changed into a folid Sediment every
time it is boiled.

⁴ The Drinks thus made by a Decoction, par-
take of the Nature of the unfermented Mafs (at
§. 53. N.   ) before-mentioned, being aceffent
and very flatulent; which latter Inconvenience ob-
taining much in the Decoction of Barley, made
Galen prefer a Decoction of Bread to it, in whofe
previous Fermentation the flatulent Parts had been
exhaled.

⁵ Ale, or the Wine of Corn, is faid to be the
Invention of *Ofiris*, who travelling round the
World, taught thofe People whofe Countries bore
Vines, the Art of making Wine from their Fruit;
and inftructed the more cold and depreffed Countries in the way of making Ale, which differs not
greatly from Wine, by malting and brewing their
Corn. And the Ufe of Ale is certainly of very
great Antiquity among the *Germans*. The Method of malting and brewing Corn for this Liquor
is thus: Any Sort of Corn, as Barley, being freed
from its Chaff and Stubble, is infufed whole in hot
Water till it begins to fwell; the Grain is then
freed from its Water, and flung into Heaps, where
it is fuffer'd to lie till it ferments and grows fo hot
as to be fcarce tolerable to the Hand, continuing
thus till every Grain begins to grow or thruft forth
its Blade; but to prevent the Vegetation from going any farther, the Heap is fpread abroad to dry,
and is afterwards further dry'd, or flightly roafted
over the Fire in a Kiln; after which it takes the
Name of *Malt*. The Grain thus treated becomes

sweet and glutinous, easily communicating its Virtues to Water; the ground Malt is therefore cast into scalding Water, and all its fine, mealy and saccharine Part is by that means extracted. If this Tincture of the Malt is boiled, inspissated, decanted off clear, and then drank, it does not inebriate or affect the Head, but attenuates the Fluids, and runs off either in a Diarrhæa or Dysentery. If it be thus set by in Casks, it ferments and turns to Vinegar; but to prevent that, it is deposited, with some bitter Plant, as Hops, in a Heat of about 60 Degrees; and thus the Fermentation is restrained, to the Production of a vinous, inebriating Liquor, which affords an Alchohol, or inflammable Spirit by Distillation, not at all inferior to that obtained from Wine; but such very strong Ale is not healthy for strong Constitutions.

' Wine, invented by *Noah*, is of much greater Antiquity than the Ale preceding, and has all along retained its most ancient Name *Vin*, from the primitive Languages; it is supposed to have been first contrived in the hot Countries, whose Inhabitants having but little Water, and that impure, were obliged to seek for a more agreeable Drink in the Grape. But the richest and most exquisite Wine, is that which runs spontaneously from the Grapes perfectly ripe, which being laid in Heaps, burst of themselves, and afford the Wine we call *Nectar*. Wine drank before it has fermented, is not at all spirituous, but flatulent, and productive of Diarrhæa's, Dysenteries, &c. yet a perfect Fermentation renders it uniform and pleasant, spirituous, inebriating, or acid.—The most common Method of extracting this Liquor from the Grape, is by treading with the Feet of Men, or pressing with some other Machine; by which means they afford a greater Plenty of Juice, but not at all comparable

ble

ble to the former. Wines of various Kinds may be alfo obtained by Fermentation from the Juice of Strawberries, Elderberries, and various other Fruits. Wines are generally of ufe when it is neceffary to warm and invigorate the whole Habit of Body ; but for People in Health, and thofe in Fevers, Water is greatly preferable, to attenuate the vifcid Blood, dilute and difcharge its acrimonious and ufelefs Parts.

§. 57. The confequent Effect of all thefe Preparations (§. 53, to 57.) of our Aliments, is, that their Parts are *attenuated*[1] and open'd, intimately *mix'd*[2], diluted, and render'd more *fluid*[3] and comminutable ; and by feparating their more grofs and ufelefs from their healthy Parts, they are thus made more perfectly *digeftible*[4] in the human Body ; alfo fitted for renewing its Parts, and paffing the feveral Organs for Secretion and Excretion.

[1] Attenuation is the Divifion of the Part of any Body into leffer Particles, by which means their Surfaces are increafed ; but it is the Surfaces of the Parts of our Aliments which are applied to the Powers of our digeftive Organs ; therefore by increafing the Surfaces of the Parts of our Aliments we have the fame Effect as if we augmented the Strength of our digeftive Organs, which are to operate upon the Aliments.
[2] No Operation is more neceffary to Health, than an intimate and uniform Mixture of the Parts of our Aliments ; but that can hardly be effected without the preceeding Attenuation.
[3] Fluidity arifes in a great meafure from the Lubricity, or fmooth Surfaces of the Particles, which

by

by that means flide eafily upon each other, without any confiderable Friction; that Lubricity of Parts may be alfo made by ftriking off their Inequalities or Afperities by Friction from repeated Motion.— The Common People often eat various Aliments without hardly ever drinking; which Aliments are however digefted and turned into Fluids; but that muft be done by attenuating their Parts, and giving them fmoother Surfaces.

⁴ Some Parts of our Aliments are perfectly affimilated by the Powers in the human Body, fo as to become abfolutely Part of ourfelves; but there are other Parts which refift the Force of all our Organs, and are therefore caft out of the Body unaltered; thus in the firft Digeftion we met with the Skins of Cherries, Goofeberries, &c. entire in the Fæces, and but little altered; and fo alfo, in the Urine after the fecond Digeftion; fuch Parts ought therefore to be feparated from the reft, which we find is performed by the Actions of the Parts in the human Body: but the Aliments are by thefe Preparations in a great meafure previoufly fubjected to fuch a Separation, to facilitate their fubfequent Digeftion in the Body. A Perfon that drinks Flefh Broths, does not require fuch a Force to be exerted by the digeftive Organs, as if he eat the folid flefhy Parts, whofe Fibres are to be broke in funder to difcharge their nutritious Juices. *Lower* tells us of a young Man almoft kill'd with frequent Hæmorrhages, whofe Life was fuftained by conftant drinking of Flefh Broths, who muft otherwife have perifh'd through Weaknefs.—So that all thefe Preparations of our Aliments are done in Imitation of Nature, to eafe her.

Maftication

Mastication of the Aliments.

§. 58. THE various Kinds of solid *Food* [1] (§. 49, to 52.) thus prepared *(per* §. 57.) undergo several other Changes in the Mouth; (1.) by biting, (2.) by *Mastication* [2], and, (3.) by mixing with Particles of Air the Saliva, and other Fluids discharged into the Cavity of the Mouth.

[1] Nature and Method directs us to consider, I. The Nature of the Aliments, (§. 49, to 57.) II. The Instruments of Assimilation, by which the Aliments are converted in Part of ourselves, (§. 58, to 433.) and III. The History of the Matter itself, which is by that means applied to renew the Parts of the Body, (§ 434, to 480.)

[2] By Mastication we understand the Comminution of the solid Aliment by Trituration in the Mouth, being at the same time diluted with the Saliva; the chief Object of this Operation is the solid Aliment to be comminuted, in order to give their Parts a larger Surface, that they may be more easily digested by the Powers of their proper Organs in the human Body; though as a secondary Object of this Operation, we may take in Spices, and other Sauces, which are used more for Pleasure than as Aliment. To explain the Business of Mastication, is to assign the Causes by which the Aliment is ground together in the Mouth.

§. 59. The first thing required in *biting* [1] or dividing our Aliment, is an Abduction of the lower *Jaw* [2] down from the upper, towards

I 4   the

the Breaſt, turning upon its *Condyloide* Proceſſes, which are articulated to the *Protube-*
rances 3 of the *Oſſa Temporalia* by a Ligament
inveſting the wholeArticulation, between which
is interpoſed a ſmall moveable *Cartilage* 4, concave on each ſide, and affixed to neither of the
Bones, but connected by its Margin to the circular Ligament inveſting the whole Articulation; being lubricated on each of its Concave
Surfaces with a mucilaginous Liniment preſſed
out of the Cells which inveſt the Articulation.
In the next place biting requires the lower Jaw
to be again forcibly preſſed up againſt the upper Jaw, that whatever Aliment is interpoſed
betwixt the Eight foremoſt Teeth (term'd *In-*
ciſores, and placed in each Jaw oppoſite to one
another) may be cut aſunder by them.

᾽ Biting is the Action by which the ſolid Aliment is broke into ſmall Parcels by the Teeth;
the Neceſſity of which Operation is evident in ſeveral of the harder Kinds of Food which Men eat,
ſuch as Nuts, *&c.*
  ᾽ The lower Jaw conſiſts of two Parts in the
Fœtus, that it may the more eaſily be extended in
Growth; but in the Adult it is one continued Bone.
A Fracture of the lower Jaw will obſtruct the
Action of Deglutition, as we have an Inſtance in
a celebrated Duke, who had his lower Jaw broke
by a Bullet; whenever that Nobleman ſwallowed
any of his Food, he was obliged firſt to put it upon his Tongue with his Fingers. The lower Jaw
is moved in various Directions upwards, downwards, backwards, forwards, and to each ſide, and
in all Directions compounded of theſe like a Mill-
ſtone;

stone; for as in a Mill one Stone which is moveable grinds the Corn upon another which is fixed, so the lower Jaw grinds the Aliment against the immoveable upper Jaw.

3 It has been the Opinion of most Anatomists, that the lower Jaw is articulated in a *Sinus* of the squammose Part of the *Os Temporale,* situated before the *Meatus Auditorius;* but *Ravius* first observed in himself, and in many Dissections, that this Cavity is filled with a glandulous and adipose Substance, which serves to quicken and facilitate the motion of the Joint ; and when absent, occasions a disagreeable grating of the Bones in Mastication; but he found that the *Condyloide* Processes of the lower Jaw were articulated with the Protuberances of the *Ossa Temporalia,* placed before those Cavities, to whose Figure that of the *Condyloide* Processes correspond.

4 In every Articulation of the moveable Bones, we meet with, 1. smooth Cartilages investing the Head of the Bones, and lubricated with their proper Mucilage. 2. Ligaments, and Capsulæ, which invest the Heads of the Bones, and arise from the *Symphysis* of the *Diaphysis* with the *Epiphysis* of the Bone, which *Columbus* truly remarks ; but these *Epiphyses* separate from the Body of the Bone in young Subjects, and are kept distinct from their proper Bones in *Ravius*'s Repository. 3. The lubricating Mucilage from *Havers*'s Glands, expressed from the Arteries in form of the White of an Egg. But besides all these Particulars, which are in common to every Articulation, the lower Jaw has also a particular Mechanism of its own, by which it is articulated with the upper, to prevent its Cartilages, and those of the *Ossa temporalia,* from being wore out or ground away by the daily Attrition which they suffer in Mastication ; for besides the

two

two cartilagenous Coverings which inveſt the Heads of the lower Jaw, and thoſe Parts of the *Oſſa temporalia*, to which they are connected, there is alſo interpoſed a moveable Cartilage, concave on each ſide, into which Cavities are receiv'd the Tubercles on each of the lower Jaw, faſten'd together by a circumambient Ligament.

§. 60. The lower Jaw is pulled down in this *Action*[1], by the Contraction of the two *digaſtric*[2] Muſcles, which ariſe fleſhy from a ſmall Cavity in the Baſis of the *Maſtoide* Proceſſes; and in their Deſcent form Tendons, which paſs through the *Stylo-hyoide* Muſcles, and the annular Ligament fixed to the Sides of the *Os Hyoides*; from whence again they become fleſhy, and being-furniſhed with fleſhy Fibres from the *Os Hyoides*, they aſcend to their Inſertion, in the inſide of the lower Margin of the *Os Maxillare inferior*, at the middle of the Chin, being the lowermoſt of all the Muſcles inſerted at that Part of the Chin, by which *Mechaniſm*[3] theſe Muſcles are found to act with the Power and Direction of the Pully, through which their Tendons paſs in a very artificial and ſurpriſing *manner*[4]; ſo that theſe Muſcles can perform their proper Office by the Contraction of their Parts inſerted into the Chin, and alſo by thoſe which are inſerted into the *Maſtoide* Proceſſes of the Head, without any Injury to the Parts, or obſtructing the Action of the other.

[1] The lower Jaw may be eaſily pull'd down from the upper, ſo as to intercept the ſecond Joint of the Thumb;

Thumb; but if it is pull'd down lower, there is danger of a Luxation.

² The *Coracobyoidei* Muſcles are alſo Digaſtrics or Biventres, but they have no relation to the Mechaniſm of theſe; and when they were formerly called *Biventres* by Anatomiſts, they were alſo diſtinguiſh'd by the Epithet *Colli.*

³ The Action of every Muſcle is to contract, or ſhorten in length, and by that means to draw the moveable Part of its Inſertion towards the leſs, or immoveable Part, in a Direction which approaches neareſt to a right Line. Were the digaſtric Muſcles to act in ſuch a Direction, they would not pull the lower Jaw down, but directly upward and backward; their Direction is therefore changed, by faſtening their middle Tendon to a Pulley, which in Infants is a callous Membrane, but in Adults a cartilagenous Ring; they thus paſs in an angular Direction, their fix'd Point being at the *Os hyoides*; ſo that one Part of the Muſcle being contracted, the other muſt follow, and pull the lower Jaw, not towards its Origin, at the *maſtoide* Proceſs; but downwards, toward the *Os hyoides.*

⁴ It was neceſſary that there ſhould be ſome Muſcles proper to the Abduction of the lower Jaw from the upper, tho' there was no occaſion for them to be large, nor very numerous, ſince the lower Jaw's own Weight, and free Suſpenſion for Motion, ſo facilitate its Deſcent from the upper, that in ſleeping, and in apoplectic and paralytic Perſons, it is generally found in that Poſture, but more diſagreeably gaping; yet it was neceſſary there ſhould be ſome Muſcles for this Office, to overcome the natural tonic or contractile motion of the elevating Muſcles, which conſtantly ſuſtain the Weight of the lower Jaw from ſubſiding when we are awake. The *quadratus genæ*, or *latiſſimus colli,*

colli, would not have been ſufficient to pull the
Jaw down of itſelf, if it aſſiſts in that Action ; becauſe its Force is ſpent in corrugating the Skin of
the Neck, Face, and Chin ; nor has it a ſuitable
Origin and Direction from and over the *Sternum*
and *Clavicle*; nor does it paſs along the Neck, ſo
as to be inſerted into the lower Jaw. A Muſcle is
therefore contrived by a wonderful Mechaniſm, ſo
as to perform the ſame Office which it would have
done in an oppoſite Direction to its Origin and
Progreſs. But it is alſo probable that the Elevation of the upper Jaw from the lower by the
ſtrong *Splenii, complexi, &c.* Muſcles which pull
back the Head, does alſo contribute to the opening of the Mouth ; for we find that a Dog will
growl notwithſtanding his lower Jaw be held firm
upon a Stone Table, *&c.*

§. 61. The latter Action (§. 59.) or Adducti-
on of the lower Jaw to divide the Aliment, is
performed by the Contraction, (1.) of the *Temporal Muſcles*; which ariſe by a broad, ſemi-
circular, and fleſhy Origin, from an Excavation in the *Os Frontis*, the Top of the *Sphenoides*, and *Os Temporale*, from whence the Fibres running together, are united under the *Os
Jugale*, being alſo ſtrengthened and directed
by other Fibres received from the ſame Bone,
they are inſerted, partly fleſhy, and partly tendinous, into and round the *Proceſſus Corones* of
the lower Jaw. (2.) By the Contraction of
the *Maſſeter Muſcles*, which ariſe thick and
fleſhy from the firſt Bone of the upper Jaw,
the *Os Jugale*, from whence its Fibres croſſing
each other, are inſerted into the external and
                                        lower

lower Margin of the lower Jaw, for about four
Fingers Breadth from its Angle towards the
Chin. (3.) By the Contraction of the *Pterugoideï externi* [1], which ariſe from the external
Face of the outer Wing of the *Proceſſus Pte-
rugoides*, belonging to the *Os Sphenoides*, whence
deſcending backward, they are inſerted by a
ſtrong Tendon within ſide the ſemilunar Space
betwixt the *Condyloide* and *Coronoide* Proceſſes
of the lower Jaw ; when theſe Muſcles act together, they draw the lower Jaw upwards and
forwards, and obliquely forwards to one ſide,
when only one of them acts. (4.) By the
Action of the *Pterugoideï interni* [2], which ariſe
fleſhy and tendinous from the whole internal
Surface of the outer Wing of the *Pterugoide*
Proceſs, thence deſcending to their Inſertion,
by a ſtrong and broad Tendon, into a ſmall
Excavation a little above and within ſide the
Angle of the lower Jaw, under the *Condyloide*
Proceſs ; when both theſe Muſcles act together,
they pull the Jaw very ſtrongly upwards and
backwards, like the *Maſſeters*, and obliquely
backward or to one ſide when only one of them
acts. Now if theſe eight deſcribed Muſcles
contract together, they preſs the lower Jaw a-
gainſt the upper with an *incredible Force* [3]; the
whole Force terminating in the two Rows of
Teeth [4] placed in each Jaw ; and thus the eight
Dentes Inciſores being ſtrongly preſſed together,
the Act of biting is performed.

[1] Theſe muſt pull the lower Jaw forwards, becauſe their Origin at the immoveable Bone is more
forwards

forwards than their Inſertion into the Jaw; but when they act in conjunction with the digaſtric and temporal Muſcles, they then move the Jaw backwards and upwards.

2 If only one of theſe act, it draws the lower Jaw to one ſide; but contracting both together, they elevate it.

3 The great Strength of the Lion, the *Britiſh* Maſtiff-Dog, and all Sorts of voracious Animals in general, conſiſt in theſe eight Muſcles. *Veſalius* tells us of having ſeen an Actor who took up an Iron Pin of twenty-five Pounds Weight in his Mouth, and reclining his Head backward, flung it nine and thirty Foot behind him with ſuch a Force, that it ſtuck into a Beam at that diſtance; and of another, a *Turk*, who would carry a Beam in his Mouth of a Weight ſufficient to load any ſtrong Man; and I myſelf have ſeen a Man take an empty Hogſhead in his Teeth and carry it about with eaſe; and another Man who would lift prodigious Weights by a Rope with his Teeth. Phrenitic Patients ſometimes ſhut their Jaws with ſo much Violence as to break off pieces of their moſt hard Teeth. In theſe Actions the *Dentes inciſores* ſuſtain the biggeſt Force, which are therefore made of a more compact Subſtance than the *Molares.*

4 All the Teeth may be diſtinguiſh'd into four Claſſes. I. The *Inciſores*, fix'd perpendicular with one ſolid Root, forming a Wedge or Chiſſel by a circular Excavation within, being eight in Number, four in each Jaw; the Office of theſe is to bite, cut, and tear the Aliment, not to grind it; they are the firſt that appear in Infants, at the time when they live upon fluid Aliments requiring no Maſtication. II. The four *Canini*, placed one on each ſide the *Inciſores*, with a ſingle Root, being

very

very strong, and of a conical Figure, terminating
in a sharp Point, fit to hold fast and lacerate the
more tough Ailments.   Ruminating Animals having no Use for these Teeth, are always without
them; they are much stronger than the *Incisores,*
and serve to hold the Aliment fast, that it may be
the better divided by the rest of the Teeth.   III.
The *anterior Molares,* eight in Number, placed
two on each side of the *Canini,* having a somewhat
plain, but rougher Surface than the rest, and fastened with a double Root.   IV. The *posterior Molares,* twelve in Number, three of a side in each
Jaw, having broad, flattish Heads, with rough
Surfaces, and fastened with three or four Roots;
upon these the Aliment is chiefly comminuted into
smaller Parts, and ground into a soft uniform Mass,
like Fruits which have been ground between two
Stones in a Mill; therefore graniverous Fowls,
who have none of these Teeth to grind the Grain
they feed upon, have very strong Stomachs, which
being stuff'd with small angular Stones, performs
the Office of our *Dentes molares.*   The Substance
of the Roots and internal Part of the Teeth is
boney, but their external Covering is different
from any of the other Bones, approaching the
Texture of the hardest Marble.

§. 62. The Food being thus divided by biting, is then *pressed*[1] between the rough and
large Surfaces of the *Dentes Molares,* to be there
further comminuted by grinding.   'Tis forced
in betwixt the Grinders, (1.) by the Contraction of the *Buccinator*[2] Muscle, which (arising broad and fleshy from the anterior Part of
the *Processus Corones* of the lower Jaw, adheres
fast to the Gums of each Jaw by direct Fibres,
which

which paſſing along the Cheeks, are inſerted
into the Angles of the Lips, and preſs the
Cheeks cloſe to the outſide of the grinding
Teeth: (2). By the *Orbicularis Labiorum* or
Sphincter of the Mouth, which (being faſtened by membranous Ligaments to the Gums in
the middle of the upper and lower Lip, en-
compaſſes the Mouth and Lips with its fleſhy
Fibres, and) is inſerted into no Bone, but cor-
rugates, contracts, or ſhuts the Mouth. (3). By
the *Zeugomatic Muſcles*, which ariſe fleſhy from
the external Part of the *Os Jugale*, whence
deſcending obliquely, they are inſerted into the
Angles of the Lips, which they draw obliquely upwards, and preſs a Portion of the Cheek,
near the upper Part of the *Buccinator*, againſt
the Gums of the upper Jaw. (4) By the *Ele-*
vator labiorum communis, which ariſing from
the fourth Bone of the upper Jaw deſcends
obliquely to its Inſertion at the Corners of the
Lips, under the Tendon of the preceding Muſcle, and moves the Lips more directly upwards,
compreſſing them and the adjacent part of the
Cheeks againſt the Teeth and Gums: (5.) By
the *Elevator labii ſuperioris proprius*, which is
a double Muſcle, one Part ariſing above the o-
ther from the fourth Bone of the upper Jaw,
and deſending obliquely, terminates in an Expanſion under the Skin of the upper Lip; the
other Part of the ſame Muſcle ariſes from the
anterior Part of the upper Jaw, about the middle of the Baſis of the Noſe, and is diſperſed
into the middle of the upper Lip, theſe Muſcles

acting

acting together, press the upper Lip, contracted
by the Sphincter Muscle, against the anterior
and superior Teeth and Gums: (6.) by the *Depressor labii inferioris proprius,* which arises
from the lower Part of the Jaw-bone at the
Chin, and is inserted into the lower Lip. (7.)
By the *Elevator labii inferioris proprius,* which
arises from the anterior Part of the Gums and
lower Jaw, about the *Dentes Incisores,* and is
inserted into the Skin of the lower Part of the
Chin. These Muscles, by the Assistance of
(8.) the *Depressor labiorum communis,* which
arises fleshy from the inferior Margin of the
lower Jaw, and ascending on the Side thereof,
is inserted in the Angles of the Lips. (9.) The
oblique Muscles of the lower Lip, arising from
the middle of the forepart of the inferior Margin of the lower Jaw, ascending obliquely into
the lower Lip. (10.) By the *Platysma Myoides*
or *quadratus genæ,* which being extended immediately under the Fat, spreads almost over
the whole Breast, down to the Paps, forming
a broad membranous and tendinous Expansion
upon the upper Part of the pectoral Muscle,
from whence it is continued above the *Clavicles,* over the Neck, under the Chin, and over
Part of the Face, above the Masseter Muscles,
as high as the Basis of the Nose, strictly bind-
ing together with its tendinous Fibres all the
Muscles it passes over, and applying the Cheeks
to the grinding Teeth and Gums, and variously
contracts and moves the Integuments of the
Breast, Neck, Chin, and lower Part of the

Face.——When all the Muſcles act together, both the Cheeks and Lips are then ſo ſtrongly preſſed againſt the Gums and Teeth, that no Part of the ſolid or fluid Aliment can fall down between the Teeth, Gums, and Cheeks; but if they act ſucceſſively one after another, the Aliment is then determined to various Parts of the Mouth. The Action of theſe Muſcles is antagoniz'd within ſide the Teeth by the *Tongue* 4, which keeps the Aliment from ſlipping down on its Side, and alſo preſſes it between the Teeth, being a Muſcle the moſt voluble or nimble at Will of any in the Body, and capable of being eaſily moved to all Parts of the Mouth. The Tongue performs its Motions, (1.) by the *Geniogloſſi* Muſcles, which ariſe fleſhy from the internal Part of the Chin, and dilating as they proceed backward, are inſerted into the Root of the Tongue, ſerving to contract the Sides, and draw the Tongue forwards. (2.) By the *Ceratogloſſi*, which ariſe broad and fleſhy from the Side of the *Os Hyoides*, from whence aſcending, we perceive them diſperſing their Fibres plentifully through the Tongue, which they ſerve to pull back, preſs down, and flatten. (3.) By the *Stylogloſſi*, which ariſe ſharp and fleſhy from the external Part of the *Proceſſus Styloides* 5 of the *Oſſa Temporum*, whence deſcending obliquely forwards, they are inſerted into the back Part of the Tongue, which they elevate, draw to each ſide, or flatten, as they ſend out fleſhy Fibres to the internal Sides of the lower Jaw. (4.) By the muſcular

muſcular Fibres, which form the *Body of the Tongue* itſelf, ſome of which are longitudinal, ſhortning the Tongue, others tranſverſe, making it narrower; ſome again are perpendicular, expanding it thin, and flat; others contracting the back Part and Sides thereof, make it ſharp-pointed, and draw it inwards; others depreſs it in the ſame Figure; and laſtly, there are ſtraight Fibres, which contract the Root of the Tongue together. By all theſe various Muſcles and Fibres acting ſeparately and conjunctly, we may eaſily account for the Determination of the Aliment by the Tongue between the grinding Teeth and the Conveyance of the fluid as well as the ſolid Aliment, by the ſame Organ towards the *Fauces* and *Oeſophagus*, eſpecially when the joint Action of thoſe Fibres which paſs from the Tongue amongſt the external Muſcles, which both act together, and by that means the ſolid or fluid Aliment, which ſlips down under the Tongue, or on each ſide of the lower Teeth, is readily taken up, and laid upon its Back, in order to be ſwallowed.

The great Number of Muſcles which are here enumerated for the Office, all of them act at Pleaſure, or the Influence of the Will; and ſuch is their Connexion with each other, that if one becomes paralytic, all the Aliment will be forced by the Action of the reſt to that Part of the Mouth near the paralytic Muſcle, inſomuch that the Patient is oblig'd to ſupply the place of that Muſcle by preſſing the Cheek with his Hand; the ſame thing happens when we are about to ſwallow even ſo

much as a Drop of *Saliva,* fo that the Cheeks leave
no Cavity, but prefs all the *Saliva* upon the back
of the Tongue. Thefe Mufcles have been well
pictur'd by *Euftachius,* who was not only affifted
herein by Plenty of Bodies, but even thofe too of
the lean and various countenanc'd *Italians,* in which
Subjects it was much eafier to prepare the Mufcles
of the Face, which are interwoven with Skin and
Fat, than in the more plump-fac'd Inhabitants
of the Countries which are nearer to the North ;
and *Santorinus* has even furpaffed the Induftry of
Euftachius in his Obfervations upon this Head.

² The buccinator Mufcle is of great Efficacy, as
well in preffing the Cheeks againft the Teeth, by
which means the firft Cavity of the Mouth is clofed, as by compreffing the fmall Glands of the
Cheeks, and by that means folliciting them to a
more plentiful Secretion of *Saliva* ; if thefe Mufcles
become paralytic, the Patient cannot chew his Aliment ; for whatever he takes in his Mouth, is
thruft out on each fide of his Cheeks.

³ This Mufcle gave occafion for *Galen* to ima-
gine that there was an univerfal *Panniculus carno-
fus,* which he affirms to be extended like a Mufcle
next to the Skin all over the Body ; but tho' this
Mechanifm is-frequent in Brutes, there was no occafion for it in a human Body, becaufe Infects and
other Nuifances might be remov'd by the Hands.

⁴ The Tongue has fo many Ufes, that it is no
eafy matter to recount them all ; it is the Organ
of Tafte, the Articulator of Speech, and a great
Inftrument in Deglutition ; but it alfo fhares a
great Part in the Bufinefs of Maftication, which is
quite different from that of Deglutition ; infomuch
that if the Tongue becomes paralytic on one fide,
the Patient cannot chew his Aliment on that fide.

⁵ The

5. The *Os Styloides* is not a Proceſs of the *Os Temporale*, as Anatomiſts generally imagine; but a diſtinct Bone, which is faſtened by Ligaments to the *Os Petroſum*, as *Ruyſch* firſt demonſtrated to us in old People; indeed the Articulation is obliterated, and the *Os Styliforme* becomes continuous with the *Os Petroſum*; but even in the *Cranium* of Adults it is eaſily broken in that Part, and is hardly ever to be found entire in the Skulls of the Church-yards.

6. The Muſcles of the Tongue, of which it is chiefly compoſed, give it that exceeding Volubility or Nimbleneſs which we find in the human Tongue; for the internal Structure of the Tongue is truly an inſcrutable Muſcle, the Texture of which has been deſcribed by no Body before *Malphigius*; nor even has he expoſed the Texture of the Fibres belonging to the Tongue in a human Subject; but in that of a Calf; for the human Tongue is ſo ſmall, ſo tender, and ſo intermixed with Fat, that its Structure is obſcured, and nothing can be diſtinctly obſerved. The Tongue of an Ox exhibits the internal Structure not only more evident by its Magnitude, but its Fibres are alſo more conſpicuous, by their more frequent Action in cropping the Meadows. So various are the Directions of theſe Fibres, that there is no Arch of a Circle but what may be freely deſcribed by the Tongue; to diſſect this Part, it ſhould be firſt boiled in Water, and often ſhifted, till there remains nothing of the Fat mixing itſelf with the Water; then pinning it down, firſt remove the Cuticle, and then the perforated *Corpus reticulare*, then the papillary Covering, and their adhering *Adeps*; and thus you may have a diſtinct View of the muſcular Fibres.

K 3 §. 63. From

§. 63. From hence it evidently appears in what manner the Aliment is ground and attenuated by the Action of the Muscles moving the Jaws, (§. 60, and 61.) being first divided by opening and shutting them, then pressed on each side betwixt the grinding Teeth, by the Muscles of the Cheeks, Lips and Tongue ; where, being sufficiently comminuted, it is conveyed backwards to the *Oesophagus*.

§. 64. By this Preparation in the Mouth, the Aliment undergoes the same Changes as have been already mentioned (at §. 57.) *viz.* a farther Attenuation and more intimate Mixture of their Parts. 2. It undergoes several other Changes with being mixed with Saliva and Fluids of the Mouth; with the Mucus of the Palate and *Fauces.* 3. And lastly, it receives other Alterations from the small Particles of Air which are intermixed and retained by the viscid *Saliva.*

Of the Origin, Nature, and Mixture of the Saliva with the Aliments.

§. 65. THE *Saliva* flows into the Mouth from 1. the *Parotides*, two conglomerate Glands, situated each in a Cavity at the Root of the Ear, between the *Condyloide* and *Mastoide* Processes, belonging to the lower Jaw and *Os Petrosum*, under the *Os Jugale*;

it

it contains a *conglobate Gland* 1, within fide,
and is largely extended forwards, backwards,
and downwards, fomewhat in a triangular Figure; thefe Glands do by their Structure feparate the *Saliva* from the *Arterial Blood* 2, and
convey it when feparated, each into one *common Duct* 3, which difcharges it into the Mouth
through the *buccinator Mufcle* 4, near the third
of the upper grinding Teeth : 2. from the *fub
Maxillares*, two confiderable Glands, fituated
one on each Side, juft within the inferior Margin of the lower Jaw, being large towards the
Angle of the Jaw, and extended fmaller under
the whole extent of *Dentes Morales* ; thefe alfo
feparate *Saliva* from the arterial Blood, and
difcharge it into a long *excretory Duct* 5 arifing
from its pofterior Part, and continued almoft
to the *Dentes Incifores*, receiving the *Saliva* by
its feveral lateral Branches which communicate
with the Parts of the Glands, and difcharging
it by two of the Emiffaries under the Tongue,
near the Bafis of its *Frenulum* : 3. from the
Sublinguales of *Rivinus*, and *Bartholin*; which
are perhaps no more than a Continuation of
the laft mentioned Glands, difcharging their
Saliva in the fame Part of the Mouth by many
fmall Ducts on the Sides of the other Ducts,
under the Tongue : 4. from the *lenticular and
miliary Glandules*, whofe fmall Emiffaries perforate the *Tongue* 6, *Palate* 7, Gums, Lips, and
Cheeks, difcharging a much thinner *Saliva*
than the reft, but of the fame Nature ; and
laftly, 5. from the fmall Glands in the back

K 4   Part

Part of the Palate, or *Fauces*, of the *Uvula* and *Tonſils*, which diſcharge a more thick or mucous *Saliva*, mixing with the Aliment.——— And ſuch is the Situation of theſe Glands and Emiſſaries, that they afford their Fluids moſt plentifully when they are *moſt required* [a], *i. e.* in the Action of Maſtication and Speaking. Though there are ſome who reckon ſtill more ſalival Glands and Ducts than thoſe now enumerated; but their Exiſtence in the human Body may juſtly be queſtioned.

The Effects and Changes wrought on Aliments by the *Saliva* are very conſiderable. The ruminating Animals, as the Ox, *&c.* feeding upon nothing but dry Hay, have a remarkable Contrivance to draw out its nutritious Juices; they firſt ſwallow it entire, after rolling it up into large Balls in their Mouths, being in that State quite indigeſtible by them; the dry Hay being thus moiſtened with the *Saliva*, and conveyed into the firſt Stomach, is further ſoftened by the warm Juices of that Stomach, and its tough Fibres are thus more eaſily fitted for a farther Diviſion; the Animal then ruminates, or again throws up the round Morſules of Hay into its Mouth, where it is minutely ground by a ſlow and careful Maſtication between the grinding Teeth, and ſo intimately blended with the *Saliva*, as to make a copious Froth or Foam; ſo that the ſmall Veſſels of the Hay being thus mollified and broke, and again ſwallow'd, it eaſily parts with its nutritious Juices in the true Stomach. Were we prudently to imitate this Artifice, we might put off Hunger much longer by the ſame Aliment, extracting more nutritious Juices from it by a well chewing, than by devouring it

in

in large Mouthfuls, almoſt untouch'd by the Teeth.

[1] It is remarkable in the parotid Glands, that beſides their conglomerate Structure, they contain each a large conglobate Gland, which inſerts its Duct into the common excretory Duct of the whole Gland; but what ſhould be the Uſe of it? It can hardly be to pour a Lymph into the *Saliva*, to attenuate it in its Courſe; for Lymph coagulates with Fire, but the *Saliva* evaporates; it muſt therefore be of the ſame Uſe with the other Parts of that ſalival Gland.

[2] The ſame Blood which affords the moſt ſubtil Fluid of the Nerves in the Brain, does alſo yield the *Saliva*, by many ſmall Branches of the external carotid Artery, diſperſed thro' the parotid Glands.

[3] This Duct is conſiderably large, and upon Preſſure yields a large Thread of *Saliva*, which runs very ſenſibly cold in the Mouth, or upon the Tongue, when the Duct and Gland which lie under the Skin have been cooled by a Blaſt of cold Air upon the Face; while the internal Parts of the Mouth remain much warmer, by being ſhut; and defended by its proper Muſcles.

[4] The *Saliva* is preſſed out of this *Ductus Stenonianus* by the Contraction of the *Buccinator* and *Maſſeter* Muſcles; but the Duct did not paſs under thoſe Muſcles, leſt the *Saliva* ſhould have been wholly obſtructed by too great a Preſſure. It frequently happens after inveterate Pains of the Teeth, that theſe parotid Glands are poſſeſſed with Tumours, which ought never to be extirpated, becauſe upon dividing any of the ſalival Ducts they do not heal up, but degenerate into an incurable Ulcer, continually pouring out *Saliva*; and in the mean time thoſe Parts of the Patient's Mouth are very dry, which ought to have been ſupplied with

Saliva

Saliva by their proper Ducts.—The Duct opens itself into the Mouth by a circular and prominent *Papilla,* or Eminence, which freely admits the *Saliva* into the Mouth, but refifts a Blow-pipe, Probe, or other Body, with a confiderable Force.

⁵ Thefe Ducts were firft difcover'd by *Wharton,* and are fo large and confpicuous in a Man that is fafting, that if he looks in a Glafs while he is af-fected with a fapid Body, he will perceive them fpout out a little long watry Stream of *Saliva;* which is forced out by the Action of the *pterugoidei* and digaftric Mufcles.—In thefe Ducts there are calculous Concretions frequently formed.

⁶ The Tongue has not only a Covering of ex-ceeding fmall Veffels, which *Ruyfch* injected with Wax, but it has alfo a glandular Expanfion, made up of fmall Glands, which pour out the Humour, continually moiftening the Tongue, whofe excre-tory Duct was firft obferved by *Vaterus.*

⁷ By the Palate we intend the membranous Covering, which is full of fimple Glands, inveft-ing the Palate, and which is continued even thro' the Nofe, *Fauces,* pituitary *Sinuffes, Gula, Larynx,* Wind-pipe, Stomach, and Inteftines; this Cover-ing is ufually called from its Inventor, *Membrana Schneideriana;* in whofe fimple Glands are fepara-ted a Humour, which is at firft a very thin Fluid, but by ftanding in their *Folliculi* becomes a thick *Mucus,* to be preffed out whenever there is a Call for it. There are alfo the like mucous Recepta-cles difperfed about the *Uvula, Epiglottis,* and *Fauces.* The Diforders of this Membrane are in-cluded under one common Title, *viz. Catarrhales;* in the Nofe it conftitutes a *Coryza,* in the *Fauces* an *Angina,* and in the *Larynx* a *Cynanche.* In this Membrane is feparated all that *Mucus,* whofe Vifci-dity in a healthy Body is fometimes fo great as to be

be hardly feparable ; and which Ancients for a long
time imagined to come from the Brain. The prefent Vifcidity of this Humour is no Argument that
it was not very fluid before ; for I may be bold to
affert that there are no Humours feparated in the
human Body, but what are at their firft Secretion
perfectly thin and fluid ; but thofe which are more
thick and tenacious, become fo from a thinner
State, by Stagnation and Warmth of the Parts.
The *Semen*, Bile and Earwax, with the Fat, which
are the moft vifcid Fluids in the Body, were thin
and limpid when firft feparated from the Blood,
but become infpiffated by ftagnating in their Cells.
But provident Nature has given a mucous Fluid
for the Defence of all thofe Parts of the Body,
which are to fuffer any great Attrition, or fuftain
the Acrimony of any Fluid it is to retain or convey. Therefore not only the Paffages of the Air
and Aliments are lined with this *Mucus*, of whofe
Glands *Schneiderus* has writ five thick Volumes,
but alfo the whole Surface of the urinary Paffages,
the Bladder, *Urethra*, *Vagina*, *Uterus* and external
Parts of the *Pudenda*, abound with thefe mucous
Receptacles. But this *Mucus* is not only of an
aqueous, but alfo compounded of an oily Subftance,
that it may the better obtund Acrimony, and abate
Friction. In this refpect Sailors imitate Nature,
by oiling or fmearing their Hands with Pitch when
Ropes are to run through them, which prevents
them from being excoriated.

8. The celebrated *Nuck* found a falivary Duct in
a Dog, which paffed from its Gland in the Orbit
into the Mouth. But that excellent Anatomift was
too hafty in placing that among the falivary Ducts
of the human Body, fince neither he nor any Body
after him, could ever find it there. We are altogether certain there muft be fome Ufe for this Duct

in

in the Dog, which the human Body has no need
of ; therefore, as the Dog does not fweat when he
is very hot, but exhales Plenty of Vapours by the
Mouth when he runs panting and blowing, this
Duct feems to increafe the Difcharge that way, by
which he is freed from his fuperfluous Moifture.
However, there are yet two fmall *Tubuli* proper to
the human Body, which pafs from the lachrymal
Sacks into the Mouth, about the middle of the upper *Dentes Incifores,* through which one may thruft
a fmall Briftle or Hair ; thefe difcharge a great
Quantity, but only the thinneft Part of the Mucus
and Tears into the Mouth.

§. 66. The *Saliva* [1] is a thin tranfparent Humour, almoft void of Smell and *Tafte* [2], which
does not coagulate, but entirely evaporates
with a *ftrong Heat* [3], and upon Agitation forms
a ropy and lafting *Froth* [4], being feparated
from the *pure* [5] arterial Blood by its proper
Glands, from whence it flows more *plentifully* [6], fluid and fharp into the Mouths of
hungry People ; but after long fafting is extremely *acrimonious* [7], *deterging* [8], penetrating
and *diffolving* [9] : it will excite and augment
Fermentation [10] in Syrups, Juices, Bread, and
mealy Vegetables ; after long fafting it gently
fcowers the Membranes of the *Fauces, Oefophagus,* Stomach, and Inteftines, and is conftantly fwallowed without notice in the healthy
Bodies, as well of Brutes as the human Species, whether fleeping or waking ; when it is
fpit away too profufely there follows *a Lofs of
Appetite* [11], a bad Digeftion, and a wafting of
the whole Body ; its *Compofition* [12] being of
mauy

many aqueous and fpirituous Parts, which being intermix'd with a fmaller Quantity of Oil and Salt ftrictly united, forms a faponaceous Fluid.

[1] The *Saliva* is not all of the fame Kind; the thinneft comes from the fmall Glands of the Mouth; that which comes from the parotid and fubmaxillary Glands is ftill thicker; and the moft vifcid of all comes from the fmall Glands of the *Uvula*, the Tonfils, and adjacent Parts of the *Fauces*. To make a chemical Analyfis of the *Saliva*, one ought to chufe that of a healthy young Man, which is fpit without any Incentive in the Morning fafting, after having firft wafh'd his Mouth. That fœtid Liquor which is fpit out by the Force of Mercury in the Venereal Difeafe, ought not to be efteemed *Saliva*, but a putried animal Fluid, which has been known to kill Dogs and other Animals.

[2] The *Saliva* of a Perfon in Health is properly without any Tafte upon the Tongue; though in fome morbid Difpofitions it is fometimes difagreeably fweetifh, in People recovering of intermittent Fevers it is Salt, and in many acute Difeafes it Taftes bitter, or rank.

[3] The *Saliva* differs particularly from the Lymph and Serum of the Blood, in that it wholly evaporates by a ftrong Heat; whereas the two latter are concreted, like the White of an Egg, by a Heat equal to that of boiling Water.

[4] The *Saliva* which is fpit into Glaffes for that purpofe by cleanly People, will throw up a Froth upon its Surface, which will fometimes ftand a whole Week; which Property is an Obftacle to the chemical Analyfis of this Fluid; for when it comes to fuffer a ftrong Fire, a tenacious Froth

rifes,

rifes, and ftops up the Neck of the Cucurbit, fo as to endanger the breaking of the Veffel.

⁵ The Blood is convey'd to the Head exceeding pure, agreeable to the Principles of Hydraulics; for the *Saliva* is feparated from the Blood of the carotid Artery, which gives Branches to the Face, and from whence the parotid and fubmaxillary Glands receive their Arteries.

⁶ The *Saliva* continually flows into the Mouth of a Perfon in health, and nothing is a furer Sign to a Phyfician of Difeafe in a Patient, than his having a dry Mouth; but the Quantity of *Saliva* flowing into the Mouth at different times is various; when a Servant looks at, or carries a fine Difh of Meat to the Table, he has then a fudden and more plentiful Difcharge of *Saliva* into his Mouth without any Influence of the Mind; whence a common Phrafe of the Mouth watering. The *Saliva* alfo abounds moft plentiful in the Morning, when there is a larger Quantity of it retained in its proper Ducts and Glands, through the whole Night's Inactivity of the Mufcles ferving to Maftication, which prefs out their Contents.

⁷ The *Saliva* of the Religious, who have obferved long fafting, makes their Breath ftink, their Spittle is alfo foetid, acrimonious, and frets their Gums.

⁸ It is a known Obfervation among the Vulgar, that the *Saliva* is efficacious in cleanfing foul Wounds, and cicatrizing recent ones; thus Dogs by licking their Wounds which are acceffible, have them heal in a very fhort time.

⁹ The *Saliva* diffolves colour'd Spots, cold and hard Tumours, and greafy Spots in the Skin, &c. which are manifeft Signs of its faponaceous Quality; it even fo ftrongly affects the Coats of the Stomach by its diffolving Power, as to occafion Hunger,

Hunger, one of the moft violent and uneafy Senfations.

10 It is a common Obfervation, that the *Indians* prepare their inebriating or fpirituous Drink from a Maftication of *Maiz* by their old Teethlefs Women, who fpit out this Juice mixed with their *Saliva* into an earthen Veffel, in which after a while is converted into Ale, by boiling and fermenting, which is then a Liquor extremely acceptable for thofe People. Syrups alfo, which have been fpit in by Accident, have been known to ferment, grow turbid, and turn fower.

11 When the *Saliva* is lavifhly fpit away, we then remove one of the ftrongeft Caufes of Hunger and Digeftion; the Chyle prepared without this Fluid, is not of fo good a Condition; and the Blood itfelf is the worfe for being deprived of this diluting Liquor. I once try'd a new Experiment upon myfelf, by fpitting out all my fafting *Saliva*, the Confequence was, that I loft my Appetite; hence we fee the pernicious Effects of chewing and fmoaking Tobacco; for to allay the Drought which that Herb occafions, they drown the Stomach with other Liquors, which deftroy its Tone, and is follow'd with a Dropfy, or an univerfal ill Habit of Body. I muft needs be of opinion that the fmoaking of Tobacco is very pernicious to lean and hypochondriac Perfons, by deftroying their Appetite, and weakening their Digeftion. When this celebrated Plant was firft brought into Ufe, it was cry'd up for a certain Antidote to Hunger; thus alfo when it became fafhionable at the *French* Court to chew Paftils made of Wax, Cardamoms, and other Spices, it was obferved that the Number of hypochondriacal and confumptive People was greatly increafed by that means. The fame ill Confequences

fequences attend chewing of *Maſtich*, which is a general and received Cuſtom in *Aſia*.

12 In the Analyſis of Bodies by Fire, we are very often diſappointed of our Ends in ſearching after their natural Compoſition. The Bodies whoſe Principles we ſearch after, are generally firſt expoſed to Fermentation or Putrifaction, in order by that means to open their Subſtance; we then apply thoſe Bodies, which have been thus changed, to the Torture of Fire, and we obtain Liquors which we give out for the Principles of thoſe Bodies; thus *Alcohol*, or an inflammable Spirit, muſt be a conſtituent Part of Wheat, becauſe the Grain, after a Fermentation, and various Treatment by Fire, affords ſuch a Spirit by Diſtillation; and thus alſo when we eat the fleſhy Parts of Animals, by the ſame Rule we muſt alſo ſwallow the moſt pungent, fœtid, and ſudorific volatile Salt, which is obtainable from them by a ſtrong Fire. But beſides theſe Difficulties, which attend every chemical Analyſis, the *Saliva* is alſo ſubject to many other inconveniences, which prevent our Examination of its Nature by Fire; with a ſmall heat it is indeed not much changed, but then it will not aſcend, but ſtays in a viſcid Form at the Bottom of the Veſſel; and if you urge the Fire ſtrongly, it riſes all into Froth. A gentle heat makes the *Saliva* ſend forth a ſomewhat acid Smell, and if its aqueous Part be evaporated to Dryneſs, twenty Ounces of *Saliva* will afford nineteen of ſimple Water, like common Water, and there remains about an Ounce of a gritty or tartarous Subſtance. If that tophaceous *reſiduum* be diſtill'd with a ſtrong Fire, it then affords a little volatile and fœtid Salt, being a Mixture of both Oil and Salt, leaving black Fæces behind, which alſo contain ſome Oil; it indeed contained no Spirit, if by Spirit you mean one that is inflammable,

and

and capable of mixing as well with Oil as Water; but it contains a little Salt, which is neither of an acid nor alcaline Nature; and such is the Compofition of healthy *Saliva*; but morbid *Saliva*, which flows in mercurial Salivations, fhoots into Cryftals, almoft like Nitre, which arife from the acid Salts of the *Mercurius Dulcis*, and are of a quite different Kind from the natural Salts of the *Saliva*; for Nitre, above all Salts, conftantly refults from a Mixture of volatile Acid with the folid and fluid Part of the human Body.

§. 67. The *Saliva* then being *preffed out* [1] of its Emiffaries by the Action of Maftication, (§. 58, to 64.) and intimately mix'd with the Food during its Comminution between the Teeth, ferves, 1. to *affimilate* [2] the Aliments, or change them, fo as to nourifh the Body; 2. to form an intimate *Mixture* [3] of their oily and aqueous Parts; 3. to *diffolve* [4] their faline Parts; 4. to excite a *Fermentation* [5], and by that means, 5. to make a Change in their *Smell and Tafte* [6]; 6. to caufe an *inteftine Motion* [7] in their Parts; 7. to afford fome prefent *Refrefhment* [8] or Aliment. 8. And laftly, to ferve as the *Medium* [9] for Tafte, by applying the fapid Body to the Tongue, it being of its felf infipid.

[1] The *Saliva* is preffed out by the Contraction of the feveral Mufcles to which its Glands are contiguous, and is always difcharged into that Cavity where the Aliment is firft attenuated, that is, into the Mouths of human Species; into the firft Stomach of ruminating Animals, and into the Crops of Fowls.

L The

² The *Saliva* is a Liquor feparated from the Blood, afterwards returned again into the Blood, and then again feparated into the Mouth; it is therefore a Fluid abfolutely proper to the human Body, and of a particular Kind, fince it does not coagulate upon the Fire; but being accurately mix'd with the Aliments, it converts them into the Nature of the human Body, and forms even Bread alone, by a continued Trituration in the Mouth, into a chylous Subftance.

³ It feems to be a Circumftance abfolutely necef-fary to perfect Health, that all the component Par-ticles of the Chyle, Blood, and other Fluids, re-main uniformly and exquifitely mix'd, fo that none of their Parts may flow by themfelves. Were the faline Parts to feparate from the oily, the fmall-eft Veffels would be deftroy'd by their corroding Quality; the Oils by themfelves would render the Parts they poffefs inacceffible to aqueous Fluids, and the Water alone would defert all the larger Ar-teries and Veins, and efcape into the fmalleft Veffels. A linen Filtre, which has been dipp'd in Water, will not tranfmit Oil through its Pores, but it will readily tranfmit the fame, if it be firft well rubbed with Soap. In the fame manner the oily Parts of our Aliment would not enter the minute Orifices of the Lacteals, if they were not reconciled to the aqueous Parts by the *Saliva*, and other faponaceous Fluids. Hence it appears how pernicious fat Ali-ments would be to us, if they were not to be mixed with fomething in the Digeftion which corrects and removes their Vifcidity; thus the *Saliva* blended together with the oily Parts, not only mixes there-with, but alfo renders them mifcible with Water. So Bread and Butter with hang'd or dry'd Meat, which is the moft delectable Difh of the *Hollanders*, would of itfelf turn into a rancid Chyle, yielding

in-

inflammatory Belches; but by means of the Bread, and *Saliva*, and a perfect Maſtication, it affords a ſweet, lympid, and nutritious Chyle, which will be ſo much the better, if the Bread were Biſcuit, as that will oblige one to a more diligent Maſtication.

⁴ The Power of *Menſtrua* to diſſolve Bodies, does not always proceed from any conſiderable A-crimony in them affecting our Senſes; for the Wa-ter from Whites of Eggs is ſo mild; that our Eyes will bear it without any Pain or Uneaſineſs, and notwithſtanding we ſee it will diſſolve Myrrh, by a ſaponaceous Property, which reſults from a Com-bination of alcaline Salt and Oil.

⁵ Fermentation is drawn in by the Chemiſts to account for every Operation in Nature, while their Adverſaries as ſtrenuouſly exclude it from having the leaſt Share in any of her Appearances; but in this, both of them over-ſhoot the Mark widely; for whenever a fermentable Subſtance is excited by Heat, Moiſture, and a free Admiſſion of the Air, there muſt inevitably ariſe a Fermentation; but Bread is from its natural Texture apt to ferment and turn ſowr, which is ſtill further promoted by the *Saliva* inſtead of Water; the Air is freely ad-mitted, and the cloſe Mouth and Stomach admini-ſter Heat to it; what then can be the Conſequence, but a Fermentation? And that this is the Caſe will alſo appear from the frequent Rumblings and Belchings of Air, which is known to be generated in Fermentation. But this Fermentation is not completed in the Stomach, unleſs the Aliment ſtays there too long; becauſe neither the internal Air is retained, nor the ambient excluded, as it is in a cloſe Veſſel: But if Food ſhould ſtagnate too long in the Stomach of a weak Perſon, the Fermenta-tion may in that Caſe be extended, ſo as to change the Aliment from its proper Nature.

⁶ How

⁶ However various be the Mixture of our Aliment, Bread, Fiſh, Fleſh, and Vegetables, they all undergo the ſame Mixture by Maſtication, and do not loſe any of their Qualities in Deglutition; but in the Stomach *ad duodenum* they by degrees loſe their original Smell and Taſte, and turn to an uniform ſmooth Chyle, of a milky Smell and Taſte, retaining ſcarce any thing of what they had before. But there are ſome Aliments which do not ſo readily part with their natural Smell and Taſte, as Onions and Garlick, which ſmell intolerably a long time after they have been eaten, in fœtid Belches.

⁷ An inteſtine Motion is that latent internal Agitation of the Parts of Bodies, which is altogether neceſſary to Fermentation; without this perturbative motion of the Parts preceding, neither Vinegar nor a vinous Liquor could be made from Malt or Sugar. But the chief Spring of this inteſtine motion in Fermentation, ariſes from the included Particles of Air, agitated and expanded by Heat; which Air never exerts its Elaſticity more, than when it is confined in viſcid Bodies; and hence that laſting and tenacious Froth upon the *Saliva*. But this ſame Air being mixed with, and retained by the viſcid *Saliva*, inſinuates itſelf into almoſt every Particle of the Aliment, and exerting its Spring by the Warmth of the Stomach, is a great Inſtrument in diſſolving the Coheſion of the Parts of the Aliment.

⁸ A poor Creature that is almoſt famiſh'd, does no ſooner taſte a Biſcuit dipp'd in Wine, without ſwallowing any of it, but he is immediately refreſhed by it; for the bibulous Veins, which are very numerous throughout the whole Body, as well as in the Mouth and Tongue, abſorb the moſt fluid Part of the Aliment, which is by them convey'd

vey'd to the jugular Veins, and from thence to the Heart; and this Fact is fupported, not only by Arguments from Anatomy, but alfo from thofe Vegetables which entirely melt in the Mouth, without leaving hardly any Fæces by long Maſtication, fuch as I have obferved in the *Acmella Ceylanica.*

[9] No Nerve is fenfible without it is kept moift; fo that thofe who are diforder'd with Defluxions and Catarrhs, and thofe who fleep with their Mouths open, which dries their Tongue and Palate, do not tafte any thing which they put into their Mouths.

§. 68. Therefore as the *Saliva* is feparated with fo great Artifice from the pure arterial Blood, and is afterwards carefully convey'd to be intimately mix'd with the Aliment in the *Mouth* [1], it ought not to be extravagantly *ſpit away* [2]; it fhould rather have been fwallowed, that after having performed its Offices in the Mouth and Stomach, it may be returned into the Blood; and when improved therein by repeated Circulations, be again fecreted in a more *perfect State* [3]. And this is confirmed to be true by *Difeafes* [4], their *Crifes* [5], and Remedies.

[1] From hence (§. 67, 68, and 69.) it appears why none of the more perfect Animals are deprived of this Fluid, the *Saliva*; and why in Birds, and other Animals that have no Teeth, the *Saliva* is feparated by a particular Mechanifm at the bottom of their *Oefophagus.*

[2] The no lefs wife than bountiful Parent of all Things, has deftin'd every Part of the Creation to

fome

some proper Use ; and as the *Saliva* is only, separated in any large Quantity when we are eating, it must therefore be design'd to promote the Dissolution and Affimilation of our Aliment, and therefore ought not to be thrown away as useless, but convey'd into the Stomach, for further Use to the Oeconomy. A Patient never complains of Loss of Appetite whilst his Mouth and Stomach are properly supplied with *Saliva*, but when that Fluid is wanting, this is a constant Symptom. And the Person that spits-out his *Saliva* in the Morning, will hardly have any Appetite at Dinner-time ; but if all the Morning *Saliva* is swallow'd, he will be hungry enough by Noon. It is also allow'd by the universal Consent of the more civiliz'd Nations, that spitting in one's Discourse to any Body, is both unmannerly and nasty ; insomuch that among the Eastern Inhabitants it was held in the highest Detestation and Abhorrence.

3 The thin and aqueous *Saliva* is again absorbed by the lacteal Vessels, and from thence conveyed into the Blood ; and as these Parts of the Blood were separated by hygraulic Laws in the salival Glands of the Head, they will also by the same Rule be again secerned in those Parts in a more pure and animal State ; but this Return of the *Saliva* into the Blood, and its repeated Separations again from it, may be performed several times in the space of an Hour.

4 There are indeed many Diseases in which a plentiful Excretion of the *Saliva* is conducive to Health ; but that Fluid, tho' separated by the salivary Glands, is not at that time genuine *Saliva*. In a Salivation by Mercury in the Venereal Disease, the whole Mass of Blood is liquified, and discharges its purulent and rancid oily Parts thro' the salivary Glands ; which is also apparent from
the

the fame morbid Humours being evacuated by
Decoctum Guaici in Sweats. And in cachectic Difpofitions Sialogogues and Mafticatories are ufeful,
not fo much by promoting a Difcharge of the *Saliva*, as by expelling the fuperfluous aqueous Part
of the Blood that way, which may be alfo plentifully evacuated with ftrong Purges by the *Anus*.

⁵ A critical Difcharge by thefe Glands in the
Small-Pox may be falutary, by expelling the contagious Parts which occafion fo great Difturbance
in the Oeconomy ; for upon the ninth Day the Patient's Body is covered with a thick, and almoft
continued Scab, which arifes from a Condenfation
of the purulent Matter in the confluent Kind, fo
as to form a Cruft ; if a plentiful Salivation, or
fwelling of the Face, does not happen at that time,
certain Death ought to be expected ; for the purulent Matter finding no Vent at that time, by infenfible Perfpiration, is return'd into the Blood and
proves a certain Caufe of Death, by corrupting the
whole Mafs ; for that Excretion which equals five
Parts out of eight, of all the other Excretions
which are made in the human Body, cannot be
retained in the Habit without inducing moft pernicious Confequences ; but People of a melancholy
Habit ought more efpecially to fwallow their *Saliva*, becaufe the wafting of that Fluid would over-
drain their Bodies, already too dry.

§. 69. In the fame Operation of Maftication, a Quantity of *Air* ¹ is alfo intimately
mixed with the Food, and retained by the *Saliva* with the *Mucus* ² of the Palate and
Tongue ³, with which it *incorporates* ⁴, infomuch that by the *Weight* ⁵, Fluidity and *Elafticity* ⁶ of the included Air, joined with the

Heat 7 of the Body, and a continued Series of various Agitations by *Preffures* 8, the whole Mafs of Aliment becomes more attenuated, and fluid, and the inteftine Motion is by this means firft introduced, and afterwards continued therein.

1 No Fermentation can be perfectly made without Air, that Operation fucceeding the better as there is a larger Quantity of Air intimately confined in the vifcid Parts of an aceffent Subftance. Bakers know this by Experience, who bake their Dough with no other View than to raife and difperfe the Air thro' its Subftance into fmall Veficles or Eyes. But befides this *included Air*, which is the fame with the common *Ambient*, there is yet another kind of Air, which lies concealed from the Senfes within the Parts of Bodies, from whence it is never difengaged but by the Force of Fire, a hard Froft, or a violent Effervefcence of contrary Salts; or laftly, by taking off the Preffure of the external Air; and when this latent Air is by thofe Means extricated, it occupies a Space infinitely larger in the exhaufted Receiver than it did before; but both thefe Kinds of Air abound plentifully in the Food during its Maftication and Mixture with the *Saliva*.

2 This kind of *Mucus* is fo requifite and neceffary to Life, that no Animal is deprived of it; and there can be no furer Prefage of the fatal Event of a Difeafe, than the Abfence of that which fhould render the *Fauces* fupple and fmooth. A *Mucus* is a fomewhat oleaginous Subftance, thicker than Water, but mifcible with that Fluid, and feparated from the Blood by the moft fimple Glands. Ignorant Phyficians often rejoice to find a Difcharge of *Mucus* made by the Force of a ftrong Purge, as if

if they had done a great Exploit, but which is contrary to the Laws of Health.

3 The back of the Tongue is full of small Eminences, which difcharge a *Mucus* efpecially near its Root, which is connected with the *Epiglottis*; it is alfo furnifhed with the *Foramen cæcum* and mucous *Cryptæ*, and the glandular Expanfion of *Vaterus* covering the Tongue, continually moiftens it with a vifcid Humour ; all which Plenty of *Mucus* is not continually difcharged, but ftagnates, till it is expreffed for Ufe by the Motion of the Tongue, which ftrongly compreffes the adjacent Parts in its Action.

4 The *Mucus* of the Mouth is certainly of great Ufe to retain the Air mixed with it, by its Tenacity, that it may be tranfmitted together with the Aliment into the Stomach, and there prove the Author of various Changes in it ; for this reafon the *Mucus* has a particular Degree of Vifcidity ; were it lefs tenacious, it would not retain the Air ; and were it more fo, it would not at all part with the Air.

5 We have in another Place queftion'd whether all the Air is of itfelf naturally ponderous, which is not yet fufficiently determined ; but as for the Air which is mix'd with our Aliment, there is no doubt but that gravitates.

6 Philofophers have not yet fufficiently explained nor accounted for the intimate Nature of this wonderful Property Elafticity ; it is evidently demonftrated that the Air may be extremely compreffed into a very fmall Compafs, and very much dilated into a great Space ; when it is compreffed it fuftains a very great Weight, which upon expanding it will throw off. But the moft fagacious Sir *Ifaac Newton* feems to have come the neareft to Nature of any in this Affair, for he firft demon-

ftratcd

started that one Kind of the conftituent and leaft
Particles of the Air are not elaftic, nor do they
perform any Action like what we fee in the Air;
but if two of thefe ærial Particles come fo near
each other as is determined by the Creator, they
will repeal each other, and if any Body obftruct
their free Receffion, it will be then removed with
a confiderable Force; alfo that this repelling Force
increafes as the component Particles of the Air
approach nearer to each other, becoming almoft
infinite at the Point of Contact; much in the fame
manner as Loadftones, having their fimilar Poles
oppofed to each other; as the South Pole of one
to the South Pole of the other, they will repel each
other with a confiderable Force, the greater as they
approach the nearer.

[7] The external Air, which encompaffes the human Body, is always colder than the Body itfelf;
but if it becomes equally hot with the Blood, it
will be greatly rarified; and being received into
the Mouth, will diffipate, or break the fmall Air
Bubbles retained by the *Saliva*, *Mucus*, and Parts
of the Aliment.

[8] Was the Spring of the Air to be always of the
fame Tenor, it would not produce many great Effects; but the cold Air which is received into the
Mouth, and mixed with the Aliment, is afterwards expanded by the Heat of the Stomach. This
Expanfion of Air by Heat is fo fenfible, that I
have vifibly perceived the Liquor afcend in the
 æreal Thermometer whenever any Perfon entered
the Chamber in which that Inftrument was fufpended; fo that the Particles of Air contained in our
Aliments are alternately contracted and dilated
hereby, and the fmall Veficles which they compofe
are maintained as it were in a conftant Syftole and
Diaftole, performing various Impulfes by their

Sides,

Sides, acting upon their containing *Mucus*, and the Parts of the Aliment which are contiguous; therefore the Particles of Air in their Afcent will be beat down again, will be expanded in their Defcent, and will be alfo inflected by their expanfion, fo that the Aliment will fuffer a perpetual Attrition, and put on the Nature of the Fluids, by which they are encompaffed, or fuffer a perfect Diffolution, in fuch a manner as is requifite to convert them into Chyle in the Stomach. It is alfo evident, that the Food which has been well comminuted by Maftication, is in a manner formed into a fort of Chyle, for they are changed into a thick, white, uniform, and turbid Fluid; and its white Colour demonftrates, that its oily Parts are intimately blended with its aqueous, fomewhat like an Emulfion; whence it appears why Maftication is fo neceffary to long Life, infomuch that it was a Maxim among the Antients, that he who did not chew his Food well hated his own Life; for the weak Attrition of the Stomach would not overcome the Cohefion of the Aliment, if it were not to be firft well divided with a confiderable Force by the Teeth, and affifted by the Action of the Air, and diluting *Saliva*, without which it would not be converted into good Chyle. But good Blood can never be made of bad Chyle; and exact Maftication is therefore to be greatly recommended to every fedentary Perfon, who leads an inactive Life, as is generally the Cafe with Men of Letters, who do not exert mufcular Motion to break the Aliment. Clowns and Labourers often omit Maftication without any uneafinefs or detriment. Lyons, Tygers, and other voracious Animals do not chew their Food, and yet they quickly grow hungry again even after a plentiful Meal; they digeft indeed with a great Force, but they do not make any large Quantity of Chyle from their
Food.

Food. And thus alfo a Man might digeft his Food, which has been fwallowed whole, without any great Inconvenience, if he has firft fafted a confiderable time before ; the Acrimony of the *Saliva* in that Cafe fupplying its want of Comminution by the Teeth.

§. 70. The Food thus divided by the Teeth, varioufly agitated in the Mouth, intimately mix'd and diffolved by the *Saliva*, and lubricated with its *Mucus*, is there forced over the Tongue towards the *Fauces*, or pofterior Part of the Mouth. In this Operation all the folid or fluid Aliment is preffed by the conjunct, or elfe fucceffive Action of the feveral Mufcles (§. 62.) belonging to the Lips and Cheeks, from without and betwixt the Teeth into the inner Cavity of the Mouth, formed by the concave Part of the Palate and the Space under the Tongue; the two Jaws are then preffed clofe to each other, and the Aliment lodged upon the concave Surface of the Tongue, which is at that time expanded by its fix Mufcles, and afterwards preffes itfelf clofe againft the Roof of the Mouth and upper Teeth, making its Preffure backward fucceffively from one Tooth to another; and thus the Aliment is forced backwards from the Teeth by the Preffure of the Tongue againft the arched and furrowed Roof of the Palate, which is very conveniently formed to direct the Aliment towards the *Fauces* and Root of the Tongue, which performs this Motion by the fucceffive Action of its longitudinal Fibres, affifted by its *Genioglossi, Styloglossi,*

Styloglossi, and *Ceratoglossi* Muscles; a Cavity is
then immediately formed for the Reception of
the Aliment at the Root of the Tongue, cir-
cumscribed above by the *Uvula*, *Velum* of the
Palate, and the Tonsils; below by the *Larynx*
and *Pharynx*, and behind by the Membranes
which connect the *Vertebræ* of the Neck, and
invest the posterior Muscles of the *Pharynx*.
The Tongue is next dilated, and its Root
drawn forwards and upwards by the conjunct
Action of its *Genioglossi*, *Myloglossi*, and *Styloglossi* Muscles, so as to come into Contact with
all the upper Teeth; at the same time the *Velum* of the Palate is drawn right upwards, by
the Contraction of the *Pterygostaphylini* Musc-
cles, so as to shut up the Opening of the *Fauces*
into the Nose; the *Rima* of the *Glottis* is also
made narrower by its proper Muscles, the *U-
vula* too is drawn downward and forward upon the *Glottis* by its *Azygos* Muscle, in such a
manner, that with the Concurrence of the *E-
piglottis*, all Communication is cut off between
the Mouth and Lungs; and thus every Particle of the solid or fluid Aliment to be swallow'd,
is convey'd into this Cavity of the *Fauces*,
without any escaping into the *Larynx* and
Nose.

There is not any one Function in the whole human Body so difficult to be understood and described as that of Deglutition; nor is this at all surprising, since of all the compound Actions in the
Oeconomy this is the most complex; in this Action the Aliment ought first to be convey'd into the
Cavity

Cavity of the *Fauces*; then the *Oefophagus* fhould be opened, and at the fame time the Apertures which are near the *Oefphagus*, and lead into the *Larynx* and Nofe, fhould be both exactly clofed; after this the Food fhould flide in fuch a manner over the clofed *Rima* of the *Glottis*, and its covering Valve the *Epiglottis*, that no Particle of the Solid, nor the leaft Drop of Fluid Aliment flip into the *Trachea*, which would even be fufficient to caufe Convulfions, and danger of Suffocation. In order therefore to obtain a clear Notion of this complex and obfcure Action, it will be neceffary to divide its Hiftory into Stages, and to trace the Aliment diftinctly as it paffes through the feveral Cavities appertaining to the Mouth. The firft (1.) of thefe Cavities is that of the Cheeks or *Os externum*, which is terminated before by the Cheeks, and the meeting of the Lips above the middle of the Chin; behind by the meeting of the upper Jaw with the Bones of the Nofe on each Side, and by the middle of the lower Jaw. The next (2.) is a Cavity under the Tongue in the *Os internum*, continued from under its Lip, and on each Side to where the Membranes of the Mouth are continued to the Gums and lower Jaw. (3.) The Cavity above the Tongue, between its back and the concave Palate. (4.) The Cavity of the *Fauces*, feated behind the Root of the Tongue; which Capacity is much enlarged or dilated at the time of Deglutition: the Bounds thereof are the back of the Tongue, the Velum of the Palate (which is a membranous Expanfion continued pendulous backwards, towards the *Vertebræ* of the Neck, from the pofterior Margin of the Bones of the Palate, containing the *Uvula* in its middle) the *Ifthmia*, or Sides of the *Fauces*, defcending from the back Part of each *Foramen Narium*, the Top of the *Larynx* below, and the

the Membranes which inveft the *Vertebræ* of the Neck behind.—The Progrefs of the Aliment is from the two firft of thefe Cavities into the third, and from thence in the fourth; the Mouth of the *Larynx* is then fhut, and that of the *Pharynx* dilated; and then the Aliment paffes over the *Epiglottis* into the *Fauces* and *Pharnyx*, in order to defcend to the Stomach. Now fuppofe yourfelf about to fwallow an Ounce of Water, or a morfel of Bread, their Conveyance into the *Fauces* will be thus: 1. The Mufcles of the Lips and Cheeks being ftrongly contracted, will fuddenly protrude them to the Cavity above the Tongue; then, 2. the Tongue will be fpread flat and hollow to receive them; and, 3. it will be preffed fucceffively againft the Palate, and fo protrude the Aliment directed by its Sides into the then diluted *Fauces*, without any Part efcaping. But the Aliment is then arrived no further towards Deglutition than the *Fauces*; it may therefore now be proper to defcribe the Structure and Action of the *Pendulous Velum* of the Palate, with the other Parts of the *Fauces*, as they were by me explained fome Years ago to my Hearers.

The Mouth being opened, the Tongue depreffed, and the Light directed into the *Fauces*, we have then a View of its two anterior and lateral Columns, as alfo of its pofterior ones; and between thefe anterior and pofterior Columns appear the Tonfils on each fide; the upper Part of thefe Columns are bent into two Arches, which meeting in the middle, form the *Uvula*; all which Parts being very moveable, the *Uvula* with the Arches are fufpended freely in the Air, and fuftained by their Fibres being faftened to the pofterior Part of the arched Bones of the Palate. The conftituent Parts are, the two Membranes, one inferior, looking

ing downward, and the other superior, with its
Surface upward; the lateral Membranes, which
inveſt the Columns and Tonſils; alſo the mucous
Cryptæ, or Drains throughout the whole Extent of
theſe Membranes, eſpecially in the open circular
Sinuſſes of the Tonſils betwixt the Columns; the
Uvula alſo, furniſh'd with its mucous *Cryptæ*; with
Veſſels of all Kinds; and various Muſcles included
between the two Membranes.

The inferior and callous Integument of the Palate, which is thick, furrow'd and arched, concave
towards the ſides, but riſing into a Ridge in the
middle, is in that Part of a particular Texture,
different from any other; it inveſts the concave
Baſis of the two arched Bones of the upper Jaw,
as alſo of the Bones of the Palate, upon which latter it becomes more ſoft, thin, and ſmooth; proceeding backward from the poſterior Margin of
the arched Bones of the Palate, it forms the lowermoſt and external Coat of the *Velum Pendulum*,
being perforated thro' all that Extent with the ſmall
Outlets of the mucous Drains, being alſo connected laterally to the Membranes of the Mouth on
each ſide the *Velum*.

The ſuperior, ſoft, thin and ſmooth Integument
of the Palate, which inveſts the upper Surface of
the Palate-bones next the Noſe, becomes ſtill thinner in its Progreſs backward from the poſterior
Margin of the Arches of the Palate-bones, where
it gives an external and upper Coat to the *Velum
Pendulum*, every where perforated with the Emiſſaries of the mucous Drains, eſpecially towards the
Uvula; it inveſts the ſuperior Parts of the *Velum*,
and diſappears, by uniting itſelf into the lower Integument of the Palate, by which means they form
one common Covering, which includes all the
other Parts.

Between

Between the two Membranes which form this common Covering, are interfpers'd an infinite Number of fmall Arteries and Veins, render'd very confpicuous by Injecting, together with the Emiffaries of the mucous Drains, the Tonfils, the mucous *Cryptæ,* or Drains themfelves, and the *Uvula,* with its various Mufcles and Veffels.

The Tonfils are placed on each fide, between the anterior and pofterior Columns of the Palate, being made up of the fame mucous Integument, complicated into hollow Spires, in order to give a greater Extent of Surface for the numerous Emiffaries of the mucous *Cryptæ,* that they might remain diftinct and unobftructed, to difcharge their liquid *Mucus* at this Part ; fo that the Tonfils appear to be Bodies made up of mucous *Cryptæ,* the Veffels which convey and feparate that mucous Fluid, and the Ducts which carry out and difcharge the fame, being all plac'd diftinct in one Membrane, which is folded up by hollow Turnings and circular Windings ; and that their *Mucus* might be more freely difcharged at the time of Deglutition, we find the Tonfils are placed between the Mufcles of the Columns of the Palate ; the mucous *Cryptæ,* which are alfo remarkable in fome other Parts, are in none more large and numerous than in thefe.

The *Uvula* is of a conical Figure, and of a very fmooth or flippery, flexible and fub-pellucid Subftance, full of the open mucous Drains, and furnifh'd with long mufcular Fibres, terminating in a Point ; and the Remainder of it is compofed of an infinite Number of Veffels wove together.

The numerous Veffels of this Part are of almoft all the Orders of Arteries and Veins, ferving fome for the common Circulation, and others chiefly for fupplying the mucous *Cryptæ.*

M   The

The Muscles for the motion of the moveable
Palate have been moſt exactly deſcribed by *Fallopius*, *Valſalva*, *Morgagni*, and *Santorini*; from which
celebrated Anatomiſts we ſhall here take our De-
ſcriptions of thoſe Muſcle, which ought to be re-
cited, in order to underſtand their Actions, which
we are now going to enumerate.

If the Mouth of a healthy Perſon be held open
againſt the Light, and the back Part of the Tongue
preſſed down, we have then an Opportunity of
viewing the ſeveral Motions of the *Velum*, or
moveable Palate; which is a thing that well de-
ſerves to be obſerved and conſidered by us. For,

I. If the Perſon be not directed to any particular Action, but breathes freely in the uſual manner, the acute ſide of the connecting Membranes
will appear, on each ſide of the back Part of the
Tongue, a little before the *coronoide* Proceſſes of
the lower Jaw, being continued and diſperſed into
the *Velum*. Immediately behind theſe connecting
Membranes, we meet with the two anterior Columns of the Palate, which ariſing upward on each
ſide from the back Part of the Tongue, are inſerted into the *Velum*, where they make two narrow
Arches, which uniting in the middle, form the
Uvula. Behind theſe anterior we find the two poſterior Columns of the Palate, which reſembling
the former, ariſe upward into the *Uvula* and preceding Arches, almoſt diſappearing in their fore
Part. In a Space between the anterior and poſterior Columns are placed the Tonſils on each ſide.
And the laſt Part which offers itſelf to View, is
the back Part of the *Fauces*, ſpread upon the Front
of the Bodies of the upper *Vertebræ* of the Neck,
furniſh'd towards the bottom with very large mucous Drains, ſo conſpicuous as to reſemble little
Ulcers.

II. If

II. If the Person then endeavours to blow out his Breath thro' his Mouth only, whilst it remains wide open we shall then have an Opportunity of seeing, 1. The *Uvula*, hanging indeed pendulous, as before, but at the same time much more elongated, by being more strongly and highly lifted up. 2. The *Velum*, or moveable Part of the Palate, will then be strongly and suddenly elevated in its anterior Part; so that the before small Curvatures of the Arches will now form Segments of much larger Circles, by which means the Arches will become much wider and more open. 3. The adjacent Parts, situated behind the preceding, being at the same time lifted upwards and forwards, become more conspicuous, and appear to be archiform, like them, capable of being drawn backward and forward, and of resting, so as to be easily distinguish'd. 4. Also the lateral Columns of the Palate will be elevated at the same time, and in the same Action. 5. The back Part of the *Fauces* becomes more exposed to View in its upper Part, where it appears so beset with *Mucus*, that the Ignorant being deceived with its whitish Hue, imagine the whole to be ulcerated. 6. All these appear the more evident, as the Air is more strongly and swiftly drove exactly thro' the Mouth only; insomuch that the Prospect enlarges to near the lateral Openings of the *Eustachian* Tubes. 7. The posterior Cavities of the Nose will be also shut, by the *Velum* being drawn upwards, and then pressed forwards. 8. The Communication between the Mouth and Nose will by that means cease, because the *Velum* acts the Part of a shutting Valve.

III. These Appearances being duly observed, and the Parts yet remaining in their former Situation, let the Person endeavour to draw the Air quickly and strongly thro' his Mouth only, not

any

any thro' his Nofe, the Parts all that while keeping the Situation before defcribed II. By that
means it will appear that Refpiration may be performed barely by the Mouth only, notwithftanding the Nofe being open in its anterior Part ;
therefore the Force which at that time preffes the
Velum, fo as to prohibit the Air from paffing into
the Mouth thro' the Nofe, muft be capable of
refifting the Preffure of the whole Atmofphere.

IV. When all the preceding Obfervations have
been carefully made, let the Perfon then ceafe to
breathe thro' his Mouth only, and alfo breathe thro'
his Nofe ; at that Inftant all the Parts will be reftored exactly to the State defcribed at I. The
Uvula defcends, and becomes fhorter, the Arches
are let down, and become narrower, the pofterior
Arches defcend, and are cover'd more than before
by the anterior ones, and all the adjacent Parts defcend downwards, and are drawn more forward ;
the *Fauces* behind are more cover'd and conceal'd
by them, the Cavities of the Nofe above the *Fauces*
are render'd more capacious by the *Velum* defcending forwards ; and there is a free Communication
reftored between the Nofe, Mouth, *Fauces*, and
Lungs ; the Air may therefore pafs and repafs all
thofe ways.

V. If then the Perfon tries to draw the Air only
thro' his Nofe, and not at all thro' his Mouth, tho'
it be held wide open, and the Tongue moderately
depreffed, there will then appear to the Obferver,
1. The *Velum* of the Palate drawn downwards and
forwards clofe upon the back of the Bafis of the
Tongue. 2. The two Columns of the Palate will
be contracted downward, and clofe to the Sides of
the Bafis of the Tongue. 3. The pofterior Part
or Bafis of the Tongue will be expanded towards
the Columns on each fide, and will rife upward in
a Curve,

a Curve, fo as to come into Contact with the *Velum* of the Palate, and wholly intercept the Infight to the *Fauces.* 4. The Sides of the Bafis of the Tongue will be very much expanded towards the Columns, and elevated to near the height of the middle of thofe Columns. 5. The Paffage for Air this way is by that means exactly clofed, fo that it cannot pafs in the leaft, becaufe the ftrict Approximation of the *Velum palati* againft the Tongue, before the *Epiglottis,* is very vifible to the Eye; thus the Air, being ftopt from paffing this way into the Lungs, notwithftanding the Mouth's being wide open, and the *Thorax* dilated, will endeavour to feparate the Parts now in Contact by the Preffure of its whole Weight; fo that the Force by which the Tongue and *Velum* are clofed together muft be very confiderable. 6. The Air will then rufh with a confiderable *Impetus* thro' the Nofe and *Fauces* into the Lungs. 7. The lower Parts of the flexible *Alæ narium* will be contracted and preffed inward, by which means the Nofe will become narrower and fharper from the Preffure of the ambient Air upon the external Surface of the Nofe, which is much broader than the open Space of the Paffage thro' the Nofe; fo that, 8. The Dilators of the Nofe muft exert a confiderable Force at that time, to fuftain the *Alæ,* and increafe the *Foramina narium,* which would be otherways occluded by the Preffure of the Atmofphere; this will be fenfible to any Perfon who obferves this Experiment in another; fo that in this Action there will be a Cavity form'd about the *Fauces,* not communicating with the Mouth, but opening into the Nofe, and having a free Paffage for the external Air thro' their Cavity and the open *Glottis* into the Lungs, the Cavity being limited before by the Bafis of the Tongue, which is elevated at its Root, and alfo dilated there

M 3 towards

towards each fide; the *Velum* of the Palate is then
preffed clofe to the Bafis of the Tongue, being at
the fame time contracted downward, and on each
fide upon the back of the Tongue; the Cavity
thus formed behind the *Velum*, is limited below by
the Bafis of the Tongue, behind which is the *Epiglottis*, with the *Larynx* and *Pharynx*.

VI. All thefe Appearances being carefully obferved, let the Perfon be defired to blow all his
Breath ftrongly and quickly thro' his Nofe only,
without letting any Part efcape thro' his Mouth;
in which Cafe every Part will remain, and appear
as we before defcribed, except that the *Alæ* of the
Nofe will not then be contracted, nor compreffed
by the Atmofphere, but will be rather dilated, or
thruft outwards, and by that means be elevated.
And thefe are the furprizing, neceffary, and moft
ufeful Actions perform'd by this acceffary Organ
of Deglutition. We have been the more particular in defcribing thefe Appearances, that we may
have a better Notion of the Action of the Mufcles
belonging to this Part, which are exactly defcribed
by *Fallopius, Valfava, Morgagni*, and *Santorini*, as
follows,

1. The *Thyro-Palatinus* of *Santorini*, which draws
the anterior Part of the *Velum* forwards, downwards, and to each Side, and applies it to the Bafis
of the Tongue, then elevated and expanded, ex-
preffes the *Mucus* of the Tonfils and of the other
mucous Drains, at the fame time they draw the *Uvula*
downward and forward, make the Arches of the
Palate flatter, and in the laft Act of Deglutition
they in fome meafure elevate the *thyroide* Cartilage
and the *Larynx* towards the *Uvula*; they lubricate
the external Surface of the Aliment with the proper
Mucus, and then protrude it into the open Mouth
of the *Pharynx*; they help to enlarge the Cavity of
the

the *Fauces* in the foregoing, Action, and seem to drive the *Larynx* a little outward as well as upward, and by that means to thruft the *Glottis* under the Cavity of the *Epiglottis*, which is then thruft backward.

2. The *Pharyngo-Palatinus* of *Santorini*, which draws the *Velum* backward, upward, and to each Side, and elevates the pofterior Part of the *Pharynx*, alfo preffes the *Uvula* and *Velum* downward, in fome meafure elevates the adjacent Parts of the *Pharynx*, and applies it to the depreffed *Velum*; it alfo in many refpects confpires to act together with the *Thyro-Palatinus*, as will appear from what was before faid of that Mufcle.

3. The *Gloffo-Palatinus* of *Santorini*, which draws the anterior, lateral, and upper Parts of the *Velum* forward and downward, and preffes it againft the back of the Tongue, which is then elevated and expanded, at the fame time preffing out the *Mucus* from the Tonfils and adjacent Drains, it alfo depreffes the *Uvula* downward and forward, and renders the Arches of the *Velum* flatter; elevates the lateral and pofterior Parts of the Tongue, and preffes them againft the *Velum* towards the laft Part of Deglutition, alfo lubricating the external Surface of the Aliment; and then protruding the fame into the open Mouth of the *Pharynx*, it alfo affifts in forming the Cavity of the *Fauces* of the preceding Action.

4. The *Hypero-Pharyngæus* of *Santorini*, which by the Direction of its Fibres draws the *Velum* upwards ftrongly and equally together with its Arches towards the pofterior Margin of the Bones of the Palate, fo that when it acts with the Conjunction of the preceding Mufcles, it compreffes and increafes the Contact of the Tongue and *Velum*, it prevents the *Velum* in that Situation from being

M 4   moved

moved forward towards the Mouth, or backwards towards the *Fauces*, by the Force of the Air, and therefore determines the Paſſage of the Aliment to the *Fauces* in Deglutition, and of the Air thro' the Noſe only in Expiration and Inſpiration.

If all theſe Muſcles act together, and concur with the Action of the Muſcles which elevate and expand the Baſis of the Tongue, they then make the *Velum* immoveable, either backward or forward, whilſt there remains a free Paſſage thro' the Noſe and open *Glottis*, in ſuch a manner that Reſpiration may be performed thro' the Noſe only, without any Air paſſing by the Mouth.

5. The *Spheno-pterygo-palatini* of *Cowper*, which dilate the back Part of the *Velum*, and expand it to each Side, at the ſame time they ſtrongly move it on each Side towards the Hooks of the internal Wings of the *Pterygoide* Proceſſes backward, and in ſome meaſure depreſs the ſame as by the Direction of a Pully, by which means they draw the *Velum* backwards, ſo as to ſhut the *Foramina Narium* in that place, and direct the Aliment contained in the *Fauces* into the *Pharynx*, in the laſt Act of Deglutition.

6. The *Sphæno-palatini*, or *Spheno-ſtaphylini* of *Cowper*, which ſtrongly move the poſterior Part of the *Velum* backward, and ſomewhat obliquely upward, moving the *Uvula* together with it, they dilate and expand the *Velum*, and preſs it againſt the anterior Part of the firſt *Vertebra* of the Neck; they alſo ſtrongly and exactly ſhut up the poſterior Cavity of the *Foramina Narium* and prevent any Air from paſſing or repaſſing that way thro' the Noſe; ſo that they ſuſtain the whole Preſſure of the Atmoſphere, when the Air by its Weight ruſhes into and dilates the Lungs thro' the open Mouth and *Glottis*, they occlude the Openings of the *Euſta-chian*

chian T.ubes, and protrude the Aliment from thofe Tubes in Deglutition ; they alfo contract the Cavity of the *Fauces*, and prevent the Aliment from regurgitating out of the *Fauces* into the Nofe.

If one diligently infpects the two laft Pair of Mufcles acting together, the *Velum* of the Palate may be feen plainly ftretch'd and expanded every way; being by that means enlarg'd, it becomes better fitted for clofing the pofterior *Foramina* of the Nofe and Openings of the *Euftachian* Tubes, and to protrude the Aliment in Deglutition down into the dilated Cavity of the *Pharynx*, at that time elevated, and to direct the Air and Voice thro' the Mouth only. But when all the four mentioned Mufcles act together in their various Directions, the Bafis of the Tongue muft then be elevated, drawn back, and clofely applied to the *Velum*, the *Epiglottis* will be exactly and every way adapted to the *Rima* of the Glottis, the *Velum* drawn up tight, will prefs againft the Aliment to be fwallowed, will be re-acted upon by the Bafis of the Tongue, *Larynx*, *Epiglottis*, and *Pharynx*; fo that the Aliment will be preffed backward into the Mouth of the *Pharynx*, at which time there will be a Cavity formed in the *Fauces*, then only communicating into the *Oefophagus*; but when thefe Mufcles act fucceffively, and in various Combinations, the Air then fuffers various Agitations, by the different Motions of the *Velum*, in its Paffage through the Mouth and Nofe ; by which, with the Vibration of the *Glottis*, and other membranous Parts, the Voice is modulated, varied, and articulated in Speech.

· 7. The *Azygos* of *Morgagni* draws the *Uvula* directly forward and downward, by which means it covers the pofterior Part of the *Glottis* behind the *Epiglottis*, which Part of the *Rima*, by the Elevation of the hollow *Apex* of the *Epiglottis*, is not exactly

aftly clofed in the laft Part of Deglutition without
this Affiftance; by this means no Part of the Aliment is admitted to pafs in Deglutition under the
Epiglottis, or on either Side of the *Glottis*, but is
all protruded into the open *Pharynx*, without leaving any Part behind; infomuch that fluid Aliments, which prefs every way, cannot infinuate betwixt the *Glottis*; for if after Deglutition a fmall
Part of the folid or fluid Aliment fhould remain
upon the *Rima* of the *Glottis*, or its fmooth Sides,
it would be carried thro' the *Rima* by the Air in
Infpiration, and excite a moft violent Cough, fometimes even to fuffocation. When the *Uvula* is loft,
it occafions that Diforder, but does not hurt the
Voice. The *Uvula* is then of Service to the *Epiglottis*, and various other Ufes; it ftops out the
groffer Particles which float in the Air we breathe,
it licks up and ftops the *Mucus* of the Tongue in its
natural Defcent towards the *Glottis*, and prevents
it from being thrown upon the naked *Larynx* by
the Tongue; it ferves as an arched and flippery
Bridge, exactly fitted every way to cover the convex
Sides and *Rima* of the *Glottis*, for the Aliment to flide
eafily along in Deglutition; it prevents the Aliment
from falling out of the *Fauces* into the *Larynx* in
Deglutition; and being moved by its Mufcles, protrudes the Aliment backward into the upper Part
of the *Fauces*.

The Ufes of the *Velum* of the Palate are, to ferve
as a Valve for opening and fhutting the Cavity of the
Nofe into the Mouth, and to ferve as a Partition or
Valve betwixt the Cavities of the Mouth and Nofe;
to dilate the Cavity of the *Fauces* above, and contract
it below; to deprefs the Aliment into the *Pharynx*
in Deglutition, and to modulate the Voice, by di-
recting its Tone thro' the Nofe, Mouth, or both;
and by the Affiftance of the *Uvula*, to prevent the
Aliment

Aliment from flipping into the Lungs in Deglutition; alfo to lubricate the Surface of the Aliment.

Thus we have defcribed the Paffage of the Aliment into the *Fauces* only, the *Pharynx* being as yet not opened: fo that if a Perfon fhould laugh, talk, or fneeze at that time, the Aliment would regurgitate thro' the Nofe, or elfe flip into the *Larynx*, and excite a convulfive Cough. But to prevent thofe Inconveniencies, Nature has made good Provifion.

At the time when the Aliment is convey'd into the *Fauces*, there is a confiderable Cavity formed there for its Reception. This Cavity is limited before by the Tongue, applied to the Roof of the Mouth, and preffed againft the *Velum* of the Palate, which is alfo approximated by its proper Mufcles, (1, 2, 3, 4.) fo as to come into Contact with the Sides of the *Fauces* and Arches of the Palate. It is limited behind by the *Vertebræ* of the Neck, lined with feveral Mufcles and Membranes, and lubricated with numerous fmall mucous Glands. This Cavity is principally enlarged downwards, when the *Larynx*, *Os Hyoides*, and Tongue, are drawn ftrongly upwards, while the *Pharynx*, is relax'd, and the Aliment protruded into it. The *Cæphalo-pharyngei* Mufcles, undefervedly rejected by the Moderns, do then elevate the *Pharynx*, and expand its membranous Coats. So that while the Bag form'd by the *Pharynx* is dilated backwards, its anterior Part is depreffed, and its Sides elevated and expanded by the *Stylopharyngei*, and the mufcular Fibres which come from the *Os Sphenoides*; alfo the Parts which fhut up the Cavity of the Nofe contribute to form this *Infundibulum* of the *Pharynx*. But the Paffages to the Nofe and *Larynx* are to be at this time occluded, to prevent thofe Parts from being offended by a Regurgitation of the Aliment.

The

The *Foramina Narium* are clofed by the *Velum* of the Palate, being elevated by the *Spheno-palatini* Mufcles, and by the *Spheno-pterygo-palatini*, which move the whole *Velum* upwards, and fhut the pofterior Opening of the *Foramina Narium* with it like a Valve.———But the *Glottis* is to be alfo clofed at the fame time; which is not done, as many imagine, by the *Epiglottis*; for that is fomewhat erect, and not eafily inverted, becaufe of its Connection with ftrong Ligaments to the Sides of the Tongue; fo that it cannot fhut the *Glottis*, only prevent any thing from falling into it, in paffing from the Bafis of the Tongue. The *Ary-arytænoidei* Mufcles do thus clofe the *Glottis*, and fo clofely approximate the Sides of its *Rima*, that not fo much as the leaft Air can pafs thro'; the *Uvula* is then placed round the *Glottis*, behind the *Epiglottis*, by the Action of the *Azygos* Mufcle of *Morgagni*, by that means clofing the *Glottis*, fo that any adjacent Parts of the Aliment cannot fall into the *Larynx* with the Air in the next Infpiration. There are fome indeed who will not admit this Action to the *Uvula*; but it is apparently true from Obfervations in the Difeafes of the *Uvula*. For the *Uvula* being flit or deftroy'd, neither injures the Voice nor Deglutition, only the Patient will be perplex'd with a Cough in fwallowing, becaufe all the Aliment does not pafs clean over the *Glottis* (behind the *Epiglottis*) into the *Gula*, but fome Part adhering about the *Rima*, is thrown into the *Larynx* in the next Infpiration, where, by irritating the tender and fenfible Membranes of the *Afpera Arteria*, it will not fail to excite a convulfive Cough and Suffocation, if it be not happily ejected. Such was the Cafe of a *Danifh* Nobleman, who endeavouring to return an Anfwer while he was fwallowing a Mouthful of Meat, was fuddenly ftrangled; and upon opening his
Body,

Body, the Morfel was found ftuff'd in between the *Glottis.*

§. 71. Then the *Os Hyoides*, and Parts there-to connected, are ftrongly drawn upwards and forwards by the Action of the *Geniogloffi*, and fometimes of the *Mylogloffi*, or the lateral Fi-bres of the *Geniohyoidei*, (which latter arifing from the infide of the Chin, under the *Genio-gloffi*, are inferted about the fmall cartilagenous Horns of the *Os Hyoides*; alfo by the Action of the *Mylohyoidei*, which arifing with a broad Tendon from the middle of the Bafis of the *Os Hyoides*, is afterwards inferted by a large *Aponeurofis* into the lower Jaw, from the grind-ing Teeth too near the middle of the Chin, poffeffing all the Space betwixt the infides of the lower Jaw and *Os Hyoides*, they draw the *Os Hyoides* in all Directions towards the lower Jaw, and to each Side; they draw that Bone upwards and forwards, and elevate all the Parts connected to and upon it, as the Tongue, &c. alfo by the *Stylocerato-hyoidei*, which arife fharp and flefhy, from the *Styloide* Proceffes of the *Offa Temporalia*, and defcending obliquely forwards, they are generally perforated by the Digaftrics, (§. 60.) are inferted into the Articu-lation of the greater Horn with the *Os Hyoides*, and its Bafis, and ferve to draw the *Os Hyoides*, with all connected to it, upwards and back-wards;) the Bafis of the Tongue is alfo expan-ded, elevated, and drawn forwards; the *Os Hyoides* is preffed up againft the moveable Pa-late, the Paffage to the Noftrils is by that

means

means: fhut with the *Velum*, and the *Os Hyoides*
and *Larynx* are approximated clofe to each o-
ther in their Elevation, by the Contraction of
the *Thyro-hyoidei* (which arife flefhy from the
Side of the *Os Hyoides*; and defcending, are
inferted by a large Expanfion into the fcutiform
Cartilage, and continued to the lower and lateral Margin of the fame:) The Parts thus e-
levated, prefs back upon the Aliment to be
fwallowed, and by that means keep down the
Epiglottis from rifing, which together with
the *Uvula*, being preffed by its proper Mufcles
upon the *Rima* of the *Glottis*, clofe up the A-
perture which admits the Air in Infpiration;
they likewife fpread upon the Surface of the
Aliment a lubricating *Mucus*, preffed out of the
Velum of the Palate, *Uvula*, Tonfils, Root of the
Tongue, the *Epiglottis*, and its Glands, with
the *Glandulæ arytænoidææ*, and mucous Drains
of the *Pharynx*, much facilitating the Deglutition of the Aliment; the elevated and expanded Root of the Tongue, with the *Os
Hyoides* and *Larynx* are then drawn forwards
by the *Genioglofſi*, *Myloglofſi*, *Genio-hyoidei* and
Mylo-hyoidei Mufcles, which by that means
fufficiently dilate the *Fauces* and *Pharynx*, connected to the Root of the Tongue, *Os Hyoides*
and *Larynx*, fo far as to make room for the
Aliment to be fwallowed, efpecially when the
external *Pterygoidei* and fome Fibres of the
Maſſeter Mufcles violently draw the whole
lower Jaw forwards, by which means the Cavity is much enlarged, while the *Gloſſo-pharyn-*
gæi,

gæi, Hyo-pharyngæi, Thyro-pharyngæi, and *Crico-pharyngæi* Mufcles diftract and dilate the *Pharynx,* by drawing it forwards, and to each Side ; and thus the Aliment is convey'd into the dilated upper Part of the *Pharynx* to be fwallow'd, the Aperture of the *Larynx* is clofed, the *Oefophagus* is then relaxed, the *Stylo-pharyngei* contracted, and confequently the Aliment preffed into the upper Part of the *Gula,* but at the fame time the *Pharynx* is dilated, the *Velum* of the Palate is alfo expanded and elevated by its proper external and internal Mufcles, which clofe up the pofterior *Foramina* of the Nofe, direct the *Uvula,* and fo prevent any Regurgitation of the Aliment into the Nofe and *Glottis.*

§. 72. The very Inftant after thefe Actions have been performed, all the Mufcles (§. 71.) which were then contracted, are now relaxed, and both the *Sterno-hyoidei* begin to act (which arifing flefhy from the infide of the Clavicles near the *Sternum,* and adjoining *Sternum* itfelf, afcend ftrait upward to their Infertion at the anterior Part of the Bafis of the *Os hyoides*) and at the fame time the *Sterno-thyroidei* are contracted (which arifing from the upper and outer Margin of the *Sternum* and Clavicles, afcend to the Bafis of the fcutiform Cartilage, to which they are connected, and are inferted obliquely outwards into the lateral and external Tubercles of the fame Cartilage) together with the *Coraco-hyoidei* on each fide (which arifing round and flefhy from the upper *Cofta*

of

of the *Scapula* at the Root of the *coracoide*
Procefs, forms a digaftric Mufcle in its Progrefs, and is inferted into the anterior Part of
the *Os hyoides*), by which Mechanifm the
broad and back Part of the *cricoide* Cartilage
is preffed backwards and downwards againft
the *Pharynx*; at the fame time the depreffing
Mufcles of the Palate are contracted with a
great Force, and an almoft convulfive Celerity
(the *Gloffo-ftaphylini*, *Pharyngo-ftaphylini*, and
Azygos of *Morgagni*) whereby the *Velum* of
the Palate, then expanded and drawn tight
upwards, is now pull'd down, and protrudes
the Aliment in the *Fauces* into the Mouth of
the *Pharynx*, now elevated and dilated, the
Gloffo-ftaphylini and *Pharyngo-ftaphylini* being
at the fame time contracted; then the *Gloffo-
pharyngei*, *Hyopharyngei*, and *Thyropharyngei*
are contracted with a convulfive Motion, like
the former, by which the Tongue, *Os hyoides*,
Larynx, and back Part of the *Pharynx*, are
preffed together, and protrude the Aliment forcibly into the Mouth of the *Oefophagus*; thus
the *Pharynx* is clofed, and the *Oefophagus* contracted at the fame time; the former of which
arifes from each Side of the *coracoide* Cartilage,
and embraces or externally invefts the Mouth
of the *Oefophagus*; and thus the Aliment preffed down in Deglutition, will refide in the
Cavity of the *Oefophagus*, under the *Pharynx*.
Thus operofe or laborious is the Bufinefs of
Deglutition, which requires the Concurrence
of fo many Organs and their Actions, which
muft

muſt consequently render this Function ſubject to various Accidents and Diſeaſes; but
from a Conſideration of the Structure and A-,
ction of the ſeveral Parts concerned, we may readily underſtand why dry Food is *ſo difficult to
ſwallow* 2, the *Saliva* and *Mucus* of the *Fauces*
being not ſufficient to mollify and lubricate it;
alſo why upon a loſs of the *Uvula,* a Perſon is
troubled with a Convulſive Cough, and threat-
ned with Suffocation in ſwallowing his Aliment; and laſtly, why the Aliment regurgitates into the Noſe in ſwallowing when the
Velum of *the Palate is divided* 3 ? Whence alſo
it appears that the moveable *Velum* of the Palate performs the Office of a ſhutting Valve
with reſpect to the Noſe, and of a depreſſing
Muſcle with regard to the *Pharynx.*

1 The Morſule of Aliment is now convey'd into the *Fauces,* the Apertures of the Noſe and *Glottis* being cloſed, and the *Pharynx* dilated, to make
ſufficient room for the Food in Deglutition; it
therefore now remains for it to be protruded into
and thro' the *Gula,* which is the laſt Buſineſs of
Deglutition; in order to this, the *Pharynx* muſt
be contracted in its Diameter by the *Sterno-hyoidei,*
Sterno-thyroidei and *Coracoidei,* which draw the *Larynx* downward, and preſs it in ſuch a manner a-
gainſt the *Pharynx,* as to ſtraiten the *Gula,* eſpecially as the muſcular Fibres (which ariſe from the
Larynx and *Pharynx,* and are interwove with the
Hyopharingei, Thyropharingei, and *Circopharingei*)
contract the Capacity of the *Pharynx,* while the
Velum of the Palate, being preſſed down by its
proper Muſcles, protrudes the Aliment into the

N

Gula,

Gula, where, by the Contraction of the mufcular Fibres of the *Oefophagus,* it is further protruded down into the Stomach; all the Mufcles therefore which before elevated the *Pharynx, Larynx,* and *Os Hyoides,* will be now relaxed, and only the *Rima* of the *Glottis* remain clofed, by the Approximation of the *arytenoide* Cartilages by their proper Mufcles, in fuch a manner, that no Liquor can pafs into the *Larynx* as it defcends thro' the *Pharynx.*

² A Perfon cannot fwallow a piece of dry Bread, when the *Saliva* and *Mucus* of the *Fauces* have been before exhaufted by eating of Bread and boiled Meat, except the *Gula* be moiftened with Drink; for the exquifite Senfation of the fine Membranes which line the *Fauces* and *Pharynx,* being offended by the Roughnefs of dry Food, will not admit, but exclude the fame, as hurtful.

³ The *Velum* of the Palate is fometimes divided in venereal Ulcers, and the Fiffure being dilated by the Preffure of the Aliment, admits it into the Nofe; which Diforder is incurable, and cannot be remedied by a Plate of Metal, as may an Erofion of the Bones of the Palate; the afflicted Patient is therefore obliged to prefs the Aliment down to the bottom of the *Fauces* with his Fingers, leaning his Head backward, unlefs he had rather fuffer it to regurgitate into his Nofe. I once faw a Child, who being born with a divided *Uvula,* could not fwallow; upon opening the Mouth of the Infant, the *Uvula* appeared to be divided; and upon ordering it to fhut its Nofe when it fwallowed, the Aliment defcended without offending that Organ; this fame Child learned to fpeak, but was obliged to fhut his Nofe with his Hand at that time.

§. 73.

§. 73. The *Gula* or *Oesophagus* is a diftractile Tube, compofed of feveral Membranes or
Coats invefting each other; the firft and in-
nermoft of thefe Coats is *villous* [1] or downy,
furnifhed with many nervous Papillæ, lines
the whole internal Surface of the Tube, and
continually affords a Liquor fomewhat thicker
and more *oily* [2] than the *Saliva*, which is feparated and diftils down from the fmall Twigs
of the Arteries, diftributed through the *Oesophagus*, and ferves to lubricate the Paffage for
Deglutition, renders its Fibres fupple, and fit
for Motion, and defends them from the Roughnefs of the Aliment. The fecond Coat, which
invefts the former, is *glandular* [3], or rather
full of *Cryptæ*, or Drains, which feparate and
difcharge the forementioned Liquor into the
Cavity of the Tube; the other fide of this
Coat confifts of many fmall Veffels, which
fupply Blood to the forementioned Glans or
Cryptæ. This glandular and vafcular Coat is
invefted by a mufcular one, confifting internally of orbicular, and not *fpiral* [4] *Fibres*,
which are encompaffed externally by longitudinal Fibres; all thefe are again included in a
thin *cellular Membrane* [5], confifting alfo of Fibres and fmall Veffels, upon the back part of
which are frequently placed *two fmall Glands* [6]
on the outfide of the Tube, about the fifth
Vertebra of the *Thorax*, which prepare a mucous Juice, ferving to lubricate this Tube.

¹ A piece of the *Oesophagus* being turned inside out, and suspended in Water, in order to observe the internal Structure of this Coat, it appears villous or downy, like Velvet; but these *Villi* are nothing more than exhaling Arteries, which transmit the Injection of *Ruysch* like little Worms, the same kind of *Villi* being also found in the Stomach and Intestines, they discharge a salival Fluid which does not coagulate by Heat; between these *Villi* are interspersed many nervous *Papillæ*, whence proceeds the exquisite Sense we observe in the *Oesophagus*; these *Papillæ* are pendulous to a great length in a Tortoise, their Basis being upwards, towards the Mouth, their *Apex* towards the Stomach; it was necessary that the *Oesophagus* should have an exquisite Sense, to receive or reject the Aliment. I saw a Lad who suddenly clapt a hot Turnip into his Mouth, which had just been taken out of the Pot by his Mother, and then swallowed it; as soon as the Turnip had reach'd the Stomach, the Child presently dy'd in the utmost Misery.

² This Liquor is of a middle Consistence, between the *Mucus* of the *Fauces* and that of the Lungs; it may be separated by scraping the internal Membrane of the *Oesophagus* after Death, and may be again pressed out by scraping a second time.

³ In this glandular Membrane are numerous *Cryptæ*, or mucous Drains, called by *Duverney* lenticular *Follicules*, less than the Eggs of Silkworms, and like little Bladders, opening each with a large Orifice into the Cavity of the *Oesophagus*, which discharges their mucous Liquor, separated from their Arteries, and retained till pressed out in Deglutition; to which Action it is so necessary, that we can scarce swallow any thing when that lubricating *Mucus* is wanting. From an Obstruction of these small Glands arise a *Schirrus*, and a
difficulty

difficulty in fwallowing, which gradually increafes more and more, and is a Cafe that has frequently occured in my Practice; the only Difficulty they have in fwallowing, is from the Pain and Refift-ance of the Aliment in its Defcent. *Ruyfch* cured a Diforder of this kind by a mercurial Salivation. This Difeafe feems to arife from the indulging of fpirituous Liquors, and Drinks made very hot, which are now more in Ufe than they were with our Anceftors.

⁴ In Brutes, who have their Necks pendulous, the *Gula* is furnifhed with two Orders of ftrong fpiral Fibres, to make the Aliment which they fwallow afcend; and thefe Animals never vomit nor can Deglutition in the human Subject be explained by the Structure of this Part in them; as the Aliment in Deglutition defcends perpendicularly in the human Body, it may be fwallow'd with a lefs Force, capable of being exerted by circular Fibres; but no one ought to deny thefe Fibres to be mufcular becaufe they look pale, for the Colour of every Mufcle is of itfelf white, its Rednefs proceeding from the Blood; nor is the *Oefophagus* paffive, fo as to perform the Office barely of a Tube to the defcending Aliment; but its Fibres being ftrongly contracted on every fide, protrude the fame into the Stomach; but thefe Fibres act fucceffively one after another, the Contraction beginning at top, and defcending gradually to the bottom; nor has the Weight of the Aliment any confiderable Share in this Action, for Pofture-mafters drink with their Heads downwards, and caufe the Drink to afcend, contrary to the Force of Gravity.

⁵ The external Membrane is that which ferves as a *Stratum*, for the Paffage of the Arteries and Veins which are diftributed to this Part; for the

Veins

Veins and Arteries are diftributed freely in no Part, wherein they do not communicate with their proper reticular Cells, in whofe Cavities they. difcharge a lubricating Oil.

‘ Thefe two Glands are commonly called *Dorfalos, Verfellonius* having defcribed their excretory Ducts ; but no Body has yet been able to difcover them after him.

§. 74. The lubricated Aliment. is therefore preffed thro’ the flippery and dilated *Oefophagus,* by the Contraction of its *longitudinal and orbicular Fibres* [1] ; which at laft protrude it thro’ the broad Mouth of the Stomach, then open and relax’d, into its Cavity.

[1] Thefe longitudinal Fibres dilate the *Gula,* fhorten it, and approximate it towards the Aliment, to be fwallowed, while the orbicular Fibres contract it in diameter, and acting fucceffively downwards from the upper Part of the *Gula,* they protrude the Aliment into the Stomach.

§. 75. The Aliment being thus conveyed into the Stomach, the Mouth of that Organ and the *Gula* are naturally clofed, efpecially in Infpiration, by a thick *flefhy Mufcle* [1], rifing above and below the Level, in the middle of the *Diaphragm,* through which the *Gula* is tranfmitted, and attach’d thereto by mufcular Fibres ; by which means the Contents of the Stomach are prevented from being preffed again into the *Gula.*

[1] The *Oefophagus* does not perforate the tendinous, but flefhy Part of the *Diaphragm,* left if

　　　　　　　　　　　　　　　　there

there was an open Paſſage, the Aliment might again regurgitate out of the Stomach into the *Gula*, by the Preſſure of the *Diaphragm* in Inſpiration ; but thus the Mouth of the Stomach is cloſed, at the ſame time and by the ſame Power which depreſſes it, when we breathe in the Air.

We have now therefore a clear View of the Uſes of the *Oeſophagus*, and of the ſeveral Parts connected to it above. In ſhort, Deglutition conſiſts (1). In a Protruſion of the Aliment into the *Fauces* by the Muſcles of the Tongue. (2.) In a Depreſſure of it into and thro' the *Pharynx* (while the Apertures of the Noſe and *Larynx* are ſtrictly cloſed) by the Muſcles of the *Velum*, Tongue, *Os hyoides*, *Larynx* and *Pharynx*. And (3.) In a Propulſion of it thro' the *Oeſophagus* into the Stomach, by the Contraction of its muſcular Fibres, which is alſo facilitated in its Paſſage by the lubricating *Mucus* of the Glands.—Diſeaſes of the *Oſeophagus* generally proceed either from a Tumour of the adjacent Glands, or from a Coheſion of its Sides. I have ſeen a Tumour of the Parotids which totally obſtructed the Action of Deglutition ; and *Ruyſch* deſcribes another Caſe of this Kind from the *glandulæ dorſales*, bing indurated and ſcirrhous, which would only yield to a Cure by the Power of a mercurial Salivation ; the *Oeſophagus* coheres together, when all the oily *Mucus* has been before exhauſted from its cellular Texture by long faſting or fainting, in which Caſe Deglutition is ſuppreſſed ; a miſerable Inſtance of which has occurr'd to my own Obſervation. If it ſhould be aſked how it comes about that Liquors are ſometimes more difficulty ſwallowed than Solids ? the Anſwer is, that the Muſcles of the *Pharynx* being at that time paralytic and collapſed, the Solid has a greater Reſiſtance to open the ſame ; but then again,

Fluids are fometimes more eafily fwallowed than Solids, when the Capacity of the *Gula* is ftraiten'd by an Inflammation, or otherways.

Concerning the Action of the Stomach in digefting the Aliments.

THE Error of moft who have endeavour'd to explain Digeftion, has lain in their attributing that Function to only one or fewer Caufes than are concern'd therein, excluding the reft. To avoid falling into the like Error, we fhall confider the Stomach, 1. As a moift, warm, and clofe Veffel, in which the Aliment is receiv'd and retain'd (§. 76.) 2. As it is an Organ, fupply'd with feveral Humours, for the Diffolution of the Aliment (§. 77, and 78.) 3. As it acts upon the Food, by the Contraction of its own mufcular Coat (§. 81.) And laftly, 4. As it receives an external Force and Preffure from the adjacent *Aorta*, *Diaphragm*, and abdominal Mufcles; from the Concurrence of all which very different Caufes, the Function of the Stomach is perform'd, and ought to be explain'd.

§. 76. The folid and fluid Aliment thus fwallow'd, before diluted with the *Saliva*, mix'd with the Air, and now received into the *clofe* [1], moift, and *warm* [2], Stomach, does there quickly begin of its own accord to ferment, or *putrify* [3]; according to the different Nature of the *Aliment* [4] or Difpofition of the Stomach; and is either way wonderfully changed into an *afcefcent* [5], *alcalefcent* [6], *rancid* [7], or *glutinous* [8] Mafs.

[1] The

¹ The opening of Animals alive, and the Ructus's which afcend a few Hours after a Meal, demonftrate that the Aliment ftays fome time in the Stomach ; therefore .the Food will in this refpect fuffer the fame Changes in the Stomach, which it would have undergone by ftanding in a clean glafs Veffel, mix'd with the *Saliva*, in a warm Place ; it muft be indeed confeffed, that the Drink, and fome of the more fluid Parts of the Aliment, pafs quickly thro' the Stomach, but the more folid are retained a confiderable time.

² The Heat of the Stomach may not only be eafily render'd confpicuous by the Thermometer, but alfo fenfible to the Hand thruft into the Belly of an Animal when expiring. This Heat of the Stomach is in a great meafure communicated and heighten'd by its Contact with the warmeft Vifcera ; the Heart lies upon the *Diaphragm*, immediately above it ; the Liver invefts it before, and on the Right-fide, the Spleen on the left, the *Aorta* behind, and the *Pancreas* with the fplenic, cœliac, and mefenteric Blood-Veffels at bottom ; the whole *Abdomen* alfo conftanly adminifters the Heat of a Bath to it. But that Heat which exceeds Warmth by a few Degrees, is of all the moft efficacious in changing the Aliment ; even Water fo putrifies by the Heat under the Tropics, as to emit imflammable Vapours. The Heat of every Animal is always greater than that of the Air in which it lives, nor can any Creature live when its Blood is reduced to the fame degree of Cold with that of the Atmofphere ; for the Heat of our Air never rifes to 90 Degrees, which is almoft the perpetual Degree of Heat in the Blood of living Animals ; therefore the Heat by which the Aliment is attenuated in the Stomach, muft be nearly the fame with that under the Tropics, which fpoils the neat-

eft

eft Wines or the beft Ale. But all Vegetables grow and digeft their Aliment with a much lefs Heat, which Dr. *Grew* has fhewn to be about 50 and 60 Degrees; for that diligent Naturalift and Phyfician made Tables containing the Heat of every Day for many Years, the Medium of which was as we have now mentioned.

3 The general Error of Writers on Digeftion has been, their confidering but one fort of Change in the Aliment, as if we had never taken but one kind of Food; whence fome will have the Diffolution of the Aliment to be made wholly by Fermentation, and others barely by Putrifaction; both having fome, but not the whole Truth on their fide; for fometimes neither Fermentation nor Putrifaction are perfectly prefent in Digeftion. The flefhy Parts of Animals and fome Vegetables are naturally difpofed to Putrifaction, while Milk, the generality of Plants, and all Garden Fruits, are inclined to turn fowr. Nor are thofe to be confided in, who utterly deny Fermentation to have any Share in Digeftion; fuch ought to confider, that the Stomach adminifters the fame Heat and Moifture, as if farinaceous Aliment was mixed with four times as much Water, and fet in a digefting Heat, which would certainly turn it fowr; nor can any Reafon be given why the Stomach fhould not make the fame Change therein, tho' it may be not fo foon, or to fo great a degree, thro' its Agitation, or a Mixture of the Bile. That a fimilar Fermentation is often perform'd in the Stomach, may appear from the flatulent Diftention of that Organ, attended with Gripes and acid Ructus's, after eating of Garden Fruits; for as Fermentation is obferv'd to be the generating Caufe of this elaftic Air in fimilar Subftances out of the Stomach, the fame Phænomena muft arife from

the

the fame Caufe within the Stomach ; but then this Fermentation is not carried to Perfection in the Stomach, fince that would require the Aliment to ftand at leaft four or five Days therein, whereas it does not ufually ftay above five or fix Hours upon the Stomach ; add, that Mixture in feveral Kinds of Aliments often prevents thofe Changes ufually wrought by Fermentation or Putrifaction. Thus Milk will in a hot Summer turn fower in the Space of twelve Hours, and Blood will putrify in that time, if both are expofed to the common Air; but when mixed together, the Mixture neither turns fower nor putrid, thro' the Reftraint of their degenerating by their oppofite Subftance and Tendencies.

⁴ All the flefhy Parts, and the feveral Humours of Animals, except the Milk of Cattle feeding upon Herbs, do naturally putrify of themfelves, and will certainly do fo in the human Stomach, if thofe Powers are abfent which refift Putrifaction ; even all Sorts of Plants which come under the *tetrapetalous* and *filiquofe* Kind, putrify with a cadaverous Stench, and afford a volatile Alcaly. Thefe Appearances greatly favour the antient Hypothefis of *Pliftonicus*, or Digeftion by Putrifaction, revived by *Lifter*.

⁵ The whole Clafs of Vegetables, except a few of the aromatic and antifcorbutic Plants, turn fowre in a warm and moift Air, affording a volatile Acid ; even the fweet Meal of Oats, mixed with taftlefs Water, turns exteremely fowre in a warm Place ; and Muft, or new Wine, alfo turns fowre and corroding barely with the Heat.

⁶ By turning *alcalefcent*, we mean, to approach the Nature of a lixivious Salt, produced by Fire ; being *acrimonious*, of an urinous Smell, fermenting with Acids and tinging Syrup of Violets of a green Colour.

Colour. But lixivious or alcaline Salts are of two Kinds, 1. *Fixed*, being made from the calcined Afhes of all green Vegetables, which diffolved in Water affords a lixivious Salt. Even the fowre *Wood-forrel* affords Afhes by Fire, from whence may be made a Lixivium, perfectly endued with all the Properties of an alcaline Salt. The other fecond Kind of this Salt is volatile, obtainable by Diftillation from all the Parts of Animals or putrified Vegetables; in which Operation Part of the afcending Vapours are turn'd into volatile Cryftals, of a fœtid, urinous Smell, and fiery Tafte.

7 All Oils grow rank when taken in a large Quantity upon a weak Stomach, to which State they have a natural Tendence, putting on the Quality of a rotten Egg. If a Perfon fhould eat a good deal of frefh Butter that has been fry'd, without drinking a fufficient Quantity of fome acefcent Liquor, it turns into a putrid, acrimonous Liquid, much of the fame kind with the greenifh Cruft which is fpread over Butter that has been long expofed to a warm Air, being fo extremely rank, that it leaves an intolerable Guft for above an Hour after it has been tafted. From this Liquid ftagnating in the Stomach there afcends ardent and bitter Ructus's, and an inflammable Matter regurgitates into the Mouth, which was frequently by the Antients miftakenly called Bile. The like putrid Subftance may alfo arife from rufty Bacon or Lard, ftale Eggs, oily Fifh, &c. But that it is improperly called Bile, will appear from its flaming like Oil in the Fire, whereas Bile being caft upon the Fire, extinguifhes it; nor is this eafily produced in ftrong and bilious Habits, but rather in weak and hypochondriacal People, where the Bile is inactive.

Not

⁸ Not only glutinous, but ropy, drawing out into long Threads, and difficultly miscible with Water; like what is made by boiling the Feet, Skin and Tendons of Animals in Water, and known by the Name of *Glue.* A Substance also of the like kind, but not so firm and ropy, may be made from Meal boiled with so small a Quantity of Water that it will not turn sowre, called Paste.

§. 77. The internal *Coat*¹ of the Stomach embracing the Aliment, is *villous*² or downy, full of nervous *Papillæ*, small quadrangular Cells, *Wrinkles*³, Pores, and *tubuli*, which latter keeps it *moist*⁴ and clammy; but the convex Part of the Stomach is furnish'd with a Variety of numerous small *Glands*⁵, arising from and adhering to the vascular Coat, which receives Arteries from the *Epigastrics*⁶, and three other Branches, all from the cœliac Artery, each of whose small Branches being spent in a particular Disposition, at last send off small Twigs opening into the very Cavity of the Stomach, which is also very plentifully furnished with small *Veins*⁷ and *Nerves*⁸, surprisingly interwove with each other. This vascular Intertexture therefore supplies the Stomach with minute, pulpy and succulent Emissaries, disposed in little Heaps, of a glandular, oval, or globular Figure, whence continually distils a thin, pellucid, and frothy *Liquor*⁹ into its Cavity, *spirituous*¹⁰, and a little *saline*¹¹, being neither *acid*¹² nor *alcaline*¹³ in the most *voracious Animals*¹⁴, but *sharp*¹⁵ and scowering in such

fuch as have fafted long, being fecerned into
the Stomach by fmall Ducts ftriking off from
the gaftric *Arteriolæ*; befides which Liquor
the Stomach is alfo lined with a thick *Mucus*,
feparated by fmall Glands, collected and retained in their *Cells* [16], and afterwards expreffed
thro' proper Emiffaries into the Cavity of the
Stomach. The mufcular Coat of the Stomach
contracting as it empties, forms its preceding
vafcular and villous Lining into large *Wrinkles* [17] that are wonderfully waved in and out,
and again fubdivided into lefs, which, together with the fmall *quadrangular Cells* [18], prevent the groffer Part of the Aliment from a too
quick Paffage; alfo retain fome fmall Part,
which becomes acrimonious by *fermenting* [19],
and by this, with *Attrition* [20] againft each o-
ther, excite to hunger. Thofe Animals whofe
Stomachs are not furnifh'd with the forementioned internal Coat and its Liquors are ufually
fupplied with them in the *Crop* [21] or firft Stomach, or elfe at the lower Mouth of the *Gula*,
next the Stomach.

[1] Being the fame with, and a Continuation of,
the villous Membrane of the *Oefophagus*; being
eafily feparable in the Maw of a Hog, when it has
been inverted and dipt in fcalding Water.

[2] Confifting of *Vaginulæ*, or fmall membranous
Ducts, which direct the Courfe of and communicate with the fmalleft exhaling Arteries, and inha-
ling or abforbing Veins, thro' both which kinds of
Veffels the ceraceous Injection frequently paffes
thro' into the Cavity of the Stomach, but without
any Colour or Part of the Vermilion; which Experiment

periment happened to be made by *Ruych* about 35 Years ago, when he was endeavouring to accurately fill the Veffels of the Stomach with his Injection; the Blood fometimes efcaping thro' thefe fmall Arteries, occafions bloody Vomits in plethoric Virgins, whofe *Menfes* being obftructed below, feek to be vented upwards..

³ In a healthy living Man it is wrinkled; but in the dead Subject, whofe Parts are relaxed, they are not fo confpicuous, being fewer, more extenuated, and unequal. Thefe *Rugæ* are formed in the villous Coat of the Stomach, becaufe that is not elaftic; and the more it is filled, there are the fewer *Rugæ*.

⁴ If the Stomach of a living Dog be opened, you will find the internal Surface of it lubricated; and if the *Mucus* be abraded, it will prefently be again renewed from the numerous fmall Pores: this Liquor is of the fame nature with the *Saliva*, and wholly evaporates upon the Fire, without leaving any *Refiduum*.

⁵ Some had rather call them *Cryptæ*, after *Ruyfch*, than Glands, being lenticular Cells, which difcharge their *Mucus* at a proper time, to moiften the internal Cavity of the Stomach.

⁶ Moft of the Vifcera have but one arterial Trunk which enters its *Vifcus* in but one certain Part, yet we fee the Stomach has four diftinct Arteries; which enter it in as many different Places; it feems to have this particular Structure, that the Circulation might not be interrupted, when one Artery is compreffed in the Stomach diftended with Food, which may frequently happen.

⁷ Some of thefe Veins come from the *Cava*, thro' which the ceraceous Injection is tranfmitted, in the fame manner as it was before thro' the Arteries; a manifeft Indication that the moft fubtil

and

and spirituous Part of the Aliment are abforbed by
them in the Stomach.

[8] The numerous Nerves of this Part arife from
the *par Vagum*, in conjunction with the intercoftal
Nerves and the femilunar *Plexus*, fome of whofe
Branches terminate in the mufcular Fibres of the
Stomach; others are convoluted into various round
or pyramidal *Papillæ*, which are difperfed thro'
the villous Coat, while other Branches are furprifingly interwove in the nervous Coat of the Stomach, vanifhing at laft in that downy Subftance,
which, together with fmall Veffels, forms the villous Lining of the Stomach; whether the principal Office of this nervous Integument is to tranf-
fufe the nervous Fluid into the Stomach by their
ultimate and open Branches, we are not yet able to
determine; but it will appear that all the Nerves
terminate either in *Papillæ* for Senfation, in membranous Expanfions, or in mufcular Fibres, but
never end in clofe Cells. Thefe *Papillæ* have been
demonftrated by *Ruyfch* in feveral of his later Preparations, tho' they may be alfo proved to be in
the Stomach by Experiment. The *Vinum benedi-
ctum*, which is made by letting red Wine ftand a
Night in an antimonial Glafs, does not difcover
any uncommon *Stimulus* either to the Tongue or
Nofe, and may be fafely taken into the Stomach;
but it is no fooner arrived there, but it fuddenly
irritates the more fenfible *Papillæ* of this Organ,
and excites a Vomit; the Stomach is alfo fenfible
enough to accurately diftinguifh Poifons, whence
Wepfer well obferves, there are feveral furprifing
Phænomena produced in this Organ by the *Hem-
lock* whilft it remains in the Stomach; which immediately ceafe upon its being difcharged. It is
alfo from this exquifite Senfation of the Stomach,
that

that fome have imagined it to be the Seat of the Soul.

9 This Liquor is confpicuous when it regurgitates into the Mouth of hard Drinkers who are fafting, being not without an unpleafant Guft, which is popularly called Heart-water, being quite limpid, and very much like the Tears. When this Liquor is wanting, there arifes a great Heat and Drought in the Stomach, curable by oily Emulfions; and what is ejected by vomiting this Liquor, forms a lafting Froth.

10 That this *Succus gaftricus* is extremely fubtil, may be concluded from the Minutenefs of its Veffels, which tranfmit the ceraceous Part of the Injection without the Vermilion into the Stomach; and that it is poured into the Stomach in a confiderable Quantity, is probable from the great Number and vaft Extent of thefe Veffels, together with the great impelling Force of the neighbouring *Aorta* from whence they arife.

11 A healthy Perfon who vomits with warm Water, and after Vomiting regurgitates this Liquor, finds no other Tafte in it than that of being a little faltifh, like common Salt.

12 The Chemifts, and Followers of *Helmont*, have in general maintained, that there is an acid Liquor in the Stomach, which excites a Fermentation in the Aliment, impregnating the fame with a vital Spirit, as well as diffolving and digefting it; but this Notion is repugnant to feveral moft weighty Reafons: For, 1. No Body could ever difcover the *Succus gaftricus* to be actually fowre. And, 2. All the Fluids of the human Body are not acrimonious, but replete with a neutral Salt, like *Sal Ammoniacum*; and if they incline more to one Clafs than another, they rather tend to the Alkaline; even *Helmont* himfelf acknowledges, that

O   there

there is not any Acid in the Veins, for if there was, he thinks it would cause a Pleurify; therefore if the Blood of the cœliac Artery contains a mild muriatic Salt, and conveys the fame thro' its Branches difperfed thro' the Stomach, there is no Reafon or Experiment which will countenance a fudden Change of an alcalefcent Salt into an acid Ferment. The Argument which *Helmont* ufes, that he manifeftly perceived the Breath of a Sparrow acid, demonftrates nothing in reality, but that the Bread with which the Bird was fed turn'd fowre in its Stomach; which it will do the fooner, becaufe the intenfe Heat of that Part promotes the Degeneration of it to an Acid; hence Things which are moderately falted with Muriatics, or common Salt, may be very wholfome, fuch as Herrings, &c.

¹³ No Perfon could ever detect a perfectly alcaline Salt in any Part of the human Body; for if it were fo, Life would foon be put to an end. There is no fuch Salt in the Blood, nor even in the Bile, and much lefs fhould we expect it in the aqueous Liquor in the Stomach; but Animal Food may putrify in the Stomach, in the fame manner as it will in the open Air, and the fooner, as the Heat of that Organ exceeds the Temper of the common Air.

¹⁴ *Cofmus* III. grand Duke of *Tufcany*, gave feveral voracious Animals out of the Refervatory, where he kept uncommon Creatures, to be diffected by his Academics, among which were Falcons, Eagles, Vultures, and Swans; upon opening the Stomachs of thefe after feveral Days fafting, there was no Relicks of the Aliment found in them, in the Prefence of *Malpighi*, *Borelli*, *Read*, *Finch*, and *Steno*, who expecting to find fome fharp and corroding Liquor, met with a very mild Juice, of a muriatic Tafte, notwithftanding Eagles do not
                                                        drink,

drink, and take fo much Food at a time without
any Maftication, as will ferve them for feveral
Days, becaufe the Aliment conftantly flows to their
Stomach out of the *Gula*. They make it appear
that this Liquor is not endued with any corroding
Quality, nor does it ever confume the Sides of the
Stomach in thofe Animals in which it is found;
which would certainly be, if the Food was diffolv'd
by any Liquor approaching the Nature of *Aqua
fortis.*

[15] The Monks, after a religious Faft of twenty-
four Hours, are troubled with a ftinking Breath,
and a gnawing Pain at their Stomach. Indeed all
the Juices of the human Body do of themfelves
become acrimonious without frefh Supplies; and
this is the Cafe with Men after long fafting;
whence malignant Fevers frequently arife for want
of Provifions in Cities that are befieged. A Piece
of Copper Money has indeed been found covered
with Verdigreafe in the Stomach of an Oftrich;
but that is no Argument for accufing the Stomach
with an Acid, for that Change may be made on
Copper barely by the Moifture of the Air with
the mildeft Salts.

[16] Thefe are truly fimple Glands; for the fmall
Arteries fpringing from the Cœliac, do in their ul-
timate Branches form what *Ruyfch* calls *Penicilli*,
which are nothing more than oblong lenticular
Cells, which receive this Juice inftill'd by the fmall
Arteries, which are fpent upon the Integument of
each Cell, and by retaining the fame, render its
Confiftence thicker, till it is expreffed thro' their
patulent Mouths by the periftaltic Motion of this
Vifcus,

[17] The villous Coat being larger than the other
Membranes of the Stomach, very pliable, foft, and
inelaftic, caufes it to run into Wrinkles. This is

apparent

apparent from Experiment; for a human Stomach
turned infide out, and the *Gula* clofed by a Ligature, upon diftending it with Air forced thro' the
Pylorus, the mufcular Coat will be expanded, and
the *Rugæ* of the villous Coat, which is now outer-
moft, will be then diffipated; but upon difcharging the Air, the moft elaftic of the Membranes
will contract and wrinkle thofe which are lefs fo;
but there will always be fome Part of the Aliment
detained between the *Plicæ* of the Stomach, which
cannot be entirely difcharged by the ftrongeft Contraction of that Organ.

[18] Thefe quadrangular or quinquangular Cells
are moft confpicuous in the Stomach of ruminating
Animals, where the rough Pleats of the Stomach,
in conjunction with thefe, ferve to retain the Aliment from too quick a Paffage. In the fame manner alfo the half digefted Aliment is retained by
the *Rugæ* in the human Stomach, which is the
reafon why that Organ is hardly ever entirely emptied, but retaining fome fmall Part between the
Folds, which becomes acrimonious by its long
Stay, ftimulates the Stomach by its Acrimony, fo
as to excite Hunger or increafe the Appetite.

[19] The Aliment which is retained, and ftagnates
between the Folds of the Stomach, is fermented by
its long Stay, and changed from its natural Difpofition to an acrimonious one, either tending to
an Acid or an Alkali.

[20] If the internal Surface of the Stomach was
fmooth, it would then indeed comprefs, but not
grind the Aliment which it receives: but the *Rugæ*
or Pleats of the Stomach are foft, flaccid, and
loofe in its Cavity; fo that being agitated by the
mufcular Coat, they grind and rub againft each
other, and divide fuch Parts of the Aliment as are
intercepted betwixt them; but if there is no Aliment

ment to interpofe between the *Rugæ*, they will be
injur'd by rubbing againft each other, and give an
uneafy Senfation to the nervous *Papillæ*, which we
call Hunger.

21 The very large Clafs of graniverous Fowls
are deftitute of Teeth, and live only upon vegetable Seeds, the Meal of which only is nourifhing, tho'
they are invefted with two hard Coats. To fupply
the place of Teeth, they have therefore a particular Mechanifm in their Stomachs; in the fore
Part of the Neck, above the *Sternum*, the *Oefophagus* is dilated into a membranous Bag, the
Crop, replenifhed with fmall falival Glands, which
difcharge a Liquor to mollify the Grain; in this
Stomach the entire Seeds are macerated till they
become foft and friable; they are then protruded
into the *Abdomen*, below the *Diaphragm*, where
they are ground together by two Pair of ftrong
Mufcles, in the room of a Stomach, which receive
the Grain thro' a narrow oval Slit, and are lined
within-fide by a callous Membrane, which being
rough and wrinkled, performs the Office of Teeth
upon the mollified Aliment. Thefe Animals have
therefore diftinct Organs apart for the Performance
of what is effected in the human Body by one Machine; for in us the Aliment is both macerated
with the falival Liquor, and ground with the
Action of the Mufcles in one and the fame Stomach; whereas Fowls mollify their Aliment in
one Stomach, and grind it in another; but as the
Seeds which they feed upon cannot be ground a-
funder even when mollified, without a confiderable mufcular Force, too violent to be fuffer'd without Injury, by the villous Coat which affords the
mollifying Liquor, it was therefore neceffary that
the two Offices fhould be performed afunder. Thus
we find Beans and Tares foft, friable, and fplit or

O 3

burft

burſt in the Crops of Pigeons, but in the Stomach
we find them attenuated into a pulpy Subſtance.

§. 78. If it be conſider'd that a large Quantity of *Saliva*[1] continually flows out of the
Mouth and *Oeſophagus* to the Food now arri
ved in the Stomach, together with the *Succus
gaſtricus* of the Stomach itſelf, which is conſtantly diſcharged from its villous Coat; the
Aliment muſt neceſſarily be well diluted thereby; and being mix'd with the Relicks of the
laſt Meal as a Ferment, and excited to an inteſtine Motion by the included Particles of
Air[2], expanded by the Heat[3] of the adjacent
Viſcera and Veſſels; the Conſequences hereof
muſt apparently be a *Maceration*[4], Dilution,
Rarifaction, and *Fermentation*[5], or incipient
Putrifaction of the Aliment, whereby it is
either intimately and uniformly diſſolved into
a good Chyle, fit to *ſupply*[6] the Abraſion of
the Solid, and Conſumption of the fluid Parts
of the Body, or elſe into a rancid and offenſive
Maſs.——The external or convex Side of the
villous or internal Coat of the Stomach is compoſed of all the ſame Veſſels before-mentioned
(§. 77.) which it receives from the next vaſcular and nervous Coat that inveſts it; which being nothing but an Intertexture or Network of
ſmall Arteries, Veins and Nerves, detaches
many of the ſmalleſt thro' the villous Integument, which ſupply the *Succus gaſtricus* and
Mucus before-mentioned, partly by ſtrait Ducts
or Tubes, and partly from Pores and Cells.

The

¹ The *Saliva*, tho' not a Liquor proper to the Stomach, is a principal and neceſſary Ingredient in digeſting the Aliment. The Quantity of *Saliva* ſeparated and diſcharged into the Stomach in a Day, is eſtimated to be about twelve Ounces, which is entirely ſwallowed by People in health. I have obſerved in myſelf the *Saliva* to be ſeparated in different Quantities at different Times of the Year, ſometimes not above a Drachm in an Hour, ſometimes half an Ounce, and at other times near two Ounces, tho' the *Saliva* was not ſollicited in its Diſcharge by talking or ſpitting. Hence it happens that brown Bread, which has been ſwallowed whole without chewing, may be vomited up again a few Hours after with little or no Alteration ; but if the ſame was intimately divided by the Teeth, and mixed with the *Saliva*, it will be formed into a white Liquor, like Chyle ; but the *Saliva* will appear to be ſeparated in much larger Quantities, if we add that which is mixed with the Food, and paſſes into the Stomach, to that which may be ſpit out in a certain Time ; but if we compare the Size of the Stomach with that of the ſalival Glands, the very large Surface of the villous Coat, with the great Number and Diameters of the Arteries, it will be apparent that the Proportion of the *Succus gaſtricus* is much larger than that of the *Saliva* ; whence it happens that Girls ſometimes digeſt hard Cruſts of Bread, and other dry Subſtances, without any Drink, the *Succus gaſtricus* ſupplying all the Liquor which is neceſſary to macerate and diſſolve the ſame.

² A very conſiderable Quantity of Air deſcends into the Stomach included in ſmall ſalival and mucous Veſicles, the Air having a free Paſſage into the Mouth at every Inſpiration between the Acts of Deglutition ; ſo that it not only deſcends into

the

the *Trachea*, but alfo into the *Oefophagus*; but the Efficacy of the Air to diffolve the Aliment (mentioned §. 69. N. 1.) is much greater in a clofe and warm Place than in the Mouth.

³ The great Power of Heat in diffolving many even of the hardeft Bodies, and all thofe which we eat, is demonftrated by the digefting Machine of *Papin*. Eggs alfo are converted into a putrid Mafs by 92 or 93 Degrees of Heat, infomuch that the volatiliz'd Humours exhale even thro' the Shell; but this Heat is the fame with that of the Stomach.

⁴ Tenacious Subftances ground with Water are flowly, in Procefs of Time, mollified by the Water infinuating itfelf into the Pores of the macerated Body; but Maceration is effected in Perfection in the Stomach, where there is a large Quantity of diluting Liquor, with a conftant and gentle Attrition, by which means the hard Sea Bifket-Bread becomes mollified in the Stomach, and affords good Chyle.

⁵ This is proved, in oppofition to fome of the more fevere Mechanifians; it is alfo apparent by the vinous or acetous Odour which frequently afcends in Belchings, thro' the *Fauces* of Men or ruminating Cattle; to which we may alfo add the Tumefaction of the Stomach, which frequently follows an Hour or two after a Meal, which arifes from the Air expanded by Heat; for the Air admitted and included in the Pores of Bodies, and excited by Heat, feems to be the general Caufe of Rarefaction in them; nor is it poffible for our afcefcent Food to be converted into the volatile and alcalefcent Nature of our Fluids, if they did not fuffer a Change in their fmaller Particles. Hence the adept Chemifts have ftiled Fermentation one of the operating Hands of Nature, for it is that

Operation

Operation only which produces an inflammable Spirit from Vegetables; but this Fermentation in the Stomach is ftopt in its beginning by the large Quantity of frefh fecerned Liquor which is conti-nually poured into it, and efpecially by the Ac-ceffion of the Bile, an utter Enemy to all Fermen-tation.

⁶ From what has been now declared §. 78. it appears that the Efficacy of the *Saliva* and *Succus gaftricus*, or Juice of the Stomach, is very confi-derable in changing the Nature of our Aliment to that of animal Subftance, for which it feems to be principally defigned; for it is very certain, that there is a larger Quantity of thofe Liquors poured into the Stomach than will equal the Aliment itfelf which we take; which is alfo apparent from the Confiftence of the Chyle, refembling new Cream; it is therefore in the Stomach principally that the Aliment begins to put on the Nature of animal Subftance.

§. 79. But this is not fufficient to explain how the more folid Food is intimately digefted or diffolved in the Stomach with little or no Maftication.

The folid animal and vegetable Food which is fwallowed with little or no Maftication by la-bouring, hungry, and rapacious Men, confifts of fuch hard Parts and tough Fibres, that it is incon-ceivable how the *Saliva* and Liquor of the Stomach alone fhould make that Change in them which we find in Digeftion; for we find that Food, however grofs, is at laft diffolv'd and attenuated into Chyle; and if they are of a ftrong Conftitution, they per-fectly digeft the fame into laudable Juices; there muft therefore be other Caufes than the preceding

to

to account for fo remarkable a Change of the Aliment into Chyle in the human Stomach.

§. 80. But to diveftigate the Caufe of this Change of the Aliment in Digeftion, we ought to confider the *mufcular Structure* 1 of the Stomach, and explain the Action that Organ exerts by fuch Structure.

1 We call that Part of the human Body mufcular which confifts of contractile Fibres, invefted with a Power of approximating their Extremities to each other, and of drawing the moveable Part, into which they are inferted, towards the lefs moveable, which is their proper Action, whether thofe Fibres are foft and lax, or tendinius ; whether they run longitudinally, according to the Direction of the Bone in which they are inferted, or whether they inveft fome circular Cavity ; whether they are pale, without Blood, or ftain'd red with the *Cruor* ; for neither their circular Direction nor pale Colour diminifh their Power, as appears from the Action of the Stomach, Inteftines, and Arteries.

§. 81. The mufcular Coat of the Stomach *appears* 1 to confift of very ftrong mufcular Fibres, chiefly in its external or convex Part, which beginning at the upper Orifice, pafs in a circular or *fpiral* 2 Direction to the *Pylorus*. Thefe Fibres inveft the Cavity of the Stomach in a Direction almoft perpendicular to its Length, by which means they contract the Sides of the Stomach, and make it narrower; being alfo cover'd with the cellular Subftance of *Ruyfch*, which fupplies the Oil neceffary to lubricate

lubricate and soften the muscular Fibres in Action; but the internal or concave Surface of the same Coat is compofed in its lower Part of oblique Fibres, contracting the bottom of the Stomach obliquely towards the back Part of it, and towards its upper Orifice, whereby they shorten the Length of the Stomach; whereas the second Order of Fibres, in the upper Part, are of a greater Strength, and pass in a parallel Direction, according to the Length of the Stomach from its upper Orifice to the *Pylorus*, behind which they unite and inveft its whole Length, as they alfo inveft the upper Orifice; fo that when the Stomach is empty, they draw its Orifices nearer *together* 3; but when the Stomach, being full of Aliment, keeps them diftended, fo that they cannot approximate its Orifices, they then gently clofe its upper Orifice, and very ftrongly contract the *Pylorus*.

¹ When the Stomach of a healthy Man, foon after dying a violent Death, is gently diftended with Wind to about the Size it ufually is with Food, we may then with a gentle Hand take off carefully its external Coat.

² Thefe Fibres arife from the upper Orifice, and defcend to its lower, encompaffing the Stomach in a fpiral Direction, they contract its Capacity, and comprefs the included Aliment; tho' they do not act altogether, but fucceffively, beginning from the *Oefophagus*, as *Wepfer* has obferv'd in the Stomachs of living Dogs, who do not ruminate, but have that Organ the fame as the human Stomach.

³ Thefe Fibres are twenty times ftronger than the preceding, but they form a *Stratum* of not

above

above four Fingers Breadth. In the Stomach of a
dead Subject they appear separated, relaxed, and
as if they were divided from each other; but their
State is not such in Life. The large and thin Bladder of Urine is sometimes contracted in the human
Subject to the Size of a Walnut, and the Stomach
is frequently no larger than one's Fist. They run
from the left Orifice of the Stomach to the right,
and encompass both with their strong muscular
Fibres; they act all together, contract the Length
of the Stomach, diminish its Capacity, and bring
its two Mouths to each other. All these Fibres
do not begin to act till the Stomach is moderately
full, till then they are at rest; but the more the
Stomach is diftended, the more forcibly they are
contracted; infomuch that when it is over-fill'd,
it cannot empty itfelf, but remains diftended with
exquisite Pain, till it occasions Death, or a Palsy
of the now mentioned Fibres, whose principal Service to the Stomach, is to retain the Aliment from
paffing out too soon; and when they have loft
their Tone and Action, the Food then quickly
passes thro' the Stomach with little or no Change
from its Action, causing a Lientery.

§. 82. This muscular Coat also appears not
only to be covered with the *cellular* [1] Membrane of *Ruyfch* (§. 81.) but also with another
externally, which in the convex Part is very
full of Veffels, and in the concave Part furnished
with longitudinal and parallel Fibres, ferving to
contract or shorten the Length of the Stomach.

[1] This cellular Coat invefts the whole Body, and
every Muscle and Part which moves and rubs
against others, or contains any thing acrimonious;

it

it is compofed of an infinite Number of Follicles, or little Bladders, which receive and retain the oily Part of the Blood from the ultimate Branches of the fmall Arteries, and have fuch a Communication with each other throughout the whole Body, that by gradually applying Bandages to the fwell'd Feet and Legs of dropfical Patients, the Humour will be drove up to the Head, and infomuch that a Man whofe whole Body was fwell'd with an *Anafarca*, upon burning his Foot as he flept by the Fire-fide in the Winter, was cured by the Waters running entirely out, as if it had been from a Cafk; and Wind blown into this Membrane in any Part of the Body, may be drove thro' it in all the reft, by which means Butchers endeavour to impofe lean for fat Meat upon the Buyer by inflating it. Part of this Membrane is called *Adipofa*, being one of the common Integuments of the Body, next to the Skin; but there is another much thinner Part of it, which invefts the fmaller Mufcles and their Membranes, diftinguifh'd with the Name of *cellular Coats* by their Inventor *Ruyfch*. This Membrane has many Ufes in the human Body; it lubricates the mufcular Fibres with its Oil, prevents the Mufcles adhering to their Integuments, abates the Attrition of Parts, *&c.* infomuch that when this Membrane is deftroy'd by a Gangrene, it is attended with an Immobility of the Mufcles; but when thefe Cells are diftended with too large a Quantity of Oil, it produces an oppofite Difeafe, and renders the Mufcles unfit for Motion, by clogging them; of which fat People are too well affured by Experience.

§. 83. Tho' the forementioned mufcular Fibres are very contractile, yet they are *incapable*

ble [1] of entirely emptying the Stomach; when
they act together they close the two Apertures,
where the *Oesophagus* and *Duodenum* are inserted some way into the Stomach, which are
also naturally contracted of themselves by their
own Structure; they strongly compress the distending Contents of the Stomach, mix and
grind them together by their periftaltic Motion, and Impulse from the Motion of the adjacent Parts; they keep back the more gross
Parts of the Food in the Stomach, and further
attenuate the same, expelling the more fluid
Parts into the Cavity before the *Pylorus*, and e-
ven thro' the *Pylorus* itself into the *Duodenum*,
notwithstanding the Resistance arising from the
perpendicular Ascent of the *Pylorus*, its Incurvation, muscular Contraction, greater internal
Thickness, and the valvular Insertion of the
Duodenum into it; and thus the Aliment, reduced to an Ash-colour'd thick Fluid in the
Stomach, is pressed slowly, and by a little at a
time, rather thro' the *Pylorus* into the *Duodenum*, than by the upper Orifice into the *Oesophagus*; because the latter lies much higher,
and is more firmly closed by the *Diaphragm*.

[1] The Contraction of every Muscle is limited to
a certain degree, which it cannot exceed. In the
Stomach this Contraction is limited to about four
or five Ounces of Liquor, which the Stomach cannot expel out of its Cavity; and in the dead Subject, where the Stomach is collapsed, it will admit
of five Ounces, without appearing to be distended;
the circular Fibres are no where disposed so as to
contract

contract the Capacity of the Stomach, that it will
not receive a Quantity of Aliment without Distention, which *Bernoulli* has demonstrated in a Theorem; it therefore appears that the Stomach begins
to compress the Aliment when it contains more
than five Ounces, which it cannot do when there
is less, because there is a Space left capable of receiving five Ounces of Water; like as a Cord does
not begin to contract itself, but when it is drawn
out beyond its natural Length; but when it is returned to its former Length, it then ceases to contract any more; therefore the Stomach is never entirely emptied, nor its Sides brought close to each
other; but if it is contracted beyond the above-
mentioned Capacity, it must be owing rather to
the Pressure of the *Diaphragm* and Muscles of the
Abdomen, than the Contraction of its muscular
Coat. If the Stomach be filled with Wind, and
held to the Fire to give it a greater Expansion,
upon wounding the same, the Air will be expell'd
by Contraction of the Stomach, but the whole
Quantity of Air will not be discharged, so as to
leave the Stomach quite empty; the same may also
be better perform'd if the Stomach is distended
with Water instead of Air, which will be forced
out thro' the Puncture, till the Stomach is contracted to its natural Capacity: Hence it appears
that the Action of the Stomach is not wholly to
be referred to Trituration, as some great Men have
been too easily persuaded. The Stomach of a Dog
or a Hog has the same Structure with that of the
human Body; therefore these Animals have been
chose for Experiments, by giving Vomits, by which
accurate Observation has been made of the manner
wherein the Stomach is contracted by the peristaltic Motion being increased, being sometimes elongated, and at other times shortened, by its two

Orifices

Orifices approaching each other, but yet never so much contracted as to be entirely emptied; therefore a Quantity of Aliment which is less than five Ounces, ought by this Experiment to be incapable of the digestive Power of the Stomach. But this is contrary to Experience, which assures us, that many things the most agreeable to the Palate, may be well digested in much less Quantities; for if a weak Person should take an Ounce of Food every Hour, the same would be very well digested, notwithstanding it suffered no Pressure or Trituration from the muscular Structure of that Organ. However, the Action of the Stomach in this respect seems to be weak when it contains very little Aliment, and strongest when it is half full; but when it is too much distended, the Aliment suffers hardly any Action at all from the Stomach; so that after a moderate Meal the Appetite will quickly return again at its usual times; but by immoderate eating the Appetite will be palled for several Days, by the Putrifaction of the Aliment, occasioned by its too long Stay in the Stomach.

§. 84. Some Creatures have scarce any other Power than this contractile Force of the Stomach to digest or grind their macerated Aliment, but to a much *stronger degree* [1] than what is exerted in the human Stomach; and in some of them this Motion may even be heard, as well as proved, by an Observation of its Effects; and the nervous and muscular Structure of this Organ in the human Body, compared with the like Structure of the same Organ in Brutes, demonstrates *the same* [2] in us.

The

[1] The Oftrich, and other graniverous Fowls, have been obferved to grind Glafs in their Stomachs with fuch a Force, as to occafion a grating perceptible by the Ear, and to break off the angular Parts of the Glafs without any Prejudice to the Bird ; for the Oftrich has no Crop or preparatory Stomach ; but its true Stomach is armed with very ftrong Mufcles, and it fwallows Pieces of Iron and Stones, that by the Attrition of thofe hard Bodies. together with the Aliment, the latter may be more expeditioufly attenuated or divided ; but that it feeds upon Iron, is a falfe Report.

[2] Several eminent Men have imagined, that there was the fame Attrition in the human Stomach as they had before obferved in Birds ; but they ought to have confider'd, that the Structure of that Organ in the human Body is very different, and therefore cannot be expected to perform the fame Action ; the mufcular Fibres in the human Stomach are very few and weak, and its villous Coat very thin ; whereas that of Birds is flefhy, and compofed of very ftrong Mufcles, and its rough Lining that grinds their Food is tough and cartilaginous.

§. 85. From hence we may underftand the reafon, why when but little Aliment is taken, it is *quickly difcharged* [1] out of the Stomach ; and why when the Stomach is over-fill'd, it neither digefts nor difcharges its Contents as ufual, but after retaining the fame fome time, it is vomited up *crude* [2] ; and why when *Liquors* [3] are fuddenly drank in large Quantities, thy ftay a long time in the Stomach.

[1] Becaufe the Rank of parallel Fibres, which are detach'd from one Orifice of the Stomach to the

ther, are then flaccid ; yet thofe Fibres will again
act, when the Stomach is diftended beyond the Capacity of five Ounces of Liquor ; but even after
that, the Aliment is eafily preffed out of the Stomach, not by its own mufcular Contraction, which
then ceafes, but by the Preffure of the adjacent
Mufcles and incumbent *Diaphragm* ; which laft
defcending at every Infpiration, forces out the
Contents of the Stomach.

2. A young Glutton comes home from feafting
with his Stomach cramm'd full of Varieties, which
being retained therein for about 8 or 10 Hours,
will caufe a great Digeftion of the fame, not only
by its large Quantity, but alfo much more by Fermentation and Rarefaction ; but no Part of it e-
fcapes out of the Stomach, whofe Orifices are then
contracted, and its circular Fibres render'd paralytic ; till at length, caufing great Reaching and
Uneafinefs, the Fibres between the Orifices of the
Stomach being relax'd, and its Mouths opened,
the Aliment, which was before retained with fo
much Uneafinefs, is expelled both upward and
downward, but more above than below, becaufe
all the Fibres of the upper Orifice being relaxed,
the *Flatus* generated by the Food, is ufually found
to difcharge itfelf that way. Thus the Conful
Antonius vomiting up his *Crapula* of the Day before, daubed his Alderman's Gown, and filled the
whole Seffion-houfe with the ftinking Smell of the
Wine and his gorged Varieties. But the longitudinal Fibres of the Stomach ufually hold contracted
much longer, as they lie clofer together, and exert a greater Force ; the Orifices of the Stomach
are efpecially contracted ftrongly ; for the *Oefophagus* paffing through the *Diaphragm*, is in that Part
furnifhed with ftrong mufcular Fibres, whereby it
is conftringed ; but the mufcular Part of the *Duodenum*

denum is not continuous with the mufcular Coat of
the Stomach, but inferts its mufcular Tube a little
way within that of the Stomach, fo that it may be
clofed by a Contraction of the Fibres of the Stomach; whence it happens in unactive People, that
the tranfverfe Fibres being relaxed, the longitudinal Fibres interpofed between the two Orifices of
the Stomach, perfift in their Contraction, and retain the Aliment in the Stomach with a confiderable Force, till having arrived to its greateft Diftenfion, and the Nerves and Arteries being by
that means compreffed, thofe Fibres which are fupplied by them, muft neceffarily ceafe to act; but
the Aliment thus retained will remain crude or indigefted, becaufe the Mouth of the *Oefophagus* being clofed, will not admit the *Saliva*; alfo the Stomach itfelf being greatly diftended, and its Veffels
by that means compreffed, will not feparate the
Succus gaftricus as ufual, nor fuffer its wonted Attrition; it therefore follows, that the Aliment thus
left to itfelf, will be fermented and varioufly changed, according to its different Nature, into a putrid Mafs; whence it happens, that what is vomited by drunken People, is ufually very acrimonious; and Wine itfelf, which is of an aceffent
Nature, is quickly converted into a moft fharp
Vinegar.

3 Great Drinkers, if they indulge themfelves
with large Draughts at very fmall Intervals, are
foon made fick and drunk thereby; but if they
ftay fome time between each, and do not drink
more Liquor till the preceding has been heated by
the Stomach, they will then bear much more Wine
without Injury; and if they vomit, it will be more
eafily; becaufe the Coldnefs of the Liquors contracts the Stomach, fo as to make it expel what
was in it before, and retain what came into it laft;

therefore

therefore they who drink large Quantities of cold mineral Waters at a time, are frequently troubled with Pains at their Stomach, from the Waters not finding a Paſſage either by Urine or Stool; and even Polypuſſes have been ſeen formed in the Arteries of the Stomach, from a too plentiful and ſudden drinking of cold Liquors; in which Caſe the moſt ſpeedy Remedy is to excite a Vomit, by tickling the *Fauces* and *Pharynx* with an oiled Feather; whereas if they were to drink their Waters by ſmall and repeated Draughts, they would not only purge well, but run thro' the Body as thro' an open Tube, and eaſily produce their deſired Effects.

§. 86. The Cauſes already explained may indeed ſeem *inſufficient* [1] thus to digeſt and change the Food in the Stomach; but this Difficulty will be removed, if we conſider, 1. The conſtant attenuating *Heat* [2] of the circumjacent Parts, the Heart, Liver, Spleen, Aorta, Meſentery, Arteries and Veins, by which the Stomach is expoſed on every ſide to the ſtrongeſt Heat in the whole Body. 2. The innumerable *Vibrations* [3] of the Arteries near the Heart, and which are ſpent upon the Stomach, *Diaphragm*, *Omentum*, Meſentery, Spleen, Liver, *Pancreas*, and the *Peritonæum*. 3. The violent Pulſations or Strokes of the ſubjacent *Aorta* [4]. 4. The great Force of the *nervous* [5] and glandular Juices, ſcarce more plentiful in any Part. 5. The continual reciprocal and ſtrong Compreſſion from almoſt the whole *Peritonæum* agitating and preſſing upon the Stomach, (1.) by means of the *Diaphragm*,

phragm, which is a large Mufcle arifing on the lower part of the Right-fide from the three firft *Vertebræ* of the Loins, and on the Left-fide tendonous, from the laft and laft but one of the *Vertebræ* of the *Thorax* tendonous, a-bove which it arifes flefhy, with its Fibres paf-fing directly upward, and expanding again ten-donous; fo that on the upper part it arifes thin and membranous, and afterwards flefhy, from the whole Margin of the cartilaginous Ends of the lower Ribs, and lower Part of the *Ster-num*, detaching its Fibres towards the Center, where they become tendonous with the prece-ding; fo that this Mufcle acting from a con-vex Pofition in the *Thorax*, to a plain one in the *Abdomen*, compreffes all the *Vifcera*[6] of the latter, and particularly the Stomach. (2.) By the *ten Mufcles of the Abdomen*[7] ftrongly compreffing all the Contents of that Cavity, by their united and reciprocal Contractions, and exerting a confiderable Force upon the Stomach, as we are informed by Experience and Obfervation; for, 1. the external oblique Mufcles arifing tendonous and flefhy from the lower Margin of the twelve lower Ribs, and afcending obliquely forward, are inferted by a tendonous Expanfion into the whole *Linea alba*, over the right internal oblique and tranf-verfe Mufcles, alfo into the anterior and upper Edge of the *Os Pubis* and *Ilium*. 2. The ob-lique internal Mufcles, which arife flefhy from the circular Margin of the *Os Ilium* and Liga-ment of the *Os Pubis*, confifting of Fibres

afcending

afcending obliquely forward, horizontally, and
downward, and becoming tendonous, are inferted into the *Linea alba*, and the Cartilages of
the five lower Ribs. 3. The pyramidal Mufcles, which arife flefhy from the upper and anterior Part of the *Os Pubis*, and are inferted
tendonous into the *Linea alba* and Navel. 4.
The tranfverfe Mufcles of the *Abdomen*, arifing
flefhy from a tendonous Expanfion, fixed between the tranfverfe Proceffes of the *Vertebræ*
of the Loins, Spine of the *Os Ilium*, Ligament
of the *Os Pubis*, and the cartilaginous Ends of
the Ribs below the *Sternum*, and are inferted
by a broad Tendon into the whole *Linea alba*,
under the right Mufcles of the *Abdomen*. 5.
And laftly, the *Recti*-Mufcles, which arifing
flefhy from the enfiform Cartilage, and the
Cartilages of the two lower true, and two upper baftard Ribs, are afterwards divided into five
mufcular Portions by as many tendonous In-
nervations, being at laft inferted into the upper
and fore Part of the *Os Pubis*.

[1] Becaufe a fmall Quantity of Food is quickly
and perfectly digefted, and paffes out of the Stomach into the Inteftines without the Affiftance of
the mufcular Fibres.

[2] *Galen* compares the Stomach to a Pot, under
which is placed the Fire of the Liver; and indeed
if there is no Fire under it, there is a very great
Heat conftantly adminifter'd to it by the adjacent
Parts; for the Stomach is encompaffed above by
the Heart, feparated from it only by the inconfiderable Thicknefs of the *Diaphragm*; the *Omentum*,
and Mefentery, keep it warm below; behind it the
Aorta

Aorta diftributes its large Stream of warm Blood; the thin and warm Exhalation of the *Abdomen* communicates to it the gentle Heat of a vaporous Bath, and then no Heat refolves Subftances more powerfully than that of the human Body; too ftrong a Heat often compacts Things together, but the Heat of the Atmofphere, which is lefs than that of the human Body, refolves Flefh itfelf into a liquid Mafs within the Space of three Days. And under the Equator, where the Sun is directed perpendicularly to the Earth, Muft is converted into Wine by a Fermentation within the Space of twenty-four Hours. The Baker's Dough is render'd agreeable to the Palate by no other Artifice, than by fermenting it fome time at the Mouth of the Oven before baking. Eggs, which are turned hard in a ftrong Heat, are in a fhort time converted into a very thin Fluid by the Heat of the human Body; whence it appears that the Effect of Heat in digefting the Aliment is very confiderable, tho' Digeftion is not wholly performed thereby, as was imagined by the Ancients.

³ The Vibrations of the Arteries, which are diftributed fo plentifully, and fufficiently large about the Stomach, being agitated alternately by Dilatation in their *Diaftole*, and Contraction of their *Syftole*; when they are contracted, they prefs againft the Sides of the Stomach, and fhake the contiguous Aliment. This Vibration of the Arteries is communicated to every Part of the Stomach, encompaffed by the other *Vifcera*, which are full of the like Veffels. The Vibrations of thefe numberlefs Arteries are communicated to the Stomach three thoufand and fix hundred times in an Hour, for fo often are they dilated and contracted in that Time. But we find the alternate and repeated Action of Water will make Excavations in Stone; and in

like

like manner the Vibrations of the innumerable
fmall Arteries may perform the fame Effect, as if
contracted into one ftronger and fhorter Impulfe.
A Drop of Water falling from an Height upon a
Marble, will by being repeated 1000 times, ftrike
off a Piece of the Stone equal to what a like Body
a thoufand times greater would ftrike off by one
Fall from the fame Height. In the fame manner
the Vibration of the fmall Arteries repeated three
thoufand times, will exert the fame Force upon
the Stomach, as would have been exerted by a
greater Impulfe in a fhorter time, especially as we
find that fo fmall Arteries as thofe of the *Dura
Mater*, make their ftrong Impreffions upon the
hard Bones of the *Cranium*; in Proportion to
which, the Arteries of the Stomach, which are fo
much larger, muft exert a very great Power upon
the Sides of the Stomach, whih is fo much fofter.
Nor ought it to be objected, that the Arteries
make their Impreffions upon the Bones of the *Cranium* in the tender infantine State, for the Arteries
were then fofter than the *Cranium*, and their Impreffions grow ftronger as the Animal becomes
more adult; but the weaker any Perfon is, the
more frequent is his Pulfe, infomuch that the Artery
fometimes beats fix thoufand times in an Hour; and
fo the Vibration of the Arteries upon the Stomach is
ftronger in Health, but more frequent in Difeafes;
nor do I think their Action can ever be fo weak,
as not to equal the Contraction of its mufcular
Coat.

4 The *Aorta*, which conveys the ardent and vital
Stream, refifted behind by the *Vertebrae* of the
Back, violently agitates the Stomach, which lies
before it; and if the Mufcles of the *Abdomen* prefs
the Stomach backward, as they generally do, it is
in a manner fqueez'd between two ftrong Preffes;
but

but the great Force of the *Aorta* may be judg'd of
from its having a Power more than equal to the
Refiftance of all the other Arteries put together;
and even the Artery in the Ham, which is none
of the largeft, will elevate not only the whole Leg,
but alfo an additional Weight; we may alfo judge
of it by the Force with which one's Finger is compreffed when inferted into the *Aorta* of a living Dog.

' Concerning the Nature of the nervous Juice,
and Termination of the Nerves, we fhall fpeak
more largely hereafter ; where it will appear, that
none of them are clofed, but pervaded by the nervous Juice, which is extremely fubtil and moveable, fo as to exceed the diffolving Power of any
other Fluid in the Body; but if one may guefs at
the Action of this Fluid in the Stomach by its
Nature and Affufion, by the vaft Number of its
Nerves, it will appear to be very confiderable, becaufe the nervous *Papillæ* of the Stomach are very
plentifully fupplied with their Branches; therefore
the diffolving Power of this Juice in the Stomach
is very great.

⁶ The Stomach is fituated in the *Abdomen*, which
is a kind of a Machine, fixed behind, but moveable
in its upper and anterior Part, fo that by the *Diaphragm*, abdominal Mufcles and *Aorta*, the Stomach is perpetually agitated upward and downward, backward and forward, the more ftrongly
as it is more full. The Cavity of the *Abdomen* has not any Part empty, nor is the Stomach
fufpended among its *Vifcera* as in a Fluid ; but
being mov'd in a Place that is already full, it preffes againft the adjacent Parts, and that Preffure is
alfo returned again upon the Stomach; it defcends
with the *Diaphragm*, and is again preffed upwards
with that Mufcle, by which means the Food fuffers a Divifion, like that of boiled Peas in a Bladder,

der, compreſſed alternately with a conſiderable Force by the Hands of a Man. The *Diaphragm* in Expiration aſcends to the Line at the bottom of each Breaſt, which is obſerved by few, nor is it drawn in that Poſition in anatomical Figures; but when it is flattened towards the *Abdomen*, it preſſes the Stomach downward and forward; and as the Muſcles of the *Abdomen* re-act in Expiration, it will be again by them preſſed upward and backward; thus by the continued Action of theſe two Powers, the *Diaphragm* and Muſcles of the *Abdomen*, the Viſcera contained in that Cavity are perpetually agitated upward and downward; the Conſequence of which will be, an Attrition in the Stomach, and a Diviſion of the Aliment into minute Parts; and this Force is the ſtronger upon the Stomach, as it reſiſts by a greater Diſtenſion; but the Force of the *Diaphragm* in this reſpect may be judged of by Inſpection, as when the abdominal Muſcles of a living Dog are divided, and the Viſcera of the *Abdomen* are forcibly preſſed down by it, and endeavour to come out of the Wound; but when the *Peritonæum* itſelf is divided, the Inteſtines are then protruded with a conſiderable Murmuring and *Impetus*; and if the Finger is inſerted at the Wound, it will be preſſed with a conſiderable Force; all which Preſſure is owing to the *Diaphragm*, by whoſe Action in vomiting the Contents of the Stomach are expelled with great Violence upwards; but downward, if it is to be diſcharged *per Anum*.

' The Muſcles of the *Abdomen* are ſo diſpoſed, that there is always ſome fleſhy Part of them ſubjected under the tendonous, by which means the whole Capacity of the *Abdomen* is equally contracted; the fleſhy Part of the oblique deſcending Muſcle lies almoſt entirely above, but becomes tendon-

ous

ous below ; and then the oblique afcending Mufcle
arifes flefhy below, and tendinous above, and fo
fills up the Inequality which would have been occafioned by the preceding Mufcle alone ; but then
in the middle of thefe Mufcles backward there is
a Deficiency, which is again fupplied by the flefhy
Belly of the tranfverfe ; but then all thefe are converted into a thin Tendon in their anterior Parts,
which is therefore fupplied, fo as to be equal, by
the flefhy Recti-mufcles ; which if inferted broad at
the bottom, have no Addition, as *Riolan* obferves ;
but if they are inferted narrow, they are ufually
fupplied with the pyramidal Mufcles.

§. 87. If we therefore confider the united
Force of thefe feveral concurring Caufes (§. 76,
to 87.) acting together upon the mix'd Aliment (§. 49, to 57.) which is then become fufficiently *foft* [1] and foluble, being compofed of
vegetable and animal Juices, clofely confined
and mixed together by gentle Caufes, and of
their own Nature apt to ferment, putrify, and
turn rancid in a warm and clofe [2] Place, we
may evidently perceive that the Alterations the
Aliment undergoes in the Stomach, muft be
fuch as follow.

(1.) That the finer Part of the Aliment is mixed,
ground or diffolved [3], and attenuated by the Juices
in the Stomach, puts on the Form of a [4] grey-co-
lour'd Pulp, which paffes out of the Stomach, where
there is the leaft Refiftance [5].

(2.) That the groffer and more tough [6] Parts of
the Aliment are retained in the Stomach, after the
more fluid have been difcharged ; and by continuing to fuffer the fame Caufes, they are at length
digefted,

digefted, prepared and difcharged, like the former.

(3.) That the Fibres [7], Membranes, Tendons,
Cartilages, and Bones [8] of Animals, with the Skins,
Threads, and more folid Parts of Vegetables, are
difcharged out of the Stomach in their natural
Form, after the Tincture and juicy Parts [9] have
been extracted.

(4.) That by a Diffolution [10] of animal and vegetable Food in this manner, is form'd a Liquor approaching the Nature of our animal Juices [11], fitted
to fupply their Wafte, and fupport the whole Body.

(5.) How People are fuddenly refrefhed [12] and
ftrengthened, after they have been reduced to a
languid State by long fafting, by the fubtle and more
fluid Part of the Aliment being inftantly received by
the *Vafa inhalentia*, or fmall reductory Veins which
open into the Mouth, *Oefophagus*, and Stomach,
and difcharge themfelves into the lymphatic Veins,
from whence it paffes immediately into the fanguiferous Veins, and is afterwards diftributed by the
Arteries thro' all Parts of the Body, and fuddenly
refrefhes or recruits the whole Animal.

[1] If the Food is not well divided by the Teeth,
and diluted by the *Saliva*, it paffes thro' the Body
whole and indigefted. If the ftrongeft Man in the
World fhould fwallow dry Currants whole, he
could not digeft them, but they would be difcharged intire in his Fæces but little altered ; and
even fo ftrong an Animal as the Horfe, does not
fo perfectly digeft his Oats, but that frequently
fome of them will retain their vegetative Power,
fo as to grow.

[2] While the upper Orifice of the Stomach is clofed, by the Contraction of the mufcular Fibres in
its upper Part, below its opening into the *Pylorus*
is ftopt by a diftinct Valve.   Since

³ Since Glafs itfelf is ground fmooth by the Attrition of the Coats of the Stomach, the Effect of that Attrition will be much greater upon Animal Food. *Pyerus* found that Iron was not corroded in the Stomach of an Ox ; and *Borelli* made the fame Experiments. The Diffolution of the Aliments is alfo in part promoted, whilft they are infenfibly attenuated by the Interpofition of a diluting Fluid, in which the nourifhing Particles or folid Elements are fufpended.

⁴ The Food after a long Maftication looks white, and reflects the Rays of Light unalter'd ; even if a Perfon fhould eat red Beet and brown Bread, the *Chymus* of it made in the Stomach is always of an Afh-colour, occafion'd by the Levigation and fmooth Surface of the Parts ; by which means the mafticated Aliment is ground finer in the Stomach, and reduced to a more uniform Mixture ; but the Chyle is never vomited out of the Stomach, nor found in it of a perfect white Colour.

⁵ The more the Stomach is diftended, the more it is compreffed by the Action of the *Diaphragm*, and the Contraction of the mufcular Fibres of the Stomach itfelf, if they were not over diftended ; but the comprefs'd Aliment endeavouring to efcape, will pafs out where there is the leaft Refiftance, not at the *Oefophagus*, becaufe that is ftrictly clofed and contracted by the *Diaphragm*, with the Refiftance of the Weight of the Aliment itfelf ; the Aliment will therefore pafs out of the Stomach thro' the *Pylorus*, which is relaxed to receive the Aliment, and eafily tranfmits it thro' its large Aperture, which is yet not fo open as to admit the more grofs and folid Parts, but only the more fluid; which are of the Confiftence of Cream, preffed out by the Force of the *Diaphragm* and Contraction of the Stomach, which overcome the Refiftance of the *Pylorus* ; from whence they pafs thro' a narrow

row Aperture to the *Duodenum*, where the groffer
Parts are more intimately diffolved.

'When the Stomach is full it cannot difcharge
any of the groffer Part of the Food ; therefore fuch
Parts as cannot pafs thro' the narrow *Pylorus*, are
retained in the Stomach, and drained of their Juices,
tending towards the *Duodenum* ; till being at laft
fufficiently attenuated, they alfo are preffed through
the relaxed Orifice of the *Pylorus* by the Contraction of the Stomach and *Diaphragm*. Dr. *Wallis*
has demonftrated by Experiments, that the Aliment which is firft taken into the Stomach, is alfo
firft expell'd out of it into the Inteftines ; but the
Time required by the Stomach to make fuch a
Difcharge cannot be accurately determined.

'The ftrongeft Man does not entirely diffolve
the more folid Parts of the Aliment, nor change
them into Chyle ; for to diffolve the folid Fibres
of Beef into thofe primary fmall Particles of which
the Fibres were originally formed, would require
the Action of a greater Power than that by which
thofe Particles were formed into Fibres ; but it is
evident fuch a Power is not prefent in the human
Body, nor is any other Part of the Aliment digefted befides the Juices, which are drained out of the
divided Veffels and hollow Fibres of the Parts of
Animals and Vegetables, which Juices are afterwards chang'd to the Nature of the animal Fluids ;
but fuch Juices make up much the greater Part
of all Flefh-meats, equalling feven Parts out of
eight of the whole Subftance.

'It has been the Opinion of many, that even
the Bones of Animals were diffolved and ground
in the Stomachs of fome Creatures, as *Helmont* was
formerly of opinion, and as I myfelf once imagined ; but to be fatisfied in this Refpect I made feveral Experiments, by which it appeared that the

more

more tough Parts of the Aliment are not diſſolved in the Stomachs of Animals. I gave the Guts of an Animal to be ſwallow'd by a hungy Dog, who devoured them inſtantly with hardly ever touching them by his Teeth ; they were diſcharged not in the leaſt digeſted, but entire by him, trailing after him out of the *Rectum* in a miſerable manner. To another hungry Dog was given butter'd Bones, which were diſcharged unaltered in his *Fæces.* The furfuracious Part of Bread is alſo diſcharged entire, no Part of it being digeſted but what is diſſolvable in Water ; and the ſolid Fibres of the Fleſh of Animals are return'd whole, only drain'd of their Juices. Ligaments which were given to a Dog, were diſcharged without Alteration, after ſtaying three Days in him ; and in that kind of the Dog's Feces which is called *Album græcum,* Fragments of Bones were diſcernible to the naked Eye not much altered, the whole Subſtance being no more than the ſmall Particles of Bones which were broke aſunder by the Teeth of the Dog, and exhauſted of their ſucculent Parts.

⁹ The Horſe, who is an Animal not much ſtronger than a Man, living upon Graſs and Hay, diſcharges the entire Leaves of Graſs and Stalks of Hay, viſible to the naked Eye, after they have been macerated in the Stomach, drained in his Inteſtines, and turned to dry Balls of Dung. The Ox, who ſwallows the Graſs greedily in little Balls, never diſſolves it in his firſt Stomach, but is oblig'd to ruminate the ſame and grind it again by the Teeth, which being attenuated and macerated by the *Saliva,* afterwards ſwallowed, and the Maſtication again repeated, yet the entire Stalks and Fibres of the Graſs and Hay are no leſs diſcernible in their Feces ; in human Feces the ſolid Fibres of Fleſh are alſo diſcernible ; and the ſame alſo holds

true

true of the folid Parts of Vegetables, the Skins of
Peas, Beans, Cherries, Currants, Grapes, &c. for
all thofe are difcharged, 'fwelled indeed, and mollified, but not attenuated and diffolved.

¹⁰ An eminent Phyfician has ftarted the Queftion,
why the human Stomach is not wore away itfelf in
the Diffolution which it makes of the Stomachs
and Inteftines of thofe Animals upon which we
feed; but the Anfwer is not fo difficult as that
Gentleman imagined; for the human Stomach is
impaired by the fame Heat, and the fame Trituration which is fuffered by the Aliment, but then
it is perpetually renewed, which the Parts of the
Aliment are not. Such Parts of the Aliment as
are incapable of being diffolved by the Air and the
the Teeth, *Saliva*, Mixture of the Air and the
Juice, Heat, and Attrition of the Stomach, ftay in
that Vifcus till they are drained of their moft fluid
and moveable Particles; and then the Stomach is
relaxed, and the *Pylorus* is more inclined downwards; fo that by the Preffure of the *Diaphragm*
they are at laft alfo expelled thro' the relaxed *Pylorus*, except they fhould be vomited up with a ftimulating acid or putrid Vavour.

¹¹ It is a furprifing and almoft incredible Change
in the Nature of Things, that the very fame Chyle
fhould be made as well from the different vegetable
as animal Food; but if we confider the Matter a
little more attentively, we fhall find all Animals
reducible to two Kinds. (1.) Thofe which live upon Animals. And, (2.) Thofe which live upon
Vegetables. In the latter Clafs of Animals, which
are moft frequently in ufe for Food amongft us,
their animal Juices are the Juice of Grafs, and o-
ther Vegetables, prepared by the Efficacy of the
Stomach, Inteftines, and Liquors flowing into them:
But in the carniverous Clafs of Animals, their Fluids

are

are vegetable Juices firft converted into animal
Fluids by grameniverous Animals ; and now again
tranfmuted into another more exalted kind of animal Juices. All our Nourifhment is therefore vegetable Juices prepared by the Action of one or
more Stomachs, according as they are drawn either
immediately from the Vegetables themfelves, or
from the broken Fibres and Veffels of Animals :
So that the Fluids of thofe Animals which feed upon Vegetables approach nearer to the Nature of vegetable Juices ; whereas in carnivorous Animals they
are more exalted and attenuated, as thofe vegetable
Juices undergoing the Action of the natural and vital Organs of two Animals, are alfo more inclined
to be alcaline ; and therefore the Milk of Bitches
and She-Lyons does not eafily turn fowr. In the
fame manner our Fluids are form'd out of the Juices
of the Parts of Animals upon which we feed, and
are again digefted, and more exalted by the Action
of our *Vifcera* ; if we therefore confider, that every
thing which we eat is really vegetable Subftance,
either at firft or fecond hand, as having undergone
the Action of one or more Stomachs, it will be no
fuch difficult Matter to conceive that the fame Blood
fhould be made out of the feveral Kinds of Food.

¹² The firft Father of Phyfic, *Hippocrates*, has
told us formerly, that all the Parts of the human
Body are perfpirable ; or which is the fame, are
every where furnifhed with exhaling Arteries and
abforbing Veins. An infinite Number of fmall Arteries difperfed thro' the whole Skin, exhale an invifible Vapour, by which we are encompafs'd as
with a Cloud, and which is carried off from us by
the Air ; if this be condenfed againft the Side of a
Looking-glafs, it turns into watery Drops ; this
Vapour is never perceived in hot Weather, nor under the Tropicks ; but in a cold Air it is condenfed

into

into vifible Clouds, fo that we breathe out a fenfible Vapour as well from all Parts of the Body as
the Mouth : This Tranfpiration is very much diminifhed by a denfe Cuticle, and the repelling Force
of a cold Air ; upon which account it is probable
that this Vapour exhales in much larger Quantities
in the internal Cavities of the Body, which are all
kept moift with thefe Vapours ; but if we are thus
affured that there are exhaling Veffels which difcharge thefe Vapours, we are not much lefs certain
that there muft alfo be *Vaffa inhalentia* to draw in
Effluvia at the fame Parts; which is confirmed by
Experiments. *Bellini* having filled an inverted Stomach with Water, found it was abforbed, fo as to
diftend the Veins of the Stomach, and the Skin itfelf of the human Body will abforb the Water retained in a Veficle formed by a Separation of the
Cuticle in a Blifter. The Particles of *Mercury* and
Cantharides are alfo abforb'd upon their Application to the Skin of the human Body, and diftribute
their Action thro' every internal Part: And the
Experiment of *Ruyfch* is ftill a ftronger Argument,
by which the Injection being forced thro' the Valves
of the Veins, paffes thro' the fmall Veins into the
Cavity of the Stomach in as large or a greater Quantity than what paffes by the Arteries. I had alfo an
Opportunity of obferving the fame in the Hand of
a Child, where the Injection tranfuded thro' the
innumerable fmall Pores of the Veins like Dew.
To thefe abforbing Veffels, is owing that Refrefhment which is fo fuddenly perceived in the Maftication of our Food; which feems to favour the
Affertion of *Paracelfus*, that the ancient *Sophi*, or
wife Men, lived only by chewing their Food, without fwallowing any Part of it. A-kin to this is the
common Story of *Democritus*, who at a Hundred
and five Years of Age, is faid to have been kept
alive

alive, the Space of three Days by the Vapour or
Scent of new Bread, that he might not die within
the Time of the Feast of *Ceres*, and disturb their
Ceremony. However, we have no room to doubt
that there are very small absorbing Veins, which
convey the most subtle and vapoury Parts of the
Aliment into the lymphatick Veins, from whence
they are transmitted to the sanguiferous Veins, thence
to the Heart and Arteries, and by them in a little
time to the Brain itself; upon which follows a sud-
den Recreation of the whole Body.

§. 88. From hence we may judge, whether
Heat [1] is the only Author of Digestion in the
Stomach? Whether there is a *vital Acrimony
or Spirit* [2] which inspires a native Action to
the Stomach? Whether Digestion will be imperfect without, or promoted by *an acid* [3]?
Why a *viscid, saline, acid or bitter Humour* [4]
is often belched up by a healthy Man, upon
stooping when his Stomach is empty in a
Morning? And from whence they proceed?
Whether there are more Causes than one, and
what, to excite *Hunger* [5]? Why the Stomach
is frequently *tumified* [6] in digesting the Aliment? And why at times there is occasion'd a
Difficulty of Breathing, Flushings of the Face,
and Laziness of the Body? Why the *Omentum* [7] is connected to that Part of the Stomach,
which, upon its Distention, is elevated and
applied to the *Peritonæum?* Of what Service
is the large Quantity of Fat which adheres to
the umbilical Vein, incumbent upon the Stomach? And how will the manifold Action of

the

the Stomach is intelligible, by confidering how far it is concern'd as a Veffel to receive and retain the Food, afterwards by mixing the feveral Fluids which pafs into the Stomach, and, by acting upon the Air, and then, as it performs the Office of a hollow Mufcle, and a Veffel in *Balneo*; and laftly, as it communicates and receives the Concuffions or Agitations of the adjacent Parts.

⒈ The generality of Phyficians after *Galen*, have attributed the Digeftion of the Aliment in the Stomach only to Heat, comparing that Organ to a Pot, heated (inftead of a Fire) by the Heat of the Heart, Liver, and Spleen; but thofe Notions have been well refuted long ago by *Helmont*, efpecially by his firft Argument, that the Blood of the moft voracious Fifh is very little warmer than the Water itfelf, in which they live: But Fifh digeft their Food in a different manner from Men, for their Aliment ftays a long time in their Stomach, and diffolves very flowly; they have alfo a very large Quantity of Bile; and in general, the more Fifh breathe, the lefs Bile they have; befides, fmall Fifh devour'd by other voracious ones, are the more readily digefted, as they naturally putrify and diffolve into a *Mucus*; nor was the Food ever obferv'd to be digefted into Chyle barely by Heat, becaufe that is very ftrong in Fevers, in which the lighteft Aliment is fcarce digeftible; not to mention many other Arguments which might be drawn from the Nature of the Thing itfelf.

⒉ This is a falfe Notion of *Helmont*, which was receiv'd by *Sylvius*, and the generality of the *Chemico-Cartefian* Sex; to wit, that the Digeftion of the Aliment is performed by the Power of an acid Ferment;

Ferment; which Acid is of a very different Nature from any chemical or vegetable Acid, being peculiar to the human Body only: And that by the Action of this Ferment the Food is turned to Chyle, and receives the vital Impreffion from the Soul, which was imagined to refide in the Stomach; alfo that this Acid was convey'd from the Spleen to the Stomach by the *Vas breve.* Thus, for Example, fay they, Gold is not diffolved by any acid Spirit, but the Spirit of common Salt only; which however will not diffolve Silver, &c. But the Arguments to confute this Notion are almoft infinite; the *Vafa brevia* are Veins which convey Blood from the Stomach to the Splenic Vein, but return nothing from the Spleen to the Stomach; befides, the Blood is far from poffeffing any Acid, its Salts are of the neutral or ammoniacal Kind, and all the Juices feparated from the Blood, except Milk, afford a volatile alcaline Salt only; alfo a perfect Fermentation was never yet obferved in the Stomach. The Falcon, Eagle, Wolf, and other voracious Animals, are replenifh'd more with an alcaline than an acid Juice. And I myfelf have obferv'd a diffolved Fifh fwimming in a kind of alcaline, fœtid, and mucous Pickle in the Stomach of a Dog-fifh. The *Caffowar*, a Bird more voracious than the *Oftrich*, is found to have no Acid in its Stomach, but a muriatic Liquor; and Men who are never troubled with any acid Belchings, have a ftronger Appetite and better Digeftion than others. Upon opening the Stomachs of Animals who have fafted two Days, the Liquor found therein is mucous, faline, fharp, and bitter, being compofed of the *Saliva*, Bile, and pancreatic Juice; alfo in hungry Men in Health, there is a Liquor often regurgitated, not acid, but falt and bitter, which occafioned *Celfus* to fay that Bile is increafed by fafting.

Acids

; Acids are not fo pernicious to the human Body as many of the Moderns have imagined, and their Acrimony is quickly overcome by the Addition of any alcaline Salt. Thus *Homberg* demonftrates, that five Ounces of the ftrongeft Vinegar does not contain more than three Drams of acid Salt; for by faturating that Quantity with an Ounce of Salt of Tartar, the neutral Salt produced from them both, weighed only an Ounce and three Drams, the reft being fimple Water: Yet Acids affift the Appetite fo far, as they deftroy any alcaline Rancidity which might pall the Stomach; but if a Lofs of Appetite proceeds from a Weaknefs of the Bile, then Acids are hurtful, and Alcalies ufeful, particularly the *Sal. Vol. oleof.* of *Sylvius*, Tincture of Myrrh, Extract of Wormwood, and the like, *&c.* But if Vifcidity is the Caufe, then all Kinds of Salts promote the Appetite and Digeftion, whether they be acid, alcaline, or medial; therefore Acids will not always reftore the Appetite; nor can an acid Ferment be demonftrated from an Acid having fometimes that effect.

4 In a Man that has fafted longer than ufual, after rifing out of Bed in a Morning a bitter yellowifh Juice will rife into his Mouth, if he fupp'd upon Flefh or fat Meat; but an Acid, if he made his Supper upon Milk or vegetable Food; which mucous Liquor will alfo rife into his Mouth more eafily upon ftooping, and removing the Refiftance from the perpendicular Weight of the Fluid; the Bitternefs of it proceeds from the Bile, which *Celfus* has long before obferved to come into the Stomachs of fafting People. The fame alfo happens in Brutes, from a Mixture of the Bile, Juices of the Stomach and *Pancreas*, together with the Relicks of the Food retained in the Stomach, which are expelled upward by the Preffure of the abdominal Mufcles, whenever the

.Mouth

Mouth of the *Oesophagus* is more open than the *Pylorus*, or when the latter is closed or contracted.

' The Sensation which we call Hunger is somewhat surprising; it is not the same as Pain, and yet it gives equal Uneasiness, being sometimes so violent as to compel Mothers to kill and eat their own Children for Food. This uneasy Sensation was wisely bestow'd by the bountiful Creator upon Mortals, to inform them of the great Danger and Injuries which the Body would undergo, particularly the Fluids of it, by continual motion, which would quickly become acrimonious and alcaline, so as to destroy the whole, if they were not frequently renewed and diluted with fresh Chyle. It is also another Providence of the Creator, that we have not an Appetite for Food in Diseases, when the Powers of Digestion are too weak to operate upon the Aliment. Another considerable Use of Hunger, is, for restoring the Consumption of the Fluids, made by the *Santorian* Perspiration, and other Excretions; these are the Ends for which we have an Appetite to Food: but the Causes thereof are various; as first, the perpetual Attrition of one Part of the empty Stomach against the other; whence the nervous *Papillæ*, plentifully dispersed thro' its *Rugæ*, receive an uneasy Sensation. Secondly, the sharp Quality of the Liquors which pass into the Stomach, such as the *Saliva*, *Succus gastricus*, and sometimes the Bile and pancreatic Juice, by their retrograde Passage into the Stomach. Thirdly, the Relicks of the last Meal retained in the Stomach, and degenerating into an acrimonious Ferment; for the Stomach is never entirely emptied (*per* § 83.) some Part of the Aliment will therefore remain in the Interstices of its *Rugæ*, and vellicate its nervous *Papillæ*. Hunger is removed, 1. By filling the Stomach with

new

new Food, which is the Intention of Nature. 2.
By diluting and difcharging the acrimonious Fluid
and Relicks in the Stomach by warm, watery, and
oily Liquors. 3. By violent Paffions of the Mind
and Frights. If you fhould convey one Grain of
a rotten Egg into the Stomach of an hungry Perfon, his Appetite will be gone in a Moment, and
a Vomiting will follow, whereby what was offenfive to the Stomach, will be rejected from it.

⁶ This Tumefaction of the Stomach proceeds
from the Fermentation or Putrifaction, whereby
the Particles of Air included in the Aliment are
fet at liberty, and reftored to their Elafticity.

⁷ The *Omentum* is thus connected to the Stomach, that it might interpofe between that and the
Peritonæum, left the diftended Stomach fhould be
injured by the Preffure or Refiftance of the *Abdomen*, which is by this means commodioufly prevented by the Softnefs of that fat Body.

§. 89. When the Stomach is almoft empty,
it contracts, grows flaccid and wrinkled, retaining only the groffer Parts of the Aliment,
which at length are alfo expelled by the Force
of the *Diaphragm* in Refpiration, while the
Pylorus is relaxed; yet the Stomach is feldom
entirely emptied, fo far as not to retain fome
Part of the Aliment, and not be capable of receiving more, without Diftention.

The Remainder of the Aliment frequently ftays
a long time in the Stomach; the grofs Parts of the
Food were found in the Stomach of a Hog after
they had been eat three Days; this is occafioned
much by the narrow Orifice of the *Pylorus*, which
is hardly wider than a Goofe quill; therefore many

ny Diforders of the Stomach may be remedied barely by fafting twenty-four Hours, efpecially if a large Quantity of warm Emulfion or falt Water be drank afterwards, whereby the Stomach and Bowels will be cleanfed.

Concerning the Action of the Intestines on the Aliment.

THE Inteftines perform more exactly the Attenuation of the Aliment, which was before begun in the Stomach; the fmall Inteftines only form and feparate the Chyle from its excrementitious Part, while the large Inteftines receive, change and difcharge the grofs excrementitious Part of the Aliment, for the Chyle is never found in the large Inteftines, naturally, nor the fetid Excrement in any of the fmall ones. In examining the Action of the Inteftines upon the Aliment and Fæces, we are to confider them, 1. As a Canal, receiving and retaining the Food. 2. As a fecretory Organ, conveying various Fluids, to be mixed with the Aliment in them. 3. As a hollow Mufcle, agitating and compreffing the Food. And laftly, 4. We are to confider the Alterations fuffered by the Chyle in the Inteftines from the Actions of the adjacent Parts; to which we may add, the Alteration made in them by the Bile and pancreatic Juice.

§. 90. To underftand what happens to the Chyle of the Stomach, and its Fæces, in the Inteftines, we ought firft to confider the Structure of that membranous Tube, the feveral

Juices

Juices conveyed into it, the abforbing Veffels,
which convey the Chyle from it, with its own
vermicular Motion, and that received from the
Preffure of the circumjacent Parts.

§. 91. The firft and internal Coat of the
fmall Inteftines, which immediately embraces
the Chyle, is villous, rough, and full of *Papillæ*[1], of *a grey or afh Colour* [2], perforated
with many fmall *Tubes* [3], difcharging an aqueous and a vifcid Liquor into them; it is alfo
perforated by the Mouths of the lacteal Veffels,
and fome *large Pores* [4], diftinct from all its
others; it is three times as long as the nervous
Coat, by which it is invefted, efpecially in the
Inteftine called *Jejunum* [5], where rifing up in
Duplicatures, it forms Valves, and is full of
Wrinkles, efpecially where it is connected to
the Mefentery; the external or convex Surface
of this Coat is full of fmall Glands, Veffels,
and Nerves. By this Structure of the inner-
moft inteftinal Coat, the Chyle and *Fæces* are
retarded [6], and continually intercepted in their
Paffage, its internal Cavity is *lubricated* [7], and
defended, and the groffer Parts of the Chyle
conftantly diluted; where the fecal Part of the
Chyle becomes more infpiffated and hardened,
it is there moft lubricated, efpecially towards
the End of the *Ilium* [8], where the exquifite
Senfation [9] of the lacteal Orifices makes their
Sphincters *contract* [10], and exclude fuch *acrimonious* [11] Parts as would be injurious to the
Blood, Lymph, and internal Parts of the
Body; by which Irritation the Inteftines are
alfo

alfo excited to contract and drive forward their Contents.

¹ If a frefh Stomach or Inteftine be turned infide out, fo as to render the villous Coat confpicuous, by wafhing it and fufpending it in warm Water, the whole Surface of that Coat appears befet with *Papillæ* fticking out; thefe in the Preparations given me by *Ruyfch*, are fome of them of an Afh-colour, others red, whitifh, or nervous, and appear like a Rug: between the *Villi* of this Coat terminate the fmall Arteries, Veins, Nerves, and lacteal Veffels.

² They are indeed of a cineritious Colour in a healthy State, but in Inflammations and Injections of the Veffels, which is a kind of artificial Inflammation, they appear red.

³ Thro' which the ultimate fmall Branches of the Arteries difcharge their Liquor into the Cavity of the Inteftines, where their Openings are fo numerous, that there is hardly any vifible Point which does not contain fome of thofe Pores and Openings of the excretory Ducts.

⁴ Thefe were difcovered about 40 Years ago by *Ruyfch*, while he was wafhing an human Inteftine, which he before had injected in warm Water, at which time he perceived remarkable large Pores in the villous Coat of the Inteftines, which had till that time lain concealed from him. From a ftrict and repeated Examination of thefe Pores by myfelf in the Preparations of *Ruyfch*, they appear to be Follicles or Cells, into which the Arteries depofit their falival Juice, which by ftagnating there, becomes more vifcid, till it is at laft expreffed, for the Ufe of the Inteftine or Aliment, by their vermicular Motion and Preffure. The whole internal Surface of the Inteftines is conftant-

ly

ly moiſtened by this Liquor, and if it be wiped off, it is quickly renewed again, either of itſelf, or by a gentle Preſſure.

ʼ The internal Coat, above the Inſertion of the *Duĉtus communis Cholidocus*, is almoſt three times as long as the nervous Coat; below the Inſertion of that Duĉt it is ſix times as long; and in the *Jejunum*, according to *Feldman*, it is nine or ten times longer, eſpecially when the nervous Coat is contraĉted by the Cold and its Elaſticity; but the villous Coat being conſtantly flaccid, and ſo much longer than the nervous, is by the Aĉtion of that Coat drawn into Wrinkles; which are the larger, as the Inteſtines are leſs diſtended; but when ſtretch'd with Wind, they diſappear: at the End of the *Jejunum* theſe *Rugæ* grow leſs, and the villous Coat alſo becomes thinner; but the *Rugæ* are largeſt on that ſide conneĉted to the Meſentery, being formed into larger Pleats, by the Smallneſs of the Curvature there, and ſtronger Contraĉtion: theſe *Rugæ* are not circular, but make up about a quarter, or a third Part of a Circle, the remaining Part of the Circle being ſupplied by other *Rugæ* at ſome diſtance; by which means the Cavity of the Inteſtine is divided into as many ſmall Cells as there are *Rugæ*, or *Valvulæ conniventes*, thro' each of which the Chyle is ſucceſſively tranſmitted. In this Coat are ſituated mucous Drains or glandular Cells, which more properly belong to the nervous Coat.

ꞌ The Aliment being intercepted by the *Rugæ*, or Valves of the Inteſtines, is agitated, attenuated, and retarded in its Progreſs, that it might not paſs thro' the Body before it is ſufficiently drained by the Mouths of the Laĉteals. If it were not for the *Rugæ*, the Aliment would run thro' the Body with little or no Alteration, producing a *Lientery*,

tery. It is by the Efficacy of the Valves, that 5 Quarts of *Spaw*-water being drank in a Morning, do not difcharge any Part by Stool; but being entirely abforbed by the Veffels, return into the Blood, and pafs off by Urine. I knew a Gentleman who drank feven Pints and a half every Day, and yet he had fcarce a Stool in a Week; from whence it appears, that the Inteftines of a healthy Perfon are contracted, and more readily tranfmit their contained Juices into the Blood by the Veins, than difcharge them by Stool.

⁷ The vermicular Motion of the Inteftines never ceafes whilft there is any Life remaining in the Body; and even when they are taken out of the *Abdomen* after Death, they have been obferved to creep or move upon a Table; the fenfible *Papillæ* in their villous Coat are therefore conftantly rubb'd againft each other; and if they were not defended by the *Mucus* difcharged from the *Cryptæ* and fmall Glands, it would produce an intolerable painful or uneafy Senfation. Therefore provident Nature has carefully furnifhed the whole Surface of the Inteftines with a *Mucus,* which tranfudes thro' every Point of their internal Coat, that the nervous *Papillæ,* and other Parts, might not fuffer too ftrong an Attrition from the groffer Parts of the Aliment. Nature has wifely placed the fmall Glands, for the Separation of this *Mucus,* under the mufcular Coat of the Inteftines, by which Mechanifm their Contents are expreffed when moft wanted, by their periftaltic Motion; upon the Ceffation of which they are again filled; but when this *Mucus* is injudicioufly abraded, by the unfkilful Exhibition of a violent Medicine, a Dyfentery is produced, and the Roughnefs of the Aliment gives intolerable Pain, frequently followed with an Inflammation or Mortification.

The

⁸ The moſt fluid, Part of the Aliment, which paſſes out of the Stomach into the Inteſtines, is quickly drained off by the Lacteals in the *Ileum*, by which means it would become ſo indurated, as not to paſs eaſily thro' them, if it were not for a Juice which perpetually diſtils into them from the exhaling Arteries; which diluting and mixing with the Chyle, renders it more fluid, moveable, and capable of tranſmitting its moſt ſubtil Parts into the bibulous Lacteals. Theſe exhaling Arteries are principally ſeated in the firſt Part of the ſmall Inteſtines; but where they terminate, the ſmall Glands of *Pyerus* become gradually more nume-rous; from both which is afforded a thin *Mucus*, to dilute the Chyle and lubricate the Inteſtines. In the large Inteſtines theſe mucous Glands are alſo very remarkable, affording a much thicker *Mucus*, for the Lubrication and Defence of their villous Coat; and that the Quantity of Juice tranſ-mitted by them into the Inteſtines is very conſide-rable, may be concluded from the Quantity of Water which paſſes by Injection thro' the meſen-teric Artery into the Inteſtines in a ſhort time, and from its being the moſt extenſive ſecretory Organ of the whole human Body; as alſo from the large and ſurpriſing Quantity of Water evacuated by the ſame Organ in Diarrhæa's, and by Virtue of ca-thartic Medicines.

⁹ The exquiſite Senſibility of this Part proceeds from the great Number of nervous *Papillæ* diſper-ſed thro' it, upon which account People are quick-ly carried off by Inflammations and Excoriations of the Inteſtines; and when attended with the moſt acute Pain, will kill the ſtrongeſt Man in the ſhort Space of an Hour. To this Structure is alſo owing the great Senſibility of the Stomach and Inteſtines, whereby they are enabled to diſtinguiſh

pernicious

pernicious and poifonous Subftances from good Aliment, the firft ufually producing violent Convulfions and Irritations, whereby they are ejected upwards and downwards.

10 The Acrimony which the Fæces contract within the Space of twenty-four Hours is fo great, as to excite the Parts to an Expulfion of them, notwithftanding the greateft Reftraint of the Mind to the contrary.

11 Every Part of the human Body is fo wifely contrived by the great Architect, that the fmall abforbing Offices and Sphincters of the lacteal and other Veffels, contract their Openings upon the Approach of any acrimonious Subftance; fo that they will not admit any offenfive or fharp Liquor. The Skin upon the Approach of cold Air is contracted into innumerable little Tubercles, like the Skin of a Goofe, whereby the perfpirable Matter is obftructed thro' a Contraction of the exhaling Orifices. The Bladder for Urine is furprifingly contracted upon the Contact of an acid Spirit, or the Point of a Needle; but the fame contractile Power was more neceffary to no Part of the Body than the Inteftines; for without that they would give a free Admiffion to noxious Particles into the Blood, whereby the whole Body would be infected, and its Fluids corrupted; but to prevent that, we learn from the Experiments of *Wepfer* and *Pyerus*, that upon touching them with the Oil of Vitriol they contract like little Worms. From no more than a Defect or Abfence of the *Mucus* lubricating the Inteftines, the dry Feces will meet with fuch a difficult Paffage, as not to be capable of being difcharged, but the Inteftine is contracted; and occafions the Iliac Paffion. After taking of Arfenic, the Parts which are firft in contact with the Poifon, are violently contracted; and thence

the

the Air is retained forcibly in the Stomach, so as
to produce enormous Swelling and a Gangrene in
that Viscus.   It is by the same contractile Power,
exerted by the abforbing Veins, that the Arteries
diſcharge and pour forth their diluting Liquor into
various Cavities, Tears in the Eye, *Saliva* in the
Mouth, *Mucus* in the Inteſtines, and other Parts,
ſerving to defend the tender Fibres from the Action
of the Air, and foreign Bodies, alſo to moiſten
and keep them fit for motion.   If a Man ſhould
by Accident have taken a Quantity of *Scammony,*
his Inteſtines will quickly perceive the Acrimony
of that Reſin, which diſſolves the Blood into a
putrid Maſs with the same Force as *Mercury*; the
ſeveral Fibres therefore and ſmall Veſſels of the
Inteſtines will be ſtrongly contracted, diſcharging
a large Quantity of Juices to dilute the acrimonious Body, whereby it will be eaſily drove forward
and expell'd, as pernicious to the Body.   We barely relate theſe Appearances, without accounting for
their Cauſes by latent Properties.

§. 92. The preceding villous Coat is inveſted by a thinner vaſcular one, which encom-
paſſes the firſt *every where* [1], excepting the
Valves, this Coat being not valvular, but conſiſting of an Intertexture of innumerable ſmall
Arteries and Veins [2], which terminate partly
in ſoft and pulpy Penicilli, in the form of a
ſmall Bruſh *Pencil* [3], partly into the ſmall
Glands of *Pyerus* [4], and partly into the ſmall
excretory Ducts, diſperſed thro' the Cavity of
the Inteſtines; it is alſo furniſhed with *Veins* [5],
whoſe Extremities are either continued to the
preceding Arteries by Inoſculation, as a continual

nual Tube, or are ſpent in the ſmall Glands of
Pyerus, or elſe open, with ample bibulous
Orifices, into the villous or downy Subſtance
lining the Inteſtines; to theſe Veſſels is alſo
added a *nervous Intertexture* [6], to which the
Glands of *Pyerus* are connected near their
Roots, and are advantageouſly placed under
the muſcular Coat of the Inteſtines, to diſcharge their Mucus by Ducts opening thro' the
villous Lining; theſe Glands are but few in
Number in the two firſt of the ſmall Inteſtines,
but become larger, more numerous, and cluſter-
ed together towards the beginning of the larger
Inteſtines; their Office is therefore to dilute
the *Fæces,* lubricate and moiſten the internal
and ſenſible Fibres of the Inteſtines, defend
them from the Acrimony and Roughneſs of
the *Fæces,* and adminiſter a digeſtive *Heat* [7] to
their Contents.

[1] The ſecond Coat of the Inteſtines is not extended between the *Rugæ* of the firſt or internal Coat
of them, but is only extended over the ſame in an
equal Cylinder.

[2] The Inteſtines are ſo very full of ſmall Veſſels,
that, one would be perſuaded they were nothing
elſe, from inſpecting ſome Preparations of them given me by *Ruyſch*; one would take them to be nothing but Arteries, if they only were fully diſtended; and for nothing but Veins coming from the
Vena Porta, if they were injected by that Veſſel at
the Liver, or coming from the *Vena Cava,* if the
Injection was thrown in by that Veſſel; and by
theſe numerous Veſſels ſpent upon the villous Coat
is preſerved the Heat of the Inteſtines.

R   When

3 When a small Branch of an Artery, diftributed to the nervous Coat of the Inteftines, comes to terminate, it is fuddenly fubdivided into an infinite Number of other fmall Twigs, refembling the Hairs of a Brufh Pencil fticking out of a Quill. Thefe *Penicilli* terminate two ways, fome difcharging their Liquor into the Cavity of the Inteftines, others tranfmit their Liquor to the fmall Glands of *Pyerus*, which retain it till it becomes more infpiffated before it is difcharged.

4 Thefe are very fmall Cells, receiving a Humour from the Arteries, which is retain'd in the membranous Follicles till they are full, and then difcharged; the fmalleft of thefe Glands inveft the *Pylorus*, and grow gradually larger, and more aggregated, as they approach nearer the *Cæcum*; becaufe the Chyle is not acrimonious after it is juft paffed out of the Stomach, but becomes fo by its long ftay; and therefore *Pyerus* does not well conclude the Action of his Glands to be for diluting the Chyle, for they are more numerous where the Chyle is thickeft and more excrementitious.

5 There are feveral Sorts of Veins which abforb Liquors from the Cavity of the Inteftines. 1. Veins from the Mefentery. 2. From the *Cava*. 3. Lacteal Veins. 4. Lymphatic Veins. The Paffage of Water into the Cavity of the Inteftines, by injecting it at the mefenteric Artery or Vein, or at the *Vena Cava*, demonftrate the abforbing Faculty of thofe Veffels.

6 The Nerves of the Inteftines are very numerous; but for what End are they thus diftributed, it may be afk'd? Whether they do not convey Part of their Juice in the manner of Arteries with their correfponding Veins? And whether the *Refiduum* is not poured into the Cavity of the Inteftines in the Form of a Vapour? Both thefe feem probable,

ble, tho' they do not admit of Demonſtration.
This is certain, that moſt extreme and ſudden
Weakneſs is occaſion'd by Diarrhæa's. I have had
Patients from the *Indies* who have been miſerably
extenuated to mere Skeletons by ſerous Diar-
rhæa's.

⁷ Heat from the innumerable ſmall Veſſels which
encompaſs the Inteſtines, by the Action of which
Heat, being the ſame as (at §. 86. N. 2.) the Aliment continues to be further attenuated and digeſted to a much greater Degree, by the greater Extent of this Organ. The Inteſtines never grow
cold whilſt there is any Life in the Body ; and as
ſoon as ever they are cold after Death, their periſtaltic Motion ceaſes, and the Coats of the lacteal
Veſſels collapſe ; to this we may add that the Pulſations of the Arteries cauſe a perpetual Attrition of
the Chyle in the Inteſtines, different from that occaſioned by their periſtaltic Motion or their Heat.

§. 93. The preceding vaſcular Coat is inveſted by another *muſcular* one ¹, conſiſting on its
Inſide of thick and ſtrong annular Fibres, inſerted into the Edge of the *Meſentery* as into a
Tendon ² ; at which Part the Fibres receive
their Nerves; by theſe the whole Cavity of the
ſmall Inteſtines is, Part after Part, ſucceſſively
contracted, the Valves at the ſame time *riſing
upwards* ³ ; their Contents are alſo reciprocally
preſſed *upwards* ⁴ and downwards, againſt the
Side of the villous Coat, according to the Direction of the Inteſtines, by which means the
Chyle is ground together, more intimately
mixed, attenuated, and prevented from running into *Concretions* ⁵, at the ſame time deter-

ging

ging the Sides of the Inteftines. The convex or external Surface of this mufcular Coat is compofed of *longitudinal Fibres* [6], which run crofs the former, ferving to contract the Length of the Inteftines, whereby they are corrugated and ftraiten'd, especially on that Side annex'd to the *Mefentery*.

[1] A mufcular Expanfion or Membrane, which arifes from the *Pylorus*, and terminates at the end of the *Ilium*; the Action of which is, to fhorten the Length of the Inteftines by its longitudinal Fibres, and to contract their Diameter by its circular Fibres, whereby the Capacity of the Inteftines is fo far diminifhed, as to have no empty Space; the Action of this mufcular Coat is therefore ftronger than that of the Stomach, for that never applies the Sides of the Stomach clofe to each other, fo as to leave no Space in the fame. The Thicknefs of the mufcular Coat of the Inteftines is fo remarkable, that it caufes the Inteftines to creep like a Worm, even after they have been taken out of the Animal and laid upon a Table. The fame Motion is alfo performed in the fmall Inteftines of a living human Body by virtue of this Coat, which is quite different from the Motion of them, which frequently arifes from their being diftended with Wind, as is fometimes obferved in dead Bodies. In all living Diffections the Inteftines are conftantly obferved in a vermicular motion, being fucceffively contracted and relaxed, one Part after another; and that the Relaxation and Diftenfion of them proceeds from their contained Air and Aliment, but their Contraction from thefe mufcular Fibres. This periftaltic Motion of the Inteftines continues even a confiderable time after

the

the Death of an Animal; for upon opening Rabbits, which have been kill'd by breaking their
Necks, the Inteſtines continue to creep a long
while after they have been pull'd out and thrown
away. This Motion is demonſtrated to ſubſiſt in
the human Body for the Space of two whole Days
after Death, during which time the Chyle paſſes
by the lacteal Veſſels; the Effects therefore of this
Action muſt be very conſiderable from. ſo ſtrong
and laſting a Contraction, continued conſtantly
thro' ſo long a Tube as the Inteſtines.

 ² A Muſcle is a Subſtance compoſed of red moving Fibres, but a Tendon is a Continuation of
the ſame Fibres, which are neither red, nor yet
contract; the Fibres of the Inteſtines are therefore
muſcular, diſpoſed upon each other in ſeveral *Strata*, the outermoſt of which ſerves as an Integument
for the ſeveral included *Strata*; there is no neceſſity that theſe Fibres ſhould appear equally red with
thoſe of the larger Muſcles, for Redneſs is not a
characteriſtic Mark of a Muſcle, becauſe every
muſcular Fibre appears white and pellucid, like a
Snail's Horn, after the Blood has been waſhed out
with Water; but in the Muſcles of Inſects, even
in their natural State, there is no Appearance of
Redneſs, notwithſtanding their muſcular Motions
are performed with a greater Strength in proportion, than thoſe of the human Body, as *Rober-
vallius* has demonſtrated in his Treatiſe *de ſaltu
Pulicis*. Thoſe muſcular Fibres of the Inteſtines
which are annular, become tendonous towards the
Meſentery; which has been rightly obſerved by
Willis, and they afterwards are continued with the
Nerves, which are diſtributed to the Inteſtines thro'
the Meſentery; and every Muſcle is nothing more
than an Expanſion of ſmall Nerves.

The

³ The mufcular Coat of the Inteftines being contracted, and their whole Capacity by that means diminifhed, there muft neceffarily follow a Contraction of their more lax villous Coat into large Folds, which will ftill further diminifh and divide the internal Cavity of the Inteftines; and thus they are divided into as many Cells as there are projecting Valves, formed by the Corrugation of their internal Coat ; but when the Aliment endeavours to pafs from one Cell to another, it is retarded, preffed againft the bibulous Pores of the villous Subftance, and its moft fluid Part is by that means abforbed by the three Orders or Kinds of Veins ; and thus the Aliment will receive a fecond, third, and more than a hundred fucceffive Triturations, Dilutions, and Abforptions ; which will at leaft be repeated as often as there are Valves in Number. The whole inteftinal Tube is therefore not always open, but contracted in one Part, and relaxed in another ; in which repeated Actions the perfpirable Matter and mucous Liquor of *Pyerus* will be difcharged in larger Quantities into the Inteftines at the time of their Relaxation, and intimately mixed with the Aliment at the time of their Contraction ; and laftly, the oily Part of the Blood, which was received by the cellular Coat of the Inteftines during their Relaxation, is preffed out in the Contraction of their mufcular Coat, and lubricates every flefhy Fibre.

⁴ We are taught by the repeated Experiments of *Wepfer* and *Pyerus*, that the Inteftines are not only contracted downwards from the Stomach towards the *Anus*, but alfo in a contrary Direction from the *Anus* towards the *Oefophagus*, whereby the Aliment is drove back by this vermicular Contraction, affifted in its motion by the Preffure of the abdominal Mufcles ; thus the Aliment receives

a very

a very confiderable *Remora*, or Retenfion, Attrition, Divifion, and Mixation, by the repeated
Actions of this mufcular Coat of the Inteftines,
which not only continues during the whole Life
of the Animal, but even after Death, when the
Heart has ceafed to move for many Hours.

   ⁵ A Dram of Turpentine will fo ftick to the
Fingers and Hands of a Perfon, that it can fcarce
be wafh'd off; but when the fame is made into
Pills, it will not adhere to the Sides either of the
Stomach or Inteftines, and yet it will prefently
tranfmit many of its Particles into the Blood, and
pafs off by Urine : This extraordinary Effect proceeds partly from the continual Effufion of faponaceous and diluent Juices into the Inteftines, in conjunction with their periftaltic Motion, which prevent the leaft Particle of the Turpentine from ftay-
ing two Inftants in one Place ; but the exhaling
Arteries efpecially pour out a thih Liquor, by numerous fmall Ducts, into every Part of the Inteftines, which repels and wafhes off fuch vifcid Parts
of the Contents, as might otherwife adhere too
ftrongly to each other, and to the villous Coat of
the Inteftines ; fo that if the Inteftines fhould be
deftitute of this Defence, by an Excoriation, Inflammation, or Suppuration, the Patient muft inevitably perifh, as no Aliment would then be of
any Service to him. The Inteftines have even
been obferved to grow together from thofe Caufes,
and produce a furprizing and fatal Iliac Paffion ;
otherwife the Fæces are feldom obferv'd to adhere
to the Inteftines, notwithftanding they are fometimes form'd into fuch bituminous and hard Lumps,
beginning to ftick to the Sides of the *Rectum*, as
not to be capable of being difcharged without the
Affiftance of the Fingers, or fome other Means.
And even in the Heart, which performs fuch a

strong and perpetual Contraction, we frequently find that Polypusses are form'd by a Coagulation of the more viscid Parts of the Blood adhering to the Sides and other Parts of that Organ.

⁶ The Mechanism of these longitudinal Fibres is very particular, they being intermix'd with the circular Fibres interfecting them in various Directions, and that chiefly in the small Intestines. There is the same Reason for these Interfections, as for the tendonous Interfections in the Recti-muscles of the *Abdomen*, the *Complexi*, &c. i. e. that by the frequent Interposition of new Tendons, towards which each end of the Fibres are to contract, the Strength of the Muscles may by that means be increased; whereas if the Contraction was to be continued without Intermission through the whole Length of these Fibres, they would quickly be tired by a slight Action. We may also add, that by the Contraction of these longitudinal Fibres, the posterior Part of the Intestines is drawn closer towards their anterior Part; the Curvature of the Intestines is straitened by them, their internal *Rugæ* increased, and their Valves brought nearer to each other; they also assist the Action of the orbicular Fibres, in forming the Cells of the Intestines; but their Contraction is not performed at once thro' the whole Tract of the Intestines, but unequally, sometimes in one Part, and sometimes in another.

§. 94. The preceding muscular Coat is invested externally by the *cellular Membrane* ¹, lately discover'd by *Ruyfch*, being a Continuation of the adipose Membrane of the *Mefentery*, very serviceable to the muscular Fibres in their Action, by lubricating them with the contained Oil, and keeping them moveable upon

upon each other, being the Seat of many Diforders of the Inteſtines, and in lean People, ſo
thin, as to be hardly viſible; and this cellular
Coat is again inveſted externally by the outermoſt Integument, continued from the *Peritonæum*, which covers all the preceding, connects
the Inteſtines in their convoluted Order to the
Meſentery, and binds down their Veſſels.

ᴵ The elegant Structure of this Membrane de-
ſerves our particular Attention; in order to which
we are to obſerve, that the Meſentery proceeds
from a Reduplication of the *Peritonæum*, which
paſſing forwards from the *Vertebræ* of the Loins,
is reflected back again in the ſame Courſe, ſo as to
form two Plains, between the middle of which is
contained the Inteſtines; and further backward
from the Inteſtines are diſpoſed the Arteries, Veins,
Nerves, and lacteal Veſſels, paſſing between the
two *Laminæ* of the Meſentery, to and from the
Inteſtines. The ſmall Arteries and Veſſels, which
are ſpent upon the cellular Subſtance, depoſit an
oily Fluid, to be preſſed out again by lubricating
the Parts. This cellular Subſtance of the Meſentery forms a ſomewhat fibrous Body, together with
the contained Fat interpoſed between the two *Laminæ*. When the two *Laminæ* of the Meſentery
have both reach'd the Inteſtines, they depart from
each other, and embrace or encompaſs the Body
of the Inteſtines. This Structure may be eaſily demonſtrated in a dead Subject that is much emaciated, by making a ſmall Inciſion in the external
Membrane of the Meſentery, and inflating the ſame
with a Blow-pipe, whereupon the *Flatus* will paſs
by Preſſure between the two *Laminæ* of the Meſentery, and even round the Inteſtines, next to their
muſcular

muſcular Coat. And in great Part of the Inteſtines, the two Plates of the Meſentery are firmly
connected to their muſcular Coat, moſt ſtrongly
to that Part of them which is oppoſite to the Meſentery ; but in that Part where the Plates of the
deſcending Meſentery firſt apply themſelves to the
Inteſtines, there is little or no Coheſion between
the muſcular Coat of the Inteſtines and the *Laminæ*
of the Meſentery. Alſo in thoſe Parts where the
Veſſels of the Meſentery paſs into the muſcular
Coat of the Inteſtines, there the cellular Subſtance
of the Meſentery alſo inſinuates itſelf together with
the Arteries, and paſſes between their external Coat
from the *Peritonæum* and their Muſcular Coat; and
this is the cellular Coat of the Inteſtines which
Ruyſch diſcover'd by Inflation. In Oxen and fat
Animals it is the Receptacle for Fat, and is called
Adipoſa ; but in lean Animals, being compoſed
barely of the *Laminæ* and an Intertexture of Fibres,
it is denominated *Celluloſa*, being of the ſame Nature with the common Adipoſe, or cellular Membrane, which is diſtributed between all the Muſcles. In the Inteſtines indeed it is very thin, in
proportion to the thin muſcular Coat underneath ;
and it is alſo ſo thin in the Forehead, *Scrotum* and
Penis, that ſeveal Authors deny its Exiſtence there ;
which is yet demonſtrable in thoſe, partly by *Anafarca*'s, or hydropic Swellings, as alſo by emphy-
ſematous or windy Swellings, when the Cells of
the Membrane are diſtended by extravaſated Fluids.
The Uſe of this cellular Membrane is, to lubricate
the Veſſels with its oily Contents, keep them flexible
and fit for Motion, and to prevent the muſcular
Fibres from becoming dry, and growing to each
other, which they are very apt to do. If a Muſcle
is deſtitute of this Membrane, it adheres to the
adjacent Skin, or to its own looſe Integument, ſo as

not

not to be moveable; but if on the contrary this Membrane is too much diftended with Fat, the Mufcle then becomes weaken'd, relax'd, and unfit for Motion ; as is obfervable in Hogs which have been fatten'd for fix Months together, at which time if they were not to be kill'd, they would be fo ftuffed up with Fat, as to be incapable of breathing ; and by compreffing the Veffels, would intercept the Motion of the Blood and Life of the Animal. This Membrane is alfo the Seat of Tumours, mention'd in the Obfervations of *Bonnetus*, which frequently rife in the Inteftines themfelves, fo as to obftruct their Capacity. The fame cellular Membrane feems to be alfo infinuated between the infide of the mufcular Coat and the internal villous Coat of the Inteftines.

§. 95. The whole continued and *long* [1] Tube of the Inteftines beforemention'd, is connected to the complicated and wrinkled Edges of the much fhorter *Mefentery*, fo as to hang pendulous, in various Convolutions and Folds, in all manner of Directions; they are lubricated, warmed, mollified, and render'd fit for Motion by the adjacent Fat of the *Omentum* [2], which is incumbent on them, and infinuating between their Convolutions, emits oily and lubricating Vapours, prov'd by undeniable *Experiments* [3], and feparating them from the *Peritonæum*, prevents them from adhering to that Membrane and to each other, and defends them during the repeated Contractions and Preffure of the abdominal Mufcles; the Inteftines are alfo advantageoufly expofed to thofe Parts of the *Peritonæum*, which communicate the

the reciprocal Succuſions from the *ambient Parts* 4 : Their Contents in Health being always fluid and *diluted* 5, and growing gradually thicker as they arrive nearer their Exit; being alſo *conſtantly* 6 in ſucceſſive *Contractions* 7 and various Agitations by the periſtaltic Motion, which perpetually exiſts in a ſurpriſing manner in all healthy living Animals. The Inteſtines are therefore exquiſitely adapted to further, grind, *macerate* 8, *dilute* 9, *attenuate* 10, *volatilize* 11 and *ſeparate* 12 the Parts of our Aliment or Chyle, to *preſs* 13 the ſame into the Orifices of the Lacteals, and to *retard* 14 the Paſſage of thoſe Parts, which are yet crude, or half digeſted, till they are more perfectly diſſolved; and theſe Offices are in common to the whole Tract of the Inteſtines indifferently.

1 The Inteſtines are four or five times as long as the Perſons from whom they are taken, and yet they are folded together in ſo ſmall a Compaſs as the Meſentery, without any Diſtortion, or even Compreſſion of any one of the many thouſand ſmall Nerves and Blood-Veſſels which are ſpent upon them; thus ſurpriſingly are they connected by the Meſentery, which ſuſtains all the Inteſtines in their Convolutions. But the Inteſtines are ſhorter in the living Animal than they appear in a dead Subject.

2 The fat Body of the *Omentum* is a membranous Bag, compoſed of two *Laminæ*, between which paſs the adipoſe and epiploic Veſſels; it inveſts the Inteſtines down to the Navel, and inſinuates between their Convolutions, ſo as frequently

to

to adhere to them; it every where defends the Inteſtines from being injur'd by the Impulſe of hard Bodies, or by the tenſe *Peritonæum*, between which it is interpoſed; and by keeping them both lubricated, prevents the Inteſtines from adhering to the *Peritonæum*, or to each other; which is apparent from the Inteſtines growing to the *Peritonæum* when the *Omentum* has been cut out. There was a Madman at *Paris* who made many and dangerous Wounds in his *Abdomen*, of which notwithſtanding he recovered; and the following Year threw himſelf from the Top of a Church; upon opening him, his Inteſtines were found adhering to all the Parts of the *Peritonæum*, which had before been wounded by him. The Uſe of the *Omentum* in warming the *Abdomen* is very remarkable, in the Hiſtory which *Galen* gives us of a Swordſman which he ſaw, who had his *Omentum* cut off thro' a Wound of the *Abdomen*; after which that Part became always ſo cold, that he was obliged to defend it with warm Cloths. But the reaſon why the *Omentum* is not extended lower than the Navel, is becauſe there the Force of the abdominal Muſcles is very much diminiſhed, and ſo there is leſs danger of their adhering to the *Peritonæum*, and of being injur'd by Preſſure: but even below the Navel provident Nature has not been wanting, for in that Part the cellular Membrane of the *Peritonæum* is gradually more and more diſtended with Fat.

³ The oily Fluid contained in the Cells of the *Omentum*, is reſolved into a ſubtil Vapour by the conſtant Motion and Heat of the Parts, and become ſo volatiliz'd, as to paſs thro' its ſmall Pores and lubricate the Inteſtines. That the Oil of the *Omentum* does exhale thro' its Pores, is confirm'd by many Experiments: *Ruyſch* ſaw innumerable ſmall Orifices by a Microſcope in the *Omentum*,

after

after he had waſh'd off the Oil by a long Maceration; the Oil of the *Omentum* alſo paſſing thro'
theſe Pores, makes the Fingers of the Anatomiſt
feel greaſy upon handling the ſame in a dead Subject. To theſe we may add, that the Injection of
Ruyſch has made its way thro' the ſame Pores, by
which the oily Vapour exhales; and the ſame alſo
ſeems to be proved by the rancid Vapour which
appears upon opening the *Abdomen* of live Animals, as alſo from the ſudden Decreaſe of the Fat
in Animals which have been ſtuff'd or fed; which
if fatigued with ſudden and violent Exerciſe, become three times leaner than they were before; as
is experienced in Horſes, whoſe oily Cells, placed
between the two Membranes of the *Omentum*, are
diſcharg'd of their Contents; inſomuch that a real
Oil has been ſeen forced out of the *Omentum* by
ſudden and violent running, and retained in the
Cavity of the *Abdomen*, which has been the death
of many fine Horſes.

⁴By the Action of the ſeveral Muſcles of the *Abdomen*, the oblique aſcending and deſcending Muſcles, together with the Recti, Tranſverſe Muſcles
and the *Diaphragm*, do all alternately preſs upon and
agitate the Viſcera of the *Abdomen*.

⁵ This appears from Anatomy, whereby is demonſtrated, that no Part of the Chyle is found in-
craſſated in the ſmall Inteſtines, from the *Pylorus*
down to the *Cæcum*; at which Part it ſuddenly begins to put on a more firm Conſiſtence; and in the
Cæcum and Cells of the *Colon* it firſt begins to turn
fetid, and put on a ſolid and globular Figure.

⁶ It is a common Error to imagine that the Inteſtines are a Tube as thin as Paper, diſtended
with Air; but whoever has ſeen the Inteſtines of
a live Animal, or in a human Body ſlipping thro'
a Wound of the *Peritonæum*, will be certainly aſſu-
red

red that they are neither fo thin nor fo pellucid, but thick, narrow, and having very little Cavity, unlefs they fhould be diftended by *Flatus* or morbid Relaxation.

.⁷ The periftaltic Motion of the Inteftines is perpetual, and continues even after Death ; and when it then ceafes, it may be eafily renewed ; as the Heart itfelf may be excited to its Motion by forcing Wind thro' the thoracic Duct. Nor am I fenfible of any other reafon why we can recall a Patient to Life who is in a deep *Deliquium*, without any Pulfe, but by communicating new Motion to the Chyle in the Inteftines, whereby it is propelled by their vermicular Contraction into the thoracic Duct ; which being thus drove forwards, will alfo give the Blood a Tendence to the Heart, and recall it to its preftine Motions. But this periftaltic Motion begins at the *Oefophagus*, and terminates at the end of the *Ilium* ; the large Inteftines not being agitated in the fame manner, it gradually defcends from the *Pylorus* to the beginning of the *Cæcum* ; and fometimes afcends circularly from the *Colon* toward the *Pylorus*, being always performed in but one Part of the Inteftines at a time, and never continued at once thro' the whole Tract.

⁸ The very tough and flippery Skins of Animals, and many vegetable Fruits, are fo opened by Maceration only, that after parting with all their alimentary Juice, they are caft out dry in the Fæces.

⁹ The Quantity of diluent Liquor afforded by the Inteftines to the Chyle, may be eftimated from the great Extent of that Tube, from the great Number and Size of the mefenteric Arteries, which has been calculated by *Borelli* ; alfo from the Experiments of *Ruyfch*, whereby the ceraceous Injection

 action paffes thro' the excretory Ducts of the mefenteric Veffels into the Cavity of the Inteftines;
alfo from the Appearance of the Aliment, which
is found not much thicker at the end of the *Ilium*,
than it was in the Stomach, even after it has parted
with fo much of its lacteal Juice; which is a manifeft Argument that it is fupplied with a confiderable Quantity of new Juices, equal to what was
abforbed by the lacteal Veffels; for if it was not
equal, the Relicks of the Aliment would become
indurated in the fmall Inteftines; but this Juice
can only be transfufed into the Cavity of the Inteftines by the mefenteric Arteries.

10 Thus the Juices which are contained in the
fmall Veffels of Animals and Vegetables, are poured out of their broken Tubes, and abforbed by the
lacteal Veffels. *(Vid.* §. 87. N°. 7.) for Nature
now applies the fame Force to diffolve their Parts,
as fhe formerly did to unite them; yet the tough,
Skins and Membranes are not diffolved by the digeftive Powers of a living Animal, becaufe Nature was employed conftantly for four or more
Months together in framing them; but the digeftive Powers act upon them but a very fmall Space
of that Time in order to diffolve them.

11 The Particles of the Aliment are fo far attenuated, as to be capable of paffing the fmall Orifices of the Lacteals, and afcend thro' them and the
thoracic Duct into the Blood, without forming
Obftructions or running into Concretions. Bodies
are volatilized according to Mr. *Boyle*, either, 1.
by increafing their Surface fo far, that their Weight
cannot overcome the Refiftance of the Medium
in which they afcend. Thus a Wedge of Gold
may be extended into fuch an immenfe Surface, as
to fwim in Water, and very difficultly defcend
even in Air, notwithftanding that Metal exceeds

by

by its fpecific Gravity the Weight of all other Bodies; or, 2dly, by applying a volatile and very
moveable Subftance to one that is fixed; fo that
the lighter Subftance adhering to the heavier, carries it up with itfelf in a Sublimation. Thus Iron,
which is fo ponderous a Metal, is render'd fo volatile by mixing with *Sal Ammoniacum*, as to fub-
lime in the Form of Flowers. Both thefe Methods
are made ufe of by Nature to volatilize or attenuate the Chyle, whofe Particles are expanded by
Heat, and their Surfaces increafed by Dilution; and
the Liquor with which they are diluted being very
fubtil and moveable, elevates with itfelf the more
heavy and fixed Particles of the Aliment, and fo
makes them volalile. The Change this way
wrought in the Parts of the Aliment is fo great,
that an Ox or a Man that feeds only upon Vegetables, which contain an acid and fixed Salt, will
thence make Blood, whofe Salts are volatile, and
naturally turn into an Alkali. The volatile Nature of Animal Subftance is confirmed by a remarkable Argument of *Bernier*, when he relates
that the Carcafe of that vaft Animal the Elephant
turns all into Vapours in a few Days by the Heat
of the Weather at *Indoftan*, leaving nothing but a
dry Skeleton. And thus alfo the human Excrements which are thrown about the Streets at *Ma-
drid* in *Spain*, are in one Day dry'd by the Heat of
the Weather into an inodorous Powder, without
infecting the Air with any Putrifaction.

[11] There can by no means be made a better Separation of the more fubtil Parts of a foft pulpy
Subftance in an Emulfion, than by this Method of
continually pouring in frefh Supplies of new Juices
in a confiderable Quantity; but this Juice poured
into the Inteftines, is again ftrongly expreffed, feparated, poured into them afrefh, and then again

expreſſed and conveyed into the Blood : and this
Emulſion is more perfectly performed by the ſoft
Parts of the Aliment being admitted into the numerous Cells of the Inteſtines, in order one after
another, in each of which it is compreſſed, attenuated, and opened, meeting with a Reſiſtance in
every Part, except at thoſe Orifices which lead to
the Lacteals ; by which means is obtained a com-
pleat Separation of all the more fluid Parts in the
Chyle.　But this Emulſion of the Aliment is alſo
the more exact, by being performed in ſo long a
Tube as the Inteſtines, through which it is many
Hours in paſſing, whereby all the more fluid and
nutritious Parts of the Aliment are drained off the
more compleatly.　In like manner a Separation is
made of the more ſubtil and uſeful from the leſs
ſerviceable Parts of oily and farinaceous Seeds, by
pouring on a large Quantity of Water, then beating
them into a milky Emulſion, then decanting and
expreſſing the milky Liquor, and pouring on freſh
Water, repeating the Operation as before ; by
which means nothing will be left but the hard,
earthy, and inſoluble Parts of the Seeds.

¹³ The Orifices of theſe Veſſels being ſo ſmall
as to eſcape the Sight, even when armed with a
Microſcope, has occaſioned many to imagine that
the Paſſage of the Chyle thro' ſo ſmall Veſſels,
can be explained no other way than by Suction ;
which is ſtill further countenanc'd by the Inteſtines
taken out of a dead Subject, and ty'd at each end,
not tranſmitting any of the Air or Water with
which they were diſtended ; which ſeems to argue,
that there are no Pores in the Inteſtines capable of
receiving any Liquor ; but that is a Falacy ariſing
from the Loſs of the periſtaltic Motion, and the
Stricture of the abſorbing Orifices, which are now
empty and collapſed.　So thick a Fluid as Milk
would

would never pafs the Lacteals, if it were to fuffer
a free Paffage, without Refiftance or Preffure, thro'
the Tract of the Inteftines; but its Paffage is retarded, and moft fluid Parts expreffed, by the periftaltic Motion, as many times as the Chyle is fucceffively applied to frefh lacteal Orifices, through
which fome of the more fluid Parts find a ready
Admittance; for if a thin Tincture of Indigo Blue
be injected into the Inteftines of an Animal juft
kill'd, while they are yet warm and contracting,
and you affift it with a gentle Preffure, like what
the Chyle fuffers in the *Abdomen*, the Tincture will
then vifibly enter the Lacteals, and tinge them of
a blue Colour; which is proved by an Experiment
of the Royal Society, *Phil. Tranf. Abr. Vol. 3. p.* 101.
feq. Nor is it any Wonder that the Lacteals fhould
fo collapfe after Death, as to render their Orifices
invifible by any means, fince the excretory Ducts
of the mefenteric Veffels do the fame; for Wind
cannot be preffed thro' them into the Blood, notwithftanding they are fo large as to emit the ceraceous Injection thro' their Orifices into the Cavity
of the Inteftines.

¹⁴ In four Ounces of Bread eaten by a fafting or
hungry Perfon, there will always remain fome nutritious Parts, capable of being abforbed by the
Lacteals, even after it has been digefted in the Stomach, and drained in the Inteftines for a whole
Day and Night; it is therefore advantageoufly retarded for that Purpofe by the retrograde periftaltic Motion, with the numerous Valves, Convolutions, and great Length of the Inteftines, whereby
one Drachm of the fame Aliment is fucceffively
applied to, and drained at leaft above a hundred
times by frefh Orifices of the Lacteals, before it
arrives at the large Inteftines. This Artifice of
Nature's protracting the Inteftines to a confiderable

S 2 Length,

Length, is continued almoſt univerſally thro' all
Sorts of Animals, but with a ſurpriſing difference
in their particular Diſpoſitions, according to their
different Nature, and the Structure of their other
Parts. The Inteſtines of a Hare are ſhort, that
they might not obſtruct the Swiftneſs of that Creature; but then it has a large *Cœcum*, whoſe Cavity is ſo divided by a ſpiral Valve, that it performs
the Office of the longeſt Inteſtines, tho' commo-
diouſly wound up in ſo ſmall a Space. The voracious Dog or Wolf-fiſh has Inteſtines not above
a Foot long, but then their Cavity is lined internally with a beautiful ſpiral Valve, or Reduplication of their inner Coat, which retards the Aliment from a too quick Paſſage. The Range-deer
of *Lapland* has very long Inteſtines, but then they
are ſmall or narrow, to facilitate the running and
long faſting of that Animal.

§. 96. The *Duodenum* [1], or firſt of the ſmall
Inteſtines, has this in peculiar to itſelf, that it is
diſpoſed in a *ſtreight* [2] Direction, being alſo
narrow, and without Inequalities or Valves,
connected to the Back by a Proceſs of the *O-
mentum* [3], and but very looſely, if at all, to
the *Meſerœum*; it is perforated near the End
of its ſtreight Progreſs, for the Inſertion of the
common *Duct* [4] of the Bile, and for the pancreatic Duct of *Virſungius*, which latter opens
into the villous Coat by ſometimes a ſingle,
but frequently a *double* [5], Navel-like Aperture,
either ſeparate or joined cloſe together; therefore the Chyle paſſes quickly thro' this Inteſtine, ſliding by its Perforations with but little
Alteration, and parting with but little of its
                                                    lacteal

lacteal Juice; becaufe we are taught by the anatomical Diffection of it, that there are very few Lacteals opening into it, and that the retarding Valves are much more lefs both in Size and Number than thofe obferved in the following *Jejunum* and *Ilium.*

[1] The Inteftines were very early diftinguifhed by the Ancients into *Tenuia,* or fmall; and *Craffa,* or large; the *Tenuia* they again fub-divided into the *Duodenum, Jejunum,* and *Ileum.* But the Moderns afk, what neceffity there is for impofing diftinct Names on the fmall Inteftines, when they are but one continued Tube? An Anfwer is ready, that Nature has wifely difpofed that Tube differently in different Parts; and that it was a Piece of Induftry among the Ancients to obferve and diftinguifh that difference according to Nature.

[2] It is remarkable that this is the only Inteftine, with the beginning of the *Jejunum,* that is difpofed in nearly a ftrait Courfe; all the reft being furprifingly convoluted into various Turnings and Windings.

[3] The *Duodenum* is connected to the *Pancreas,* and the *Pancreas* is invefted by the pofterior *Lamen* of the *Omentum;* by this Communication the *Duodenum* is therefore connected to the *Omentum* and Loins, and to the Liver by the common Duct of the Bile; which Connection was the more neceffary, as it ufually is not attached to the Mefentery, the common Support of all the other Inteftines.

[4] Which is about the Size of a Goofe-quill, its Aperture being furnifhed with a fort of Caruncle or Valve, which admits the Bile from the Liver into the *Duodenum,* but prevents any thing from

returning again out of that Inteftine into the Duct, which has been fometimes found dilated to an incredible Size by calculous Concretions.

⁵ There are very few Inftances of the pancreatic or biliary Ducts opening into the upper Part of the *Duodenum*; but in fome of the rapacious Animals thofe Ducts are inferted by three diftinct Apertures; as in Fifh, Lions, Tygers, &c. but their Infertion is fo oblique, paffing a confiderable way between the Coat of the *Duodenum*, that they muft of neceffity be compreffed whenever that Inteftine is diftended with Aliment; for the *Ductus Choledochus* paffes firft a little way between the external and mufcular Coat of the *Duodenum*, it then paffes about an Inch further between its internal villous and mufcular Coat; which Mechanifm performs the Office of a Valve, that the Bile may find a ready Paffage out of the Duct into the Inteftine, but that nothing might return that way back again.

§. 97. It therefore appears from hence, that three different Fluids are received and mixed with the Chyle in the lower Part of the *Duodenum*, where it opens into the *Jejunum*¹, to wit, the hepatic and cyftic Bile, with the lymphatic Juice of the *Pancreas*. The *Jejunum* is continued from the lower Part of the *Duodenum*, from whence it arifes nearly in a *right Angle*², and proceeding backwards from it, occafions a Stoppage and Mixture of the Bile and pancreatic Juice with the Aliment.

¹ The *Duodenum* arifes from the *Pylorus*, and terminates at its Incurvation, immediately below the Infertion of the biliary Duct, where it begins

to be called the *Jejunum*, becaufe it is generally found empty, and is diftinguifhable from the other Inteftines by its large Number of Valves. The *Ilium* arifes from the preceding Inteftine, where its Valves become lefs numerous; and in this Inteftine the Contents of the Stomach are found thicker as they are nearer to the *Colon*.

² When a perpendicular Cylinder changes its Courfe, fo as to become parallel to the Horizon, it forms a right Angle, which is eafily demonftrated by Geometricians, and occafions a Check to the Motion of a Fluid paffing thro' fuch a Cylinder; as this Structure is therefore found at the end of the *Duodenum*, the Chyle, pancreatic Juice, and Bile, will be in fome meafure obftructed, and be more intimately mixed before they pafs over the firft Valve of the *Jejunum*. The Refiftance which the Contents of the *Duodenum* meet with in this Angle, is fo confiderable, that in Animals which have been ftarved to death, to render them more relifhing, I have feen the Stomach full of Bile; which not being able to overcome the Refiftance of this Angle at the *Jejunum*, did yet make its way thro' the lefs refifting *Pylorus*. The Ufe therefore of the *Duodenum* appears to be for mixing the Aliment with the Bile and pancreatic Juice, which is promoted by being check'd and retain'd fome time in its Progrefs by this Angle of the *Jejunum*; for it is certain that it cannot abforb much Chyle, becaufe it has few or no Lacteals; nor can it afford any confiderable Quantity of the inteftinal Juice, fince it is not connected, like the other Inteftines, to the Mefentery.

Concern-

Concerning the Nature and Action of the cyftic and hepatic Bile.

§. 98. THE Bile difcharged into the *Duo-denum* is of two Kinds, either cy-ftic or hepatick. The Cyftic Bile or that of the Gall-bladder, is thicker, darker colour'd, and *more bitter* ¹ than the Hepatic, which flows immediately from the Liver; the Cyftic does *not conftantly* ² run into the *Duodenum*, but only in a large Stream at fuch a time as it is forced out by a *Contraction of the mufcular Coat* 3 of its including Bladder, or by fome ex-ternal *Compreffure* 4. The *hepatic Bile* 5, which flows in a *continual Stream* 6 from the Liver into the *Duodenum*, barely from the expulfive Force of the vibrating Arteries, and of Refpi-ration, is much thinner, *lefs acrimonious* 7, and more pellucid than the preceding; with thefe the pancreatic Juice alfo flows almoft conti-nually into the fame Inteftine. Thefe three Juices being mixed together with the *Saliva* and *Mucus* of the Mouth, *Oefophagus*, Sto-mach and Inteftines, form a vifcid and *frothy Liquor* 8 in the Cavity of the *Duodenum*, which is oftentimes preffed back again into the empty Stomach.

¹ This is by much the moft bitter Juice of any which circulates in the Mafs of Blood, but it has a fort of balfamic Tafte joined with its Bitternefs, hardly imitable by any other Subftance, except the
Ear-

Ear-wax, and the Bitternefs of *Elecampane.* This Bile is more acrimonious and bitter, as the Animal is more voracious, and better in Health; as we find in the Sea-Wolf, and in the Land Animal of that Name; but when the Body is difordered the Bile is then made lefs bitter.

² Hence it is, that in Animals which have fafted a long time, the Gall-bladder is fo full and diftended with Bile, as to be almoft ready to burft. And I myfelf have fometimes found the Gall-bladder furprifingly diftended with a very bitter, yellow, and vifcid Bile in Swine, which have defignedly been made to faft for feveral Days; for as the Cyftic Duct arifes perpendicularly upward out of the Gall-bladder, the Bile cannot afcend out of it, unlefs it be prefs'd by a confiderable Force.

³ By the Contraction of the Fibres of the fecond Coat in the Gall-bladder, which according to *Ruyfch* are mufcular, and varioufly interwove in different Directions, fome of them running according to the Length of the Bladder, and others traverfing the former. Thefe Fibres being contracted by the Irritation of the Bile when become too acrimonious and abundant, occafions the Gall-bladder to difcharge its Contents.

⁴ When the Stomach is diftended, it preffes againft the Gall-bladder, the Neck of which is at that time inclined; alfo the Action of the *Diaphragm* affifts the Liver and Gall-bladder to difcharge their Bile, fo that it is wifely contrived for the Bile to be preffed moft plentifully into the Inteftines when it is moft wanted; that is, during the Digeftion of the Aliment in the Stomach; tho' it may alfo be forced out by other external Caufes, and barely by compreffing the right *Hypochondrium,* as appears from the bilious *Ructus* which follows. The Bile is alfo frequently difcharged fo plentifully

by

by Vomits, as to regurgitate in the Stomach; and Paffengers who are unaccuftomed to the Toffings and Air of the Sea, are commonly feiz'd with a convulfive Motion of the *Diaphragm* and Vomiting; in which they difcharge the Bile mix'd with the Juice of the Stomach and *Pancreas*, called by the Sailors Water-gall.

ˢ There have been fome Anatomifts who have imagined, that the Bile does not come from the Liver; but that the Bile, which they think is feparated in the Gall-bladder, is conveyed to the Liver, and there tranfmitted into the Blood; but they feem to have not fufficiently confidered the Nature of this *Vifcus*; for the Liver appears, from its Number of Blood-veffels, to be intended for no other Ufe, than a glandular Secretion of the Bile, the Gall-bladder itfelf being too fmall to afford fo large a Quantity of that Juice as is daily difcharged into the Inteftines. But the Bile is properly of two Kinds; that which comes immediately from the Liver, has a ready Paffage into the *Duodenum*; but the Paffage of that from the Gall-bladder is more difficult, on account of the perpendicular Afcent, and acute Angle of the cyftic Duct; upon paffing a Ligature about the hapatic Duct, a Tumour arifes between the Liver and Ligature; there is alfo a conftant Difcharge of Bile from the Liver, when the Gall-bladder has been broke or cut out; to which we might add other weighty Reafons, that perfuade us the Bile flows from the Liver into the *Duodenum*. If any one objects, that only the more bitter Juice of the Gall-bladder ought to be call'd Bile, he is at liberty to call it *Lympha hepatica*, or any other Name; and tho' it is true that the Bile may in fome Cafe regurgitate from the *Duodenum* thro' the common Duct to the Liver, it is yet to be doubted whether it paffes thro' the

Ductus

Ductus cyſticus into the Gall-bladder; tho' it does not ſeem poſſible, if we conſider the Reſiſtance caus'd by the acute Angle made between the cyſtic and hepatic Duct. Perhaps ſomebody may anſwer with *Bohnius*, that the hepatic Bile regurgitates into the Gall-bladder when its common Duct is obſtructed; but I think ſuch Obſtruction will alſo at the ſame time much prevent the Bile from paſſing out of the common Duct into that of the Gall-bladder; for the hepatic Duct being diſtended, will contract the Diameter of the Cyſtic, which, together with the Angle formed by them, will intercept the Bile from the *Ductus cyſticus.*

[6] *Revenhorſt* opened the *Abdomen* of a Dog, divided the *Duodenum*, and faſtned the *Ductus choledocus* to a Quill, which he inſerted into a Receiver, where the Bile continually poured in, but very dilute, and not much bitter; as it is alſo found in the Liver of a living Animal, or of one that has been lately killed, being very different from the Bile in the Gall-bladder, eſpecially in Swine, whoſe Liver and three biliary Ducts have a great Affinity to thoſe of the human Body. The Mildneſs of the hepatic Bile is very obſervable in eating the Livers of Fiſh, Fowl, and Quadrupeds, in all which that *Viſcus* is very pleaſant and palatable, whereas the leaſt Drop of the cyſtic Bile communicates a very ſtrong Bitterneſs thereto; the Quantity of hepatic Bile which is continually diſcharged, much exceeds that of the Gall-bladder; which will appear from conſidering, that the Liver is a much larger Gland than any other in the whole Body, a *Viſcus* conſiſting of more Veſſels, without Fat or Muſcles, and of ſo lax a Texture, that Water readily paſſes thro' the *Vena portæ* into the *Cava*; alſo from conſidering the great Force with which the Blood is impelled into the Liver by

the

the two mefenteric Arteries, and the cœliac Artery
arifing from the *Aorta*; but that it is alfo ftill
more confirmed by Experiment; for *Revenhorft* collected it at the Rate of three Drams, or half an
Ounce in two Hours, or fix Ounces in four and
twenty Hours, in a Dog; and therefore the Quantity of Bile feparated in the human Body, where
the Liver is fo much larger than that of the Dog,
muft greatly exceed the formentioned Quantity.

[7] It is fometimes fweetifh, but always watery,
and almoft pellucid, being tinged but of a very
pale Yellow; it is taken to be more bitter by Authors than it really is, becaufe they tafte the Mixture
of it which paffes thro' the common Duct joined
with the Cyftic-Bile; but the chief of its Bitternefs
proceeds from that of the Gall-bladder.

[8] This Liquor being retained in the Cavity of
the *Duodenum*, till it is almoft beginning to putrify,
by ftagnating in fo warm a Part, is fometimes by
the periftaltic Motion, or an external Preffure, protruded into the Capacity of the Stomach, caufing a
Bitternefs in the Mouth and *Fauces*, and is vomited
up under the Name of Bile.

§. 99. The cyftic Bile efpecially corrects
Acidities [1], prevents the Chyle from turning
Sowr, and impregnates it with its own Qualities; it is of a *Saponaceous* [2] and fcouring Nature, difpofing Oil to mix with Water; it diffolves and attenuates refinous, gummy, and
other tenacious Subftances, reducing them into
an uniform Mixture; it is neither *alcaline* [3]
nor *acid* [4]; but *confifts* [5] of faline, oily, and fpirituous Parts, diluted with Water, not *combu-
ftible* [6] till it has been firft dried, being the
moft acrimonious Humour of any *Circula-*
ting [7]

ting 7 in the whole Body, eaſily putrifying;
and when putrified, very penetrating and volatile, tranſuding thro' all Parts of the Body.
The Uſe of the Bile therefore, upon being
mixed with the Chyle and Fæces, is to attenuate and diſſolve the oily Parts, intimately
mix them 8 with the watery, to *cleanſe* 9 off
Viſcidities, and *ſtimulate* 10 the muſcular Fibres
of the Inteſtines to their periſtaltic Motion;
it alſo obtunds and corrects the ſaline and acrimonious Parts of the Chyle, *diſſolves* 11 ſuch as
were coagulated, and opens the lacteal *Paſſages* 12 for the Reception of the Chyle; it
excites the *Appetite* 13, and acts as a *Ferment* 14, in aſſimilating the crude or prepared
Aliment. It is ſometimes diſcharged in healthy Perſons, by inſerting its Duct at the Bottom of the Stomach, as it uſually does in the
Oſtrich 15, which is a moſt voracious Bird.
The Effects of the Bile here deſcribed are poſſeſſed in a much ſtronger Degree by that of the
Gall-bladder 16, than that of the *Liver* 17. But
what further relates to this Subject, will be
conſidered when we deſcribe the Liver.

1 There is no Subſtance in the human Body that
putrifies ſooner, or to a greater degree, than the Bile;
nor was that Juice ever found to turn acid; but
upon ſtanding ſome time in a warm place, it preſently turns rank and putrid of its own accord,
and ſmells intolerably; but after ſtanding a conſiderable time, it contracts the Smell of Amber-
greaſe. In ardent Fevers the Bile is extremely
acrimonious, and gives the Fæces a cadaverous
Smell. From this Juice it is that the aceſſent Aliments,

ments, upon which only many Animals feed, do not put off their acid Nature in the Stomach, but in the *Duodenum*, where they become faline or fweet; and hence it is, that in young Infants and gouty People, who live only upon Milk, the Fæces caft out of the Body are not acid, but bilious and yellow; and if the acid fhould be fometimes fo ftrong as to overcome the alcalefcent Property of the Bile, the Bile by that means is rendered inactive, and incapable of performing its Office, of attenuating and mixing the Parts of the Chyle in the Inteftines. In the Stomachs of Calves there are always found acid Contents, but not the leaft of any Acid in the Inteftines; it alfo appears from Experiments, that the Bile being mixed with Acids, is coagulated, precipitated, and varioufly changed in its Nature.

It appears to be faponaceous, by rendring oily Subftances mifcible with Water; fo that the firft may be wafhed off from thofe Parts to which they have adhered by mere Water; and fuch is the Nature of Soap, a Body compofed of Oil and alcaline Salt; by whofe Action Oils, terebinthinate Balfams, Gum-Refins, and other refinous Subftances, which repel Water, are fo reduced, as to be intimately mifcible with that Fluid. In the fame manner does the Gall of Oxen wafh out Spots of Greafe from Woollen Cloaths; and thus alfo new Wool, which being covered with the greafy Sweat of the Sheep, and rank Oil of the Comber, refufes to take the Colour of any Dye, is ufually prepared by fcouring in a Lye of Urine, but fucceeds much better in one of Gall; by which means it becomes bibulous, and fufceptible of the Colour. In like manner alfo raw Silk, as it comes from the Worm, varnifhed over with a ceraceous Subftance, wou'd never take any colour, if the gummy Subftance was not to be

firft

firſt ſcoured off by a *Lixivium* made of Water and
Gall. Paints, with the hard Gums of *Juniper* and
Lac, and other glutinous Bodies, become eaſily di-
luted wirh Water, ſo as to run freely thro' the Pen-
cil, when they have been firſt well ground with
Gall upon a Marble: Therefore a Defect in the
Quantity and Strength of the Bile, will leave the
Inteſtines plaiſtered with too much of their gluey
Mucus; but if it be too abundant or acrimonious,
as it ſometimes is in Fevers, the Inteſtines are there-
by denudated or excoriated.

3 It has been aſſerted by *Sylvius* after *Helmont*,
and by moſt of the *Dutch* Phyſicians after *Sylvius*,
that the Nature of the Bile comes neareſt to that of
a volatile alcaline Salt joined with a volatile Oil;
and that the *Chymus* of the Stomach being mixed
with its acid Ferment in that Organ, and afterwards impregnated with the acid Juice of the
Pancreas, does then paſs into a Fermentation with
the Bile; upon which follows a Precipitation of
the more earthy and feculent Parts, which deſcend
thro' the Inteſtines, while the more fluid Part of
the *Chymus*, being converted into a vital alcaline
Nature, is taken in by the Lacteals. But we can
ſee nothing by this whole Hypotheſis agreeable to
Nature; the healthy Bile of the human Body is
never alcaline, nor ſo much as ſmells urinous by
the Heat of a Bath; and if it has any Odour, it is
aromatic and grateful; nor does it effervefce with
Acids; except only Oil of Vitriol, which will even
cauſe an Ebullition with Water; but the Bile is
render'd turbid and coagulated ſeveral ways, according to the different Diſpoſition of Acids. And
if it were to be allowed true that the Bile effervefces
with Allum, which was objected to me by a profound Chemiſt, even that Obſervation is of no
Force againſt us; becauſe Allum is not really an

acid

acid Salt; nor does it cause an Ebullition with Acids, nor is the Origin of Bile from Fire, which is, the common Rise of all alcaline Salts; nor does it proceed from an alcaline Liquor, since the Blood from which it was separated is far from a lixivious Nature; nor has the Bile an alcaline Acrimony, for if it had, it would corrode and destroy the small Vessels where it passes; nor will it tinge that of Violets of a green Colour, as Alcalines do. We do not indeed deny that the Bile will turn into a very acrimonious Alcali barely by Putrification; but no rational Person will esteem a found and healthy Substance to be of the same Nature as it appears after Putrifaction and Corruption. This is certain, that the Bile does not afford any volatile Salt by the Heat of boiling Water, much less will it afford any by a Heat equal to that of the human Body; and by this Rule we ought to attribute the inebriating Faculty of Ale and Spirit of Wine to Barley, because they are prepared from that Grain, by its undergoing various Treatments and Alterations. And if you should say with some, that the Bile contains a latent Alcali, even that would not be true; for we are never sensible of an Alcali in any Body, but it must arise from Fire or Putrifaction.

⁴ The *Hippocratic* Sect of Physicians formerly maintained, even in this Unversity, that the Bile was acid, in Opposition to the preceding Hypothesis; but those seem to be still farther from the Truth, because the Bile can by no Artifice or Change whatever be render'd acid. If some object, that the green Stools of Infants smell sowre from the Mixture of Bile, they will even contradict Experience; for they afford an acid Smell, thro' a Defect in the Strength and Quantity of the Bile, or from the Aliments being turned acid by

their

their too long Stay in the Stomach before their
Mixture with the Bile ; for this Obfervation no
more demonftrates the Bile to be acid, than Oil of
Tartar *per deliquium* can be proved acid from its
compofing *Tartarus vitriolatus* with Oil of Vitriol,
a Salt which is more acid than alcaline.

⁵ Such is the Compofition of the Bile from a
chemical Analyfis. The Bile of an Ox's Gall-bladder being firft applied to a gentle Heat, exhales a
watery Lymph, almoft without Smell or Tafte,
which equals three Parts out of four of the whole ;
the Refiduum in the bottom of the Veffel being
a glutinous, fhining, and bitter Subftance, of a
yellowifh green Colour, which neither effervefces
with Acids nor Alcalies, and may be kept a long
time without putrifying ; this Subftance being diftilled in a Retort with a Heat of three hundred
Degrees, affords much Oil ; and by increafing the
Heat, a fmaller Quantity of a truly volatile Salt,
leaving much Earth in the bottom of the Retort ;
from 12 Ounces of Bile there comes off 9 of Water, 2 Ounces and a half of Oil, and a Dram or two
of Salt. Nearly the fame Proportion of fixed Salt
and Oil is obferved in the making of common Soap,
about one Ounce of Lixivium being added to three
of Oil ; which Ounce of Lixivium contains about
five Scruples of fixed Salt ; fo that the Proportion
of the Oil will be to the Salt as 1920 to 100. But
in the human Bile the Proportion of the Water to
the Oil is as 10 to 2 ; to the Salt as 72 to 1, or
fomething lefs ; it was neceffary there fhould be
more Water than other Principles in the Bile, that
it might form a fluid Soap, capable of being fpee-
dily mixed and diluted with watry Liquors ; and
this is the true Compofition of recent Bile ; but
when the Bile has been putrified, it affords a larger
Quantity of a ftronger volatile Salt ; which alfo

T   holds

holds true of all the other Parts of the human Body after they have been putrified.

⁶ Recent Bile extinguishes a red hot Coal; but after its aqueous Part has been evaporated, it takes Flame and burns; the Bile does not therefore act in the human Body as Sulphur, but as Soap, or an Oil dissolved in Water; but as for the oily and bitter Substance which is sometimes regurgitated from weak Stomachs, that is indeed inflammable, but it swims upon Water, and is very different from Bile, being the oily Part of the Aliment putrified in the Stomach.

⁷ There is no Humour in the Body except the Ear-wax, and the Urine, which has an Acrimony of the same nature with the Bile; all the other animal Juices are much less acrimonious; and those two are real Excrements, deposited in their proper Receptacles, and never returned again into the Blood.

⁸ The Bile is intimately mix'd with the Aliment, after it has been first diluted with the pancreatic Juice; which Mixture is promoted by their being retained and agitated in the warm *Duodenum*, in which Intestine the alimentary Mass appears an uniform and frothy Fluid, the Bile not being capable of exerting its Force upon the Aliment without an intimate Mixture. It dissolves fat Substances, and such things as curdle with Acids; nor could oily Substances be capable of passing the Lacteals, if they were not first attenuated by the Bile.

⁹ Some Men will rashly swallow resinous, oily, gluey, and terebinthinate Substances; which sometimes adhere to the *Duodenum*, and cause an incurable Iliac Passion; but there are very few, if any, Observations of that Disorder from this Cause, because the Bile scowrs off those glutinous Substances, and renders them miscible with Water; it atte-

nuates

nuates ſuch Parts as were concreted, and renders them ſo fluid as to paſs the Lacteals. The Efficacy of the Bile in this reſpect is well known to Painters, who uſe the Gall of an Ox diluted with Water, to attenuate their grumous or concreted Paints. At the ſame time that the Bile prevents the oily and viſcid Parts from ſtagnating, and adhering to the Sides of the Inteſtines, it alſo hinders them from turning rank and cauſtic ; which frequently would do to ſuch a degree in the Stomach and Inteſtines, if it was not for the Bile, as to endanger their Excoriation. It is by the Bile only that we are enabled to digeſt Butter, Oil, and fat Meat ; of which Subſtances we may eat more plentifully, as we have a larger Stock of Bile ; but a Perſon that has little or weak Bile, would be greatly injured by thoſe Subſtances ; and ſuch Subſtances are ſo far from generating Bile, that they obtund and deſtroy it.

¹⁰ The Bile being mixed with the Fæces of the Inteſtines, ſtimulates them to their periſtaltic Motion, by which they are caſt out of the Body ; and if it regurgitates into the Stomach, it there excites Hunger ; if it is obtunded or overpowered with Acids, it ceaſes to perform its Office ; whereupon Obſtructions enſue, the Inteſtines are clogg'd up, and the Perſon is coſtive, &c. If it abound in Strength and Quantity, or becomes putrid, it occaſions a Diarrhæa, or purging, like that produced by Myrrh and Aloes, which are pretty much of the ſame Nature with the Bile.

¹¹ The Milk which is taken into the Stomach of a Calf, quickly curdles, as well from the Ferment of the preceding Milk in the Stomach, as from the natural Diſpoſition of the Milk itſelf to that State ; the ſerous Part of it is then drained off, and the remainder becomes a thick Cheeſe, which is ſtill fur-

ther

ther drained in its Paſſage thro' the ſecond, third, and fourth Stomach of the ſame Creature, till at length nothing but a tough and Cheeſe-like Maſs is conveyed to the *Duodenum*, which is of ſuch a Nature, that it will almoſt turn into a horny Conſiſtence, as we ſee in the outſide of Cheeſes; but it is no ſooner arrived in the *Duodenum*, but the whole tenacious Maſs is fuſed by the Bile, and is diſcharged in a fluid Excrement by the *Anus*. An eminent Gentleman liv'd a long time upon nothing but Milk, in order to be cured of the Gout; ſometime afterwards he was troubled with an Oppreſſion at his Stomach, almoſt to death; after which he vomited large round Lumps of a cheeſy Subſtance. I have alſo obſerved the like Diſorder to ariſe from a Defect of the Bile, and have ordered in that Caſe a mixture of Bile, with *Venice* Soap, which has quickly removed the hard Coagulations. We generally find that thoſe gouty People who have a weak Bile are very coſtive, which may be remedied by Myrrh and Aloes, or other Subſtitutes for the Bile.

[12] By attenuating tenacious Subſtances, and exciting the periſtaltic Motion, it deterges the Sides of the Inteſtines, and ſets the Mouths of the Lacteals at open liberty.

[13] Nothing excites the Appetite more than Bitters; Myrrh, Aloes, Wormwood, Elecampane, *&c.* which ſupply the Weakneſs and Defect of the Bile. The Bile even ſeems to be one of the principal Cauſes of Hunger in a healthy Perſon. We find that when the Stomach is full we have no Senſation of Hunger, though it were filled only with Water; but as ſoon as it is empty, if we are in health, we grow hungry again; becauſe when the Stomach is empty it is flaccid, and does not reſiſt the Paſſage of the Bile into its Cavity; which by irritating its nervous *Papillæ*, excites the uneaſy

Senſation

Senſation of Hunger; which is confirmed by Inſtances of gluttonous Men and voracious Animals,
in which the *Duſtus choledocus* has been found to
open into the Capacity of the Stomach.

¹⁴ It cannot indeed be term'd a Ferment ſtrictly,
unleſs by that Name we intend a Body capable of
diſpoſing other Subſtances with which it is mix'd,
to turn into its own nature; for in that reſpect the
Bile may be ſo call'd; which is alſo confirm'd from
its being a Juice the moſt animal or elaborated of
any in the Body, it being ſeparated not from the
Arteries immediately, but from the Blood which
has paſſed thro' the Arteries, and undergone more
Actions than any other Part of the Blood throughout the Animal; for having paſſed the meſenteric Arteries and Veins, with thoſe of the Stomach,
Spleen, and *Omentum*, it returns by particular Veins
towards the Liver, and is then diſtributed thro'
that Organ by a new kind of Arteries, the *Vena
Portæ*; and then paſſes thro' the reductory Veins
of the Liver, after having depoſited its Bile in its
proper ſecretory Cells and excretory Ducts; the
Bile therefore is not an excrementitious Fluid, but
a principal Inſtrument in Digeſtion; for it no ſooner diminiſhes in Strength and Quantity, but it occaſions ſome chronical Diſeaſe, becauſe the Chyle
is not rightly prepared; whence Dropſy, Cachexy,
Leucophlegmatia, &c. for a Defect in the Digeſtion
of the firſt Paſſages cannot be repaired in the reſt.

¹⁵ *Duverney* has demonſtrated the biliary Duct
opening into the Stomach of the Oſtrich, which
is a gluttonous hungry Bird.

¹⁶ Which is all, or the greateſt part, formed of
the hepatic Bile; which cannot paſs into the Gall-
bladder, but when it meets with more Reſiſtance at
the *Duodenum* than it does at the opening of the
cyſtic Duct; but the hepatic Bile, when arriv'd in

T 3 the

the Gall-bladder, is rendered more acrimonious, bitter, thick, and higher colour'd, by ſtagnating in ſo warm and cloſe a Cell, and returning many of its aqueous Parts again into the Blood by the ſmall abſorbing Veins.

" The Quantity of which is much larger than that of the cyſtic Bile ; ſo that diluting a few Drops of the latter, it forms a penetrating Lixivium, to mix with the Aliment.

Concerning the Nature and Action of the pancreatic Juice.

§. 100. THE *Pancreas* [1] is a large *conglomerate* [2] Gland, ſituated under the bottom, a little behind, and on the right Side of the Stomach ; 'tis inveſted by the poſterior *Lamella* [3] of the *Omentum,* and lies incumbent on the *Duodenum :* it is *pendulous* [4], and continually ſeparates a ſalival Humour, by its glandular Structure, from the Blood of the cæliac Arteries, which diſtilling from their infinite Number of ſmall Branches, is conveyed at laſt in one common *Duct* [5], diſcharging the ſame in the *Duodenum* (§. 96.)

[1] This Gland is call'd *Pancreas* by the Ancients, as being all Fleſh, *i. e.* entirely eatable, without any Bones or Tendons ; or elſe from its being redder than the generality of the other Glands in the human Body. It might be very properly called the largeſt conglomerate ſalival Gland of the *Abdomen,* for it agrees exactly in its Structure, Figure,

Veſſels,

Veffels, excretory Duct, and in the Nature of its Lymph, with thofe of the falival Glands of *Wharton*, feated in the Head ; the Length of this Gland is about fix Inches, its Breadth two Inches, and its Weight about four Ounces.

² It is compofed of feveral fmaller Clufters of Glands, each of which are fub-divifible into ftill fmaller Bunches, from whence arife fmall Emiffaries, which opening into each other, at laft terminate in one Duct ; by which Duct the pancreatic Juice is difcharg'd more plentifully, as that Gland is compreffed between the *Diaphragm* and the Stomach diftended with Aliment.

³ In the human Body ; for in the fmalleft Animals it is loweft, and in Fifh it almoft fills the whole of the *Abdomen* ; its Situation in the human Body is well figur'd by *Vefalius,* after him *Afellius* found a Clufter of Glands near the *Receptaculum Chyli* in Brutes, which he denominated *Pancreas,* but very improperly, fince the Pancreas of the human Body does not come near the Mefentery ; hence it is that the Clufter of Glands in the Mefentery has been called by Anatomifts the *Pancreas Afellii,* to diftinguifh it from the true *Pancreas* of *Virfungius,* which is wrapt up in the pofterior *Lamen* of the *Omentum.*

⁴ The Situation of the *Pancreas* is juftly exhibited by *Vefalius*; and therefore *Euftathius,* who compofed his Tables to correct the Errors of *Vefalius,* has neglected the Situation of the *Pancreas,* and only given us a better Idea of its Figure, refembling that of a Horfe-fhoe ; but it is connected to the *Colon* and bottom of the Stomach, and is therefore preffed up and down at every Refpiration.

⁵ This Duct may be injected, fo as to fill its remoteft Branches, after it has been firft cleanfed by injecting Water. This Duct paffes between the

cellular Coat of the *Duodenum*, then perforates its muscular Coat, and opens into its Cavity; this Obliquity of its Insertion prevents any thing from returning to the *Pancreas* out of the Intestine; which has been a Case sometimes observed. *Wirsungius*, the Discoverer of this Duct, was enviously assassinated in the Evening of the same Day when he publickly demonstrated this beautiful Discovery; so that he could not prosecute the same any further; but the Subject was afterwards taken up by *Franciscus Sylvius*.

§. 101. The pancreatic Juice is limpid, and almost *insipid* [1], or a little saltish, constantly separated and discharged in *great plenty* [2] by the Motion, Pressure, and Warmth of the circulating Blood and Parts near the *Heart* [3], especially by the incumbent Stomach, when distended with Food. It is neither *acid* [4] nor *alcaline* [5], but nearly resembles the *Saliva* [6], as well with respect to its Origin, or the Vessels and Glands by which it is separated, as in its sensible Qualities. When the pancreatic Juice mixes with the Bile in the Intestines of a living Animal, it does not appear to make any Fermentation or *intestine Motion* [7], but joins smoothly and evenly with it: Hence it serves to mix with and dilute [8] the thick Parts of the Chyle, *Mucus*, Bile, and Fæces, to make an intimate and uniform Mixture of them all, and to render the Chyle fitter to pass the *Lacteals* [9], and mix with the Blood; to obtund or weaken the acrimonious Parts of the Chyle, and those of the *Bile* [10]; to abate the Viscidity and Bitterness of the last, alter its Colour,

and

and unite it more intimately to the Chyle: It may likewise ferve both as a Vehicle and a Menftruum, to alter or change the Tafte, Smell, and other Qualities of the various Aliments into one uniform *Nature* [11]; and to be frequently returned into the Blood, and feparated in the *Pancreas* again, *many times* [12] under the fame Form and for the fame Ufes.

[1] *Brunner* and *Swalve* have obferv'd the pancreatic Juice to be almoft infipid, in oppofition to the other Phyficians of that Day, and particularly *Sylvius* ; who, to favour his Hypothefis, fuppofed it to be acid ; but the Tafte of this Gland is fo mild and fweet, that the *Italians* prefer that with the *Thymus* to any other Part in the Calf, and call it *Bocca faporita,* or *the favoury Bit.* And if the pancreatic Juice ever taftes faltifh in the human Body, it is from the large Quantity of common Salt taken in with our Food, being often equal to half an Ounce in a Day, and is never changed into the Nature of Animal Salts by the Actions of the Body ; for common Salt is extracted out of Urine, after fix Years ftanding, as perfectly endued with all the Properties of Sea-falt, as when it firft enter'd the Body.

[2] It is fo plentifully difcharged into the *Duodenum,* that *de Graaf* and *Nuck* have gather'd it in a Dog at the Rate of from two or three Drams to an Ounce in an Hour, being therefore feparated at the rate of one, two, or three Ounces in four and twenty Hours in a Dog that weighed not above ten Pounds ; notwithftanding the Secretion muft be all that time greatly retarded by removing the compreffing Force of the abdominal Mufcles, by opening that Cavity, and from a Contraction of the Veffels

fels by the Cold, and a Diffipation of the mollifying Vapours which lubricate the *Vifcera* of the *Abdomen*, together with the Difturbance of the whole
Animal Oeconomy thro' the Tortures of the Animal. Therefore if the Weight of the human Body
be compared to that of a Dog, and if the *Pancreas*
be alfo compared with the other falival Glands,
being larger than all of them put together, (yet they
feparate twelve Ounces of *Saliva* in four and twenty
Hours;) if we alfo confider the conftant Agitation
of the *Pancreas* from the incumbent *Diaphragm* and
Refiftance of the Stomach, together with the Preffure of the abdominal Mufcles, while the falival
Glands, which lie immediately under the Skin, are
neither fo conftantly nor ftrongly preffed by the
weaker Mufcles, of Deglutition and Maftication ;
to thefe we may add, the Warmth of the Cavity
of the *Abdomen*, the large Diameter of its excretory Duct, with the Force of the adjacent Heart and
pancreatic Arteries: from a Confideration of all
thefe, it will appear that a larger Quantity of Fluid
is feparated by the *Pancreas*, than all the other falival Glands ; and that the Weight of the pancreatic Juice will not be much lefs than three Pound,
feparated in the Space of four and twenty Hours ;
but in Fifh and Infects the Proportion of the pancreatic Juice to the Aliment is ftill much larger,
fince this Gland is found bigger than the Liver in
many of the former.

³ From which it is feparated only by the *Diaphragm* and *Pericardium* ; to which we may alfo add
the Vibrations of the *Aorta* behind the *Pancreas*,
with the adjacent cœliac, mefenteric, and fplenic
Arteries.

⁴ It may feem furprifing that fo ingenious a Chemift as *Sylvius*, and many other Anatomifts, fhould
have fo boldly afferted the falfe Principle of the

pan-

pancreatic Juice being acid. They gave more way
to a prejudiced Notion and Hypothefis than to
Truth and ocular Demonftration. The chemical
Definition and diftinguifhing Marks of an Acid was
then extant, and perfectly known to *Sylvius*; but
among the many Properties of an Acid they cou'd
not fhew one in the pancreatic Juice; for firft, it
is not acid in a healthy Body, but by Mixture with
the half digefted Aliment, or fome morbid Indifpo-
fition, it may have fometimes appeared to contain
fome Particles of an Acid; nor cou'd *de Graaf* fo
far relinquifh the Truth, even under the Eye of his
Preceptor *Sylvius*, but that he confeffed the pancreatic Juice was often faline, fometimes infipid,
very often faltifh, and a little acid, and fometimes
only appearing entirely acid; but the Experiment
which he made in a Sailor, that he opened while
warm, and perceived an acid Tafte in the pancreatic Juice, feems to have been performed without
fufficient Accuracy, for that fome Part of the imperfectly digefted Chyle was mixed therewith. But
the Tafte of this Juice is always faltifh in the human Body; and in brute Animals, which do not
ufe common Salt, it is always infipid; which is
agreeable with *Brunnerus*, and Nature herfelf: It
is not however to be denied, but that the pancreatic Juice may be fometimes acid in thofe Diforders
which proceed from a Redundancy of acid Parts in
the Blood, thro' an Indigeftion of the Aliment;
but the pancreatic Juice was never found by Experiment to ferment with any alcaline Salt; for it is feparated from the Blood, which immediately before
was alcalefcent in the cœliac Artery, even according
to the Confeffion of *Sylvius*, who, together with
Helmont, acknowledges the Blood to be of an oily,
volative, and alcalefcent Nature; but for an Acid
to arife from an Alcali, is a Change that was never
yet

yet heard of in Chemiſtry, nor ever ſeen in any
Experiment whatever; it therefore ſeems incredible that ſuch great Alteration ſhou'd be made in
that Fluid in ſo ſmall a time in its Paſſage thro'
ſuch ſmall Veſſels as thoſe of the *Pancreas.* Some
will perhaps anſwer, that the pancreatic Juice is ſe-
cerned from the nervous Fluid, and that according
to *Sylvius,* that Fluid is of a ſubacid Nature; but
we ſee no reaſon why the nervous Fluid, whoſe
Subtilty eſcapes our Examination, ſhou'd be rather
eſteemed an Acid than any other Fluid in the Body;
nor does it ſeem probable that this ſubtle Fluid can
be ſeparated in a ſufficient Quantity to ſupply ſo
large a Diſcharge as that of the pancreatic Juice;
and laſtly, there will be the ſame Difficulty to conceive how the nervous Fluid, which is alſo ſeparated from the alcaleſcent Blood, ſhou'd poſſeſs any
thing of an acid Quality. The pancreatic Juice
does not tinge that of Violets of a red Colour, nor
curdle Milk, *&c.* If the whole *Pancreas,* together
with its Juice and Duct, be taken out and boiled
in Milk, it will upon keeping not turn ſowre, but
putrid. *Sylvius* indeed aſſerts, that there is a latent Acid in the pancreatic Juice, but does not
prove it; for ſuch an Acid, as is not of a ſufficient
Strength to diſcover itſelf by Appearances, cannot
be the Cauſe of ſo ſtrong an Efferveſcence as is aſ-
ſigned to it by *Sylvius;* nor does there appear any
other Reaſon why *Sylvius* ſhou'd aſſign the pancreatic Juice to be of an acid Nature, than to render it conformable to his Syſtem, which required
the Suppoſition of an Acid to cauſe a Fermentation
with the alcaleſcent Bile.

ˢ One might with more reaſon affirm the pancreatic Juice to be alcaline, agreeable with the An-
tagoniſts of *Sylvius;* but even that wou'd not be
ſtrictly true; for which conſult (§. 99. N° 3.)

The

‘ The pancreatic Juice is like the _Saliva_ in all Appearances, as well as agreeing in the Structure of its small secretory Glands, which are assembled into one conglomerate and larger Gland, discharging their Contents by their proper Ducts into one common larger and excretory Duct. It has been also frequently observed, that when _Mercury_ excites a Salivation in the Mouth, at the same time there is often felt Pains in the _Abdomen_ about the _Pancreas_, and a Diarrhæa follows in the room of a Salivation ; the only Difference between the _Pancreas_ and salival Glands seems to be, in that the first is subject to the smaller and alternate Motions of Respiration, and is therefore more strongly and constantly sollicited to its Office than the salival Glands.

⁷ The whole Doctrine of the Animal Oeconomy, Diseases, and Practice of Physic, embraced by _Sylvius_ and his Followers, were founded upon this single Hypothesis, an Effervescence of the alcaline Bile with the acid Juice of the _Pancreas_. This System was quickly opposed in a ridiculing Stile by _Carolus Drelincurtius_, a Collegue of _Sylvius_, and strict _Hippocratic_ or Observator, in opposition to Hypothesis, who conceal’d himself by the fictitious Name of _Ludovicus le Vasseur_, in a Libel _de Triumviratu Humorum_ ; in which he banters and sharply runs down this Effervescence : at the same time the Hypothesis was opposed by _Deusingius_ in a different Method, rather by Facts and Experiments, than scholastic Reasoning : these were again opposed in favour of the _Sylvian_ Hypothesis by _Florent. Schuyl_, Botanic Professor at _Leyden_ ; and in a Treatise _de Medicina veterum_, he proposes an Experiment for its Confirmation, _viz._ “ That the Effervescence of the Bile and pancreatic Juice in the “ living Animal ought not to be denied, because “ those

" thofe Juices do not appear to effervefce out of
" the Animal upon Mixture : but the Experiment
" is to be made in the living Animal ; therefore
" the Right *Hypochondrium* is to be opened in a
" living Dog, and a Ligature made on the *Duo-*
" *denum* about four Fingers breadth above the In-
" fertion of the biliary Duct, making another Li-
" gature on the Inteftine as many Fingers breadth
" below the Duct ; then return the *Duodenum* in-
" to the *Abdomen*, and let the Animal reft ; and
" upon opening him a few Hours after, the In-
" teftine betwixt the Ligatures will be found tenfe,
" diftended, and hot ; and upon making an In-
" cifion in it, there is difcharg'd a Froth and great
" Stench ; fo that it is thus manifeft by ocular
" Demonftration, that the Bile and pancreatic
" Juice do effervefce upo nmixing in the Animal."
The *Sylvian* Sect triumph'd in this Experiment;
fuppofing it fufficient to put an end to the Controverfy ; but they fhould have confidered, that
the fame Appearances would have been produced
by making the Ligatures in any other Part of the
Inteftine, below the Entrance of thofe Juices, from
the Inflammation that would thence arife, and from
the elaftic Air generated by the Fermentation of
the intercepted or ftagnant Chyle. Nor is there
the leaft Appearance of any Effervefcence upon
the Mixture of thefe two Juices in the living Animal without making Ligatures, but the Bile appears to mix and unite fmoothly and evenly, without any Commotion, with the pancreatic Juice;
upon opening the *Duodenum* in a living Animal :
And upon mixing the recent Bile and pancreatic
Juice taken from an Ox juft kill'd, I have often
feen by Experiment that they unite like Water
with Water, without the leaft Effervefcence ; to
which we may add, that thefe two Juices do not
effervefce

effervesce even in those Animals where the pancreatic and biliary Duct are inserted into each other; so that they have an immediate Contact and intimate Mixture; as in Man, and several other Animals, *viz.* the Fox, Cat, Sheep, Horse, Elephant, *&c.* Nor do those Animals suffer the least Inconveniency in digesting their Food, or in performing their natural and vital Functions, who have the pancreatic Duct inserted into the *Duodenum* at a very great distance from the biliary Duct; as they are distant from each other fifteen Inches in the Rabbit, twenty in the Hedge-hog, and even three Feet in the Ostrich.

[8] The pancreatic Juice is very thin, the Chyle of the Stomach is thicker, the Juice of the Intestines more viscid, and the cystic Bile thicker than them all (for that may be sometimes drawn out into Threads;) but as Soap does not act till it has been diluted with Water, so the Bile cannot exert its Efficacy till it has been first diluted with the pancreatic Juice; and this is the chief reason why the pancreatic Duct discharges its Contents into the *Duodenum* at the same Aperture, or very near, with the Duct of the Bile, in much the greater Part of Animals, And in rapacious Birds, which seldom or never drink, this Juice seems to perform the Office of that Liquor.

[9] By mixing with the Bile, it scowrs off the Glue of the Intestines, and dissolves the grosser Particles of the Aliment, so as to render them passable thro' the smaller Orifices of the Lacteals.

[10] It so dilutes the Bile, that notwithstanding it is mixed in so large a quantity with the Aliment, yet it leaves no Bitterness either in the Chyle or Fæces, nor even in the Contents of the *Ilium*; towards its lower end, notwithstanding, it tinges the Contents of the Intestines with a manifest yellow Colour,

Colour, for the hepatic Bile is naturally much thinner, and difcharged more plentifully than the cyftic Bile ; and then the cyftic Bile is diluted with the pancreatic Juice, in the fame manner as a large Quantity of Milk, obfcures a little Bitternefs of Wormwood, or the Acrimony of Mercury fublimate ; yet we ought not to conclude from thence with *Helmont*, that the Bile does not tinge the Fæces of the large Inteftines ; for as long as it is fecerned in its due Quantity and Strength, the Fæces are tinged yellow by it, and the more intenfely as the Bile is ftronger ; but upon an Obftruction of the Bile, the Fæces are difcharged of a white Colour, as we obferve in a Jaundice : it alfo feems not improbable, that the Strength of the Bile may be overcome by the larger Quantities of Chyle, pancreatic and inteftinal Juices ; fince it is apparent from Experiment, that different Liquors do upon mixture inftantly change their Tafte and other Properties ; thus the Bitternefs of Silver diffolved in *Aqua fortis*, is fuddenly deftroyed upon mixing a little common Salt, the Silver being precipitated to the bottom of the Veffel, and the remaining Liquor render'd very faline.

" This is one of the principal Qualities of the *Saliva* ; the Cow makes the fame fweet and pleafant Milk from all forts of Herbs, both acid, bitter, and aromatic ; and a Woman gives the fame Milk from all forts of Food, except fuch as are fpirituous, and poffeffed with a particular aromatic Pungency ; which Change is owing to the Mixture of our other Fluids with the Aliment ; to wit, the *Saliva*, Juices of the *Pancreas*, Stomach, and the Bile.

[12] There is not fo much as a Dram of the whole three Pounds of the pancreatic Juice, which are daily difcharged into the Inteftines, conveyed out
with

with the Fæces of the Inteftines of a healthy Body, which are in that State very dry; it muft therefore be again abforbed 'into the Veins or lacteal Veffels; and as its Paffage with the Blood is performed in a very fhort time, it may be again fecerned and abforbed above a hundred times in a few Hours, returned with the Blood to the Heart, and again difcharged by the cœliac Artery into the *Duodenum,* under the Name and Appearance of pancreatic Juice.

§. 102. From hence one may be enabled to give a rational Anfwer, whether there are more than *two Sorts* [1] of Bile; whether the Bile is an *Excrement* [2] of the Chyle fent to the Liver, feparated while Blood is made thereof in that Part; *whether or no* [3], and *how far* [4], it is ferviceable in preferving Health, and continuing the feveral Actions of Life; whether the Juice of the *Pancreas* and Bile will admit the Hypothefis of *Helmont* or *Sylvius* [5]; or whether they were both miftaken; whether they are the Caufe of Life, by exciting and maintaining an *inteftine Motion* [6] in the Blood; what is the Nature of the pancreatic Juice, and what its Office; why it flows into the *Duodenum,* together with (or at leaft very near) the *Bile* [7]. And laftly, whether the Animal cou'd fubfift well *without it* [8].

[1] We do not enquire fo much whether there be two Sorts of Bile in the Liver, diftinct from each other, the cyftic, and hepatic, as whether there be another, diftinct from both of them, diffufed thro' the whole Mafs of Blood. The Foundation of this

U   Con-

Controverfy, which has occafioned the Moderns to depart from the Ancients, is as follows. We find that Blood difcharged in Phlebotomy, quickly turns into a hard Cake, diftinct from its *Serum*; which laft is naturally ringed of a yellow Colour, by what the Ancients called yellow Bile; the upper Part of the Cake of *Craffamentum*, which is expofed to the Air, appears of a bright Red, and is more ftrictly denominated *Cruor* or Blood; but the lower Part of the *Craffamentum*, which is next the bottom of the Veffel, appears darker or blackifh, and is called by the Antients *Atrabilis*; and laftly, the whey'ey Part of the *Serum*, which fometimes looks milky, they denominate its *Pituita*, or Phlegm. Thefe they made the four primitive Humours; among which was the two Kinds of Bile, yellow and black; but the Name of Bile was apparently abufed in that refpect; for the Yellownefs of the ferous Part of the Blood proceeds from the large Quantity of red Globules mixed with Water; the upper Surface of the Blood appears redder, and more fplendid from its Situation, being in Contact with the Air, becaufe the fame grows black again, if it be inverted towards the bottom of the Veffel; but neither Part has the leaft fign of Bile, nor is there any Quantity or Proportion of that Humour diftinct from the Blood, the difference arifing from the chief and largeft Part of the Blood itfelf.

The Ancients fuppofed that the Chyle was drawn to the Liver by the Attraction of the meferaic Veins, and elaborated by the digeftive Faculty of that Organ; by which Faculty it was alfo converted into Blood, and that the Bile was feparated at that time as an Excrement of the Blood, and conveyed into the common biliary Duct. All which might be admitted, if the digeftive Faculty of the Liver be interpretated in a proper Senfe, except that

that the Chyle is not conveyed to the Liver, nor converted into Blood there; tho' it is not to be denied, but that some Part of the Bile may pass to the Liver, after being absorbed by the meseraic Veins.

ᵌ The Bile has many considerable Uses in the human Body, insomuch that Health and a good Constitution greatly depends upon a due Secretion of this Juice; which when vitiated, either in Quantity or Quality, cannot fail of producing obstinate Disorders. The Bile is one of the principal Instruments in Chylification; for want of a sufficient Quantity of this Fluid in the Jaundice, Crudities and acid Indigestions of the Aliment, with whitish or grey-coloured Fæces are occasioned in the *Primæ Viæ*; by stagnating in the Liver, it forms *Calculi* in the common Duct of the Bile, and of the Gall-bladder; which obstructing its Passage, renders the Chyle crude and undigested; but when too much putrified or acrimonious, it occasions Diarrhæas, Dysenteries, putrid Fevers, and various other malignant Disorders.

⁴ *Helmont* wrote before the Discovery of the Blood's Circulation; and if he had lived much longer, at that Age, he wou'd have been unwilling to have changed his System, which he had once formed, nor cou'd he well have departed from it: But as there was nothing but the Circulation of the Blood which cou'd give Rise to the Heat in the human Body, and as the Food, tho' cold and inanimate, did at last obtain the like vital Heat, and as such Things as were acid were converted into a volatile Nature, that eminent Chemist was not sensible of any other Means of explaining so different a Change than by Fermentation or Mixture of contrary Principles, by which Heat and Motion might be communicated thro' the whole Body; for *Helmont* had found by

Expe-

Experience that a confiderable Heat might arife from the Effervefcence of cold Bodies, as of Oil of Vitriol with fixed Salt of Tartar, which occafions a ftrong Heat; he alfo had read in *Fernelius*, that the *Pancreas* was the Seat of chronical Fevers; that a fort of Juice was prepared in that Body, which afterwards mixed with the Aliment; and that as the Bile, which is fo extremely bitter, was alfo mixed with that Juice and the Aliment in the fame Part, he was eafily perfuaded that an Effervefcence muft be occafioned from the mixture of thofe Liquors in the *Duodenum*, which imparted Heat and Motion to all the reft of the Machine.

' Thofe Errors were more excufable in *Helmont* than in *Sylvius*, who was an expert Anatomift, and well acquainted with the Circulation of the Blood; and yet fo defirous was he of imitating *Helmont*, that he fuppofed a Fermentation, not only of the Bile and pancreatic Juice of the *Duodenum*, but alfo another Effervefcence to be made in the Right Auricle and Ventricle of the Heart, upon the Mixture of the Chyle, Lymph, and pancreatic Juice; Liquors fuppofed to be of an acid nature, with the volatile and fetid Bile and the Blood, which were alcaline; and that from this Effervefcence arofe all the vital Heat and Motion of the Heart and reft of the Body; alfo that it was neceffary for the Prefervation of Life, that there fhould be a perpetual Conflict of an alcaline with an acid Salt:-but it has before been largely demonftrated that healthy Bile is not alcaline, and that the pancreatic Juice is not acid; to which we may alfo add, that an Animal may live entirely without the pancreatic Juice, like thofe who live entirely upon aceffent Milk, or entirely upon alcalefcent Flefh of Animals; from whence it will evidently appear, that the imaginary Conflict or Effervefcence of thofe

Liquors

Liquors which they fo confidently maintained, is without any manner of Foundation.

⁶ We before obferv'd, that *Sylvius* attributed the inteftine Motion of the Blood to an Effervefcence between acid and alcali ; to wit, the acid Liquor of the thoracic Duct, formed of the pancreatic Juice, Chyle and Lymph intermix'd, and afterwards poured into the alcalefcent Blood ; which contrary Liquors beginning their Effervefcence in the *Duodenum*, did not ceafe it even in the Right Auricle and Ventricle of the Heart ; but if it did occafion fo ftrong an Effervefcence in the *Duodenum*, it is hardly intelligible by what means that Effervefcence fhould be continued thro' fo many Turnings and Windings, efpecially after being diluted with fo large a Quantity of an infipid Lymph in the Receptacle of the Chyle and thoracic Duct ; nor can fuch a Force be by any means equal to the Caufe of fo ftrong a Motion as that with which the Blood is projected by the Heart ; it rather feems furprifing that Men of fo much Knowledge and profound Underftanding fhould propofe fuch falfe Syftems, and thence deduce fuch abfurd Confequences.

⁷ The faponaceous Quantity of the Bile is affifted by being diluted with the pancreatic Juice, in order to mix the Chyle ; in the fame manner as greafy Wool is eafily cleanfed with Soap, by diluting and wafhing in warm Water, but not fo well in cold Water ; and not at all, if it were to be fcowred with hard Soap only, without the addition of fome diluent Liquor.

⁸ This feems to be countenanc'd by feveral Experiments made by an ingenious Perfon, who entirely cut out the *Pancreas* from feveral Dogs, who yet continu'd to live without any fenfible Inconvenience. The want of the pancreatic Juice in thofe

Animals

Animals feems to be fupplied by a more plentiful Secretion of the *Succus gaftricus,* and of the Inteftines, particularly the *Duodenum* ; but it alfo does not appear that thofe Dogs liv'd without any In convenience, if they furvived the Operation any confiderable Time ; but that they frequently were fubject to Obftructions, Strumous Glands, and a fort of hectic Fever. The Obfervation of *Brunnerus,* that he had more than once found the pancreatic Duct, which he had before divided, again renew'd, feems to argue, that this Juice is not only ufeful, but neceffary to the well-being of the Animal. Nor could that Liquor be deemed ufelefs, becaufe the Abfence of it does not prefently incur violent Diforders upon the Animal. Even what reafonable Perfon would affirm the Spleen to be ufelefs, becaufe a Dog may furvive after the Extirpation of that *Vifcus?* It even cannot be affirm'd, that the moft ordinary and feemingly infignificant Parts of the human Body have not their proper Ufes ; for that would be detracting from the divine Wifdom of the fupreme Architect, who has fo exquifitely built the human Body, that it feems to be the greateft Example of Perfection amongft the fublunary Beings. There are more than a few Hiftories extant of Patients furviving the Lofs of a Limb, a Lobe of the Lungs, one of their Kidnies, &c. But would any Body therefore pronounce thofe Parts to be ufelefs? *Brunnerus* proves this indeed, that the *Pancreas* is not fo immediately neceffary to Life as *Sylvius* would have it ; but does not make it appear, that the Animal from whence that *Vifcus* was extirpated, continu'd to live in as perfect Health as before it was deprived of the fame *Vifcus.*

Con-

*Concerning the Propulſion of the Chyle
into and thro' the lacteal Veſſels.*

§. 103. BY the Contraction of the *longitudinal*[1] Fibres of the Inteſtines which
are inſerted into their external Coat as into a
Tendon, the inteſtinal Tube is thereby wrinkled in that Part oppoſite to the Meſentery,
which therefore reduces them from a ſpiral to
a cylindrical, or ſtraight Form ; by this means
the Inteſtines are relaxed on that Side connected to the Meſentery, but contracted on the oppoſite Side, whereby the ſmall *Orifices*[2] of the
Lacteals, that lie next the Meſentery, are ſo
opened and dilated, as to receive the more
fluid, moveable, and ſlippery Particles of the
Chyle, which there meet with a ready Entrance : In the mean time the Valves of the Inteſtines will be enlarg'd, made more prominent,
and brought cloſer to each other by the ſame
Contraction, ſo as to intercept and ſtop the
Chymus in its Paſſage, and almoſt entirely ſhut
up that Part of the Inteſtine thus moved or
contracted. All which is more exactly performed in the *Jejunum*, where the Valves are more
frequent, prominent, and circular, the *Lacteals*[3] more numerous, the Contraction of the
agitated Stomach is more ſenſible, and the
Chyle more diluted, quickly paſſing along by
its Mixture with the *Saliva*, *Succus gaſtricus*,
Juice of the *Pancreas*, and the two Kinds of
Bile, U 4 Thoſe

¹ Thoſe longitudinal Fibres which are ſeated in that Part of the Inteſtines connected to the Meſentery, are not inſerted into the external or common Coat of the Inteſtines, ſo that there is no Contraction in that Part which is ſupplied with the cellular Membrane ; but thoſe longitudinal Fibres which are ſituated in the oppoſite convex Side of the Inteſtines, fartheſt from the Meſentery, being faſten'd to the external Coat, they contract the Inteſtines from their arch or ſpiral Form to a ſtrait cylindrical Figure ; and by rendering them ſhorter, contract them into Wrinkles ; but while the circular Fibres are contracted, at the ſame time the internal Cavity of the Inteſtines will be leſſened, and the Valves brought into mutual Contact with each other ; by which means the Chyle will be protruded into the lacteal Veſſels, much in the ſame manner as Quickſilver is preſſed thro' Leather. The muſcular Fibres of the Inteſtines may alſo be aſſiſted in their Action by the Preſſure of the abdominal Muſcles, which is ſtronger upon them where they are uncover'd by the *Omentum*, and touch the *Peritonæum* ; but leſs on that ſide of them which is connected to the Meſentery, and therefore the Chyle will be preſſed towards the lax Part of the Inteſtine.

ᵃ Beſides the lacteal Veſſels opening into the Inteſtines, the meſenteric Veſſels alſo open into the Cavity with ſuch large Apertures, as to tranſmit the ceraceous Injection of *Ruyſch* into the Inteſtines ; but the lacteal Veſſels open moſt plentifully in that Part of the Inteſtines towards the Meſentery, but fewer on the Sides, as I have frequently obſerved ; but they are ſo diſpoſed, as not to admit any thing from the Inteſtines, only in the time of Digeſtion, when they are found full in living Animals ; at which time the Lacteals have

been

been also seen by some of the Family of *Æsclepiads*,
as *Galen* informs us. *Asellius* also constantly found,
and described those Vessels in living Animals,
which had been open'd a few Hours after a Meal;
but the Ancients being ignorant of the Receptacle
and thoracic Duct of the Chyle, and being prejudiced in favour of the Liver, imagin'd that they
convey'd the Chyle to that *Viscus.* A Dissolution
of Indigo-blue in recent Urine being forced into
the Intestine of a living Animal between two Ligatures, may by Pressure be forced into the Lacteals.

3 These are real Veins, if by Veins we intend
such Vessels as return their contained Liquors towards the Heart.

§. 104. The orbicular Fibres of the Intestines,
inserted into the Mesentery as into a Tendon,
being at the same time contracted, they diminish the Diameter or cylindrical Space of the
Tube, and press the Valves together, which
were before drawn nearer to each other; by
which means the Chyle being compressed,
mixed, diluted, agitated, and intercepted in
its Passage, is by the Force of the ambient Parts
protruded chiefly towards the Mesentery, and
there driven into the Mouths of the Lacteals,
opening into every Point of the Intestine, having been before opened by the *Periftaltic Motion* 1 for the Reception of the Chyle; therefore the Chyle does not appear to enter the Lacteals by its own Weight, or by the Force of
any *Effervescence* 2.

1 Upon

Upon a Ceſſation of this Motion, the Motion and Abſorption of the Chyle alſo immediately ceaſes; which is quickly performed, ſo long as the periſtaltic Motion continues; for the Lacteals, which are viſible in opening a living Dog, do not remain ſo long, but vaniſh almoſt in the Twinkling of an Eye, by diſcharging their Contents towards the Receptacle, and being fill'd with Lymph. To this we may add, the Obſervation of the Lacteals remaining viſible a long time in ſuch as have been hang'd, from the Chyle being ſtopt in the thoracic Duct by the Compreſſure of the Ligature.

This is an Opinion of *Sylvius*, or a falſe Deduction from a falſe Hypotheſis; for the Inteſtines at that time when the Efferveſcence is made, will have their Sides diſtended into a larger Circle, their Valves will be flatten'd, their pendulous *Villi* will be contracted and ſhorten'd; therefore no Chyle will be abſorbed by the Lacteals while the Inteſtines are in their utmoſt Diſtenſion: on the contrary, it is apparent that the Chyle is abſorbed by the Lacteals, not in the contracted, but in the relaxed Part of the Inteſtine, oppoſite to the longitudinal Fibres, the Chyle being propelled into the Lacteals by the Contraction of the annular Fibres acting towards the Meſentery: it is alſo manifeſt, that the Lacteals are not filled by any internal Force, but by an external Preſſure; becauſe upon diſtending them with Wind, no Part of the *Flatus* will enter them: to which agrees the Experiment made by the Royal Society, of forcing a Diſſolution of Indigo-Blue into the Lacteals by Preſſure: it has been alſo before demonſtrated (§. 93. N°. 1.) that the moſt natural State of the Inteſtines comes neareſt to a Contraction of them.

§. 105. From

§. 105. From hence it appears, that the Chyle which enters the Mouths of the Lacte-als, is improperly efteemed to be a Compofi-tion of the folid and fluid Aliment only; for it alfo confifts in a great meafure of the *Saliva* [1], (§. 66.) and the thin *Mucus* of the Mouth (§. 65.) with the *Mucus* and thin Liquor of the *Oefophagus* [2] (§. 73.) and Stomach, in conjun-ction with the cyftic and hepatic *Bile* [3] (§. 98, 99.) the pancreatic Juice (§. 101.) with the lymphatic Humour of the *Inteftines* [4] and mu-cous one of *Peyerus*, and perhaps a more fub-tle Liquor plentifully difcharged out of the infinite Number of fmall *Nerves* [5] which ter-minate in the Inteftines; for all thefe Humours, which are either fwallowed, or are difcharged and tranfuded into the Capacity of the Stomach and Inteftines, always enter the Lacteals, either alone or mix'd with the moft fluid Part of the Chyle, notwithftanding the lacteal Veffels are only *confpicuous* [6] after a Meal.

[1] We have before obferved from *Nuck*, that 12 Ounces of *Saliva* are feparated and difcharged into the Mouth in the Space of four and twenty Hours; but the Quantity of falival Juice which is abforbed by the Lacteals in that time is ftill much larger; for all that which was fpit out in the Experiment of *Nuck*, wou'd have been abforb'd by the Lacteals, and again feparated by the falival Glands feveral times in the Space of a Day; and therefore it is probable that feveral Pounds of *Saliva* pafs daily thro' the Lacteals.

[2] That the Quantity of both thefe Juices is not inconfiderable, will appear from the Size of the

Organ

Organ and Laxity of the Veffels; which open freely into the Cavity of the *Oefophagus*.

³ The large Quantity of this bitter Juice may be eafily eftimated. The Liver is an exceeding large *Vifcus*, and its Veffels fo lax, that Water being injected by the *Vena Portæ*, finds a ready Paffage into the *Cava*, and runs thro' the common Duct of the Bile; its Veffels are alfo very large, if we confider the great Diameter of the *Vena Portæ*, and its excretory Duct very capacious; if we therefore compare the Secretion made in the Kidnies, which feparate no lefs than three Pound of Urine every Day, with the Secretion of this large *Vifcus*, it will appear that not a few Pounds of the hepatic Bile are fecerned daily in the Liver.

⁴ But the ferous Secretion made in the Inteftines from the mefenteric Arteries is ftill much greater; for thofe Veffels are not only very large, but alfo very lax and open, fo as readily to admit the ceraceous Injection of *Ruyfch* to pafs freely into the Cavity of the Inteftines: Thefe excretory *Arteriolæ* are alfo fometimes the Caufe of Diarrhæas, when no Aliment is taken, thro' a Lofs of Appetite. M. *Rede* has obferved in his Diffections of Animals in *Florence*, which have been ftarved to death with Hunger, that the Inteftines have been relaxed, and the lacteal Veffels full of Lymph, by their abforbing thefe Juices.

⁵ The Difcharge made by the fmall Nerves of this Part is not therefore inconfiderable, becaufe it cannot be demonftrated to the Eye-fight; for we fee that a ftrong Man in frofty Weather continues to perfpire a fubtle Vapour thro' the contracted Veffels of his Skin fo plentifully, as to make five Parts out of Eight of all his Difcharges in the Space of four and twenty Hours; which is evinced by *Sanctorius*, and confirmed by Experience; but the

great

great Number of small Nerves which open into the Cavity of the Inteſtines, which are conſtantly warm, and compoſe a ſecretory Organ above threeſcore Hands long, ought greatly to exceed in their Secretion of a ſubtle and moiſt Vapour.

⁶ The ſeveral Juices which we have before enumerated, are not at all diſcharged with the Fæces in a natural and healthy State of the Body, but are abſorbed, and again conveyed into the Blood; but there is only one way for them to paſs thither, *i. e.* by the lacteal and meſenteric Veins ; therefore the ſeveral Juices which are continually poured into the Inteſtines entirely paſs thro' thoſe Veſſels without any Chyle when we are faſting, by which they are convey'd to the venal Blood, with that Blood into the Heart, and thence again into the Inteſtines. It is but a ſmall Objection, that the Lacteals of a faſting Animal are not conſpicuous, for that ariſes from the Smallneſs of thoſe Tubes, and the Pellucidity of their Contents at that time; even lymphatic Veſſels, which are much larger than the thoracic Duct, are ſeldom viſible upon the ſame Account, if they are not tied ; but yet no rational Perſon will deny the Paſſage of a Fluid thro' thoſe Veſſels.

§. 106. We may therefore ask in this Place, whether the thinner, bilious, and more lymphatic Part of the Chyle is not abſorbed by *bibulous Ducts* ¹, which open into the villous Coat of the Inteſtines, and diſcharge their Contents into the meſeraic Veins, thence paſſing with the Blood of the *Venæ Portæ* into the Liver, and affording freſh Supplies of new Matter for the Secretion of Bile. This Queſtion is certainly anſwered in the Affirmative, by conſidering the great Number, *Size* ², *Structure,*

Eture 3, and *Office* 4 of all the Veins, particularly ſpent upon the Inteſtines, from the Paſſage of their venal Blood into the *Porta*, as into an *Artery* 5, from the bilious Nature or *Diſpoſition* 6 of their contained Blood; and from the large Quantity of *Juices* 7 diſcharged into the Inteſtines, which are neither obſerved to be entirely abſorbed by the Lacteals, nor yet expelled with the Fæces; to which we may alſo add the Arguments taken from comparative Anatomy in *oviparous Animals* 8, where the Chyle paſſes freely from the Cavity of their Inteſtines into the meſeraic Veins, there being no Lacteals found in thoſe Creatures; to which add the patulent Openings of the ſmall Branches of the meſenteric Veins into the villous Coat of the Inteſtines in the human Body, the Abſence of Valves in thoſe Veins in the human Subject, with the ready Paſſage of the ceraceous Injection of *Ruyſch* into the Cavity of the Inteſtines, upon injecting the meſenteric Veins; when the Inteſtines are contracted by the periſtaltic Motion, the meſenteric Veſſels are ſurpriſingly curled and twiſted.

1 It is no difficult Matter to prove a free Paſſage from the Inteſtines into the meſeraic Veins, inaſmuch as Water and ceraceous Subſtances being injected into thoſe meſenteric Veins, readily paſs thro' them into the Cavity of the Inteſtine, and tranſude thro' every Part of their villous Lining; ſo that it is more than probable that the moſt fluid and aqueous Parts of the Contents of the Inteſtines are abſorbed by them; but it is no more ſurpriſing that the ſmall Mouths of thoſe Veins ſhould not be conſpicuous.

fpicuous to the Sight, than that the Orifices of the lacteal Veffels fhou'd not be vifible even by the beft Microfcope.

² The Veins of the Inteftines are much larger, and more numerous than the correfponding Arteries; but the Arteries depofit a confiderable Quantity of a thin Fluid, by their ftrong Contraction, into the Cavity of the Inteftines; therefore the Veins ought to carry back lefs than was convey'd by the Arteries; and therefore they ought to have been fmaller, and lefs numerous, if they were not to receive other Supplies; which required the Trunks of the Veins to be much larger than thofe of the mefenteric Arteries.

³ Every Branch is convoluted into Waves or Arches, from the convex Part of which are continued fmall Branches in a ftrait Courfe to the Inteftines; which Structure being peculiar to the inteftinal Tube, feems to import, that fomething is perform'd in thofe Veins more than is ufual in thofe of other Parts; but the other Veins of the Inteftines which come from the *Cava*, take a different Courfe, and pafs in ftrait Lines to their Terminations in the Form of fmall Pencil Brufhes; but what fhould be the Caufe of this Variation in their Structure, if it is not what we have here affigned?

⁴ The common Office of the Veins is to receive and convey a Fluid to the Heart; whether that Fluid be received from the Arteries, or abforbed from fome Cavity in the human Body, or drank in from the external Air? The Veins which receive their Fluid from the Arteries, are the fanguiferous, or red Veins; thofe which abforb from peculiar Cavities, or glandular Cells, are the bibulous Veins of the *Omentum*, Ventricles of the Brain, of the Stomach, Mouth, and Inteftines, of which laft we are here fpeaking; but it is apparent that

the

the Branches of the *Venæ Portæ*, which come from
the Inteſtines, ought to be numerated among thoſe
abſorbing Veins, from the Experiment of their
tranſmitting Injections into their Cavity ; therefore
if theſe Veins open into the Cavity of the Inteſtines,
and if their Office is to convey a Fluid from their
Origin towards their Baſis, it muſt neceſſarily follow that they receive ſome of the fluid Parts of the
Chyle contained in the Inteſtines, and conveyed
with the Blood towards the Heart : nor is there
any reaſon why any Body ſhould deny the Ingreſs
of Fluids, which have a Communication with the
patulent Orifices of the abſorbing Veins ; for even
the callous Skin of the bottom of the Feet ſo powerfully abſorbs the mercurial Ointment, that this
was the firſt and moſt ancient Method of curing
the Venereal Diſeaſe by Unction ; and Inſtances
are not wanting where the *Mercury* thus abſorbed
has reſumed its globular Appearance, and ſtopt
in the *Diploœ*, between the Plates of the *Cranium*,
after having cauſed a laſting and violent Head-ach.
It is alſo the common Office of the ſanguiferous
Veins to receive thin Fluids, ſince all the Lymphatics are diſcharged into thoſe Veins ; and therefore upon tying a ſanguiferous Vein, the Lymphatics become turgid, and more viſible : but the
lymphatic Veſſels receive a great Part of their Fluid
from various Cavities or Cells in the human Body ;
for it is reaſonable to ſuppoſe, that the Liquor of
the *Pericardium*, that in the *Abdomen*, &c. are conſtantly abſorbed ; ſince if they were to be perpetually diſcharged, and not returned, a Dropſy muſt
enſue. *Nuck* infuſed two Pound of Water into the
Cavity of the *Abdomen* of a Maſtiff Dog, and upon
opening the Animal ſome time afterward, there
was none of the Water to be found ; it is therefore
nothing extraordinary or diſagreeable with the

Nature

Nature of Veins, if the abforbing Veffels of the Inteftines drink up fome of their moft fluid Contents, and tranfmit them into the fanguiferous Veins.

⁵ The *Vena Portæ* propels the Blood of the abdominal *Vifcera*, like an Artery into the *Sinus* and Veins of the Liver, by which Force the Bile is propelled into its proper Ducts, and the Blood thro' the *Anaftomofes* of the *Vena Cava*; and it feems altogether probable, that as the Heart diftributes all the Blood to the feveral Parts of the human Body, fo the *Porta* alfo diftributes the feveral Humours of the *Abdomen* to the Liver; but as the Blood is diluted with all the lymphatic and thinner Juices of the Body, before it paffes thro' the fmall Veffels of the Lungs, fo in like manner the Blood of the *Porta* feems alfo to be diluted before it enters the fmall Veffels of the Liver.

⁶ The Blood of the mefenteric Veins is of a brownifh yellow Colour; and hardly congeals, but appears fluid when extravafated, like other Blood in the Air, appearing rather the Confiftence of Lard, while the Blood of the Arteries appears of a bright fhining Red, and quickly congeals; therefore if the mefenteric Veins received nothing but the arterial Blood, it fhould, like the Blood of other Veins, become black, thick, and quickly congeal into a hard Cake; but as this is not the Cafe, and their Blood appears more dilute, thofe Veins muft confequently receive fome other Fluid befides that of the Arteries.

⁷ There are People who drink 12 Pounds of Spaw-water in a Morning, without difcharging any Part thereof by Stool, the whole Quantity being convey'd into the Blood from the Stomach and Inteftines, and paffed off by Urine; but the Nature of thofe Waters is to exert a confiderable Force

upon

upon the Liver, which is the reason why we frequently order them in the most obstinate Disorders
of that *Viscus*. As those Veins are destitute of
Valves, and have a free Communication with the
Cavity of the Intestines, they frequently occasion
purulent Diarrhœa's, discharging the whole Substance of the corrupted Liver, so as to leave nothing but its membranous Integuments behind, like
an empty Bag. If to these Considerations we also
add the immense Quantity of the several animal
Fluids which are convey'd into the Intestines, and
are not at all discharged with the Fæces, but returned by the absorbing Veins, it will appear altogether necessary that there should be more Vessels
than the Lacteals, for the Transmission of those
Fluids.

[8] Birds, and the rest of the oviparous Class of
Animals, are destitute of Lacteals, which would
have been in danger of growing together by long
fasting; all the Chyle in those Animals is taken up
by the mesenteric Veins, which are so open as to
receive the Wind with which the Intestines are distended, by means of a Ligature and an additional
Pressure, so as to pass into the Veins: but it is not
reasonable to suppose, that a Mechanism which obtains in so large, or the greatest Part of Animals,
should be entirely excluded from Quadrupeds, or
viviparous Animals.

§. 107. If we therefore distinctly and separately consider the several *Appearances* [1] and
Alterations of the solid and fluid Aliment from
their first Entrance by the Mouth, till they
have parted with their milky Juice by the Lacteals, the whole Business of Chylification will
appear to be the simple Consequence of the
Structure

Structure and Action of the several Organs and Vessels, with the known Nature and Action of the several animal Juices therein employ'd, being demonstrable by the Senses and mechanical Reasoning; so that you may be thence able to judge for yourself whether there is any necessity for calling in the Assistance of obscure and dubious *Hypotheses* or *Postulata*[2], which have neither *Reason* nor *Experiment*[3] to support them, to account for these Phænomena; such as a vital, innate, or digestive Heat and *acrid Ferment*[4] in the Stomach, volatilizing the Food; an operating *Archæus*[5], or spiritual Cook; an alcaline Bile, converting the fix'd acid Chyle into a volatile alcaline and saline Nature; a fictitious Acrimony in the pancreatic Juice *fermenting*[6] with the alcalescent Bile; a Depuration of the Chyle by a *Precipitation*[7] of its Fæces, equally false and imaginary with the *peripatetic*[8] Qualities and *galenic* Faculties, with the *Ferment, Ebullitions,* and *Effervescencies* of the Chemists; and the innumerable other false and *pernicious*[9] Hypotheses misleading, from the Truth. A Person may hence also be able to judge why the *peristaltic Motion*[10] is performed only in the small Intestines; and why that Motion continues in a *deliquium Animi*[11]; and even after Death, when the Intestines have been removed from the Body for some time; whether it is not extreamly necessary to urge the Parts in a *Syncope* to their former Action for continuing Life; and whether or no this Motion is not composed of a

Systole

Syſtole and *Diaſtole* of the Cavity of the Inteſtines as in the Heart.

[1] That is, the whole Buſineſs of Chylification,
or that Function of the human Body whereby the
ſolid and fluid Aliments are reduced to a thick,
ſweet, and milky Juice, paſſing into the Lacteals ;
the Cauſes of which Changes in the Food, reſide
partly in the Aliments themſelves, and partly in
the Action of the ſeveral ſolid and fluid Parts of
the human Body, which we have hitherto deſcribed as acceſſary to that Office.

[2] By *Poſtulata* we underſtand ſuch evident Truths
as need no Proof, and may be ſafely relied on for
certain ; notwithſtanding other obſcure and imaginary Deductions may thence be framed : which
Poſtulata in Phyſic ought to be no leſs evident,
than the Appearances to be explained by them,
otherwiſe they are to be rejected ; they differ from
Hypotheſes, in that the latter are only Suppoſitions,
without any evident Proof ; whereas *Poſtulata* are
certain and evident Propoſitions, but not yet demonſtrated ; yet they muſt be allow'd equally true
as Demonſtration itſelf.

[3] By Experiments we underſtand an Obſervation
of the Changes in natural Bodies by our Senſes,
which always appearing in the ſame manner is the
Baſis upon which all true Reaſoning is founded ;
thus we are acquainted by Experience with ſome
of the Appearances of the Body, as that it is extended in three, and no more Dimenſions, *&c.*
upon which Phænomena we build a large Part of
our phyſical Reaſoning ; but if we truſt more to
Reaſoning than Experience, we then become liable to Falacy.

[4] All the known Vegetables which are employed in human Affairs, afford a fixed alcaline Salt by
Calcination ;

Calcination ; but the same Vegetables being dissolved by the Action of the digestive Organs in a healthy human Body, do not afford one Grain of a fixed, but a considerable Quantity of volatile alcaline Salt. When *Helmont* observed this Change, which must certainly be more than a little surprising to a Chemist, apprised of the Difficulty there is in Nature of converting a fixed into a volatile Salt, he pitch'd upon an Example or Comparison of the *Sal purgans Sennerti*, where a fixed Alcali being mixed with a volatile acid Spirit, is sublimed into a volatile Salt; he was therefore persuaded that an acid Ferment must reside in the Stomach, which volatilized the fixed Salt of the vegetable Food: but this Hypothesis has before been too largely confuted; for there is no such thing as an Acid in any Part of the human Body, except what is taken in from the Food ; and many People who feed entirely upon Flesh and Fish, without any acid or acessent Substance, form the same Blood and Juices with those that feed upon Vegetables ; nor is it any Matter of consequence, whether we use acessent or alcalescent Food, since good Chyle may easily be made from both under proper Circumstances.

⁵ The Word *Archæus* among the Ancients originally signified the first Being of all Things; but the Word was formerly abused by *Basil Valentine*, after whom the Chemist used it to signify that Faculty of organic and vegetating Bodies, whereby they converted other Substances into part of themselves. In this Sense the Term *Archæus* was receiv'd by *Paracelsus*; and *Helmont* more expresly uses it to signify a Being between that of the conscious Mind and inactive or common Matter, which directed all the Functions of the human Body in health, cured Diseases, and sometimes

X 3   caused

caufed them, &c. The Philofophers thought it neceſſary to frame fuch an Hypothefis, becaufe the human Body appeared to them fo admirably and mechanically built, and fupplied with various Artifices, that they thought it impoffible fo many different Actions, varioufly depending upon one another, fhould be performed without the Affiftance and Regulation of fome intelligent Being; but they were not willing to attribute that Office to the immaterial Soul, becaufe it would from thence follow, that we muft be fenfible of every Action performed within us, and that we muft even be capable of governing the feveral Functions which we term vital. It is not neceſſary, and therefore we fhall not give ourfelves the Trouble to confure this Hypothefis. But it feems hardly credible that *Helmont* madly believ'd all to be true that he wrote upon the *Archæus*; and when he fays, that the *Archæus* craves, chufes, digefts and expels the Aliment, he feems to intend no more, than that the Food is defired, felected, digefted, and expell'd by fome unknown Power. But one might as well confefs their Ignorance of the Caufe of any Action, as attribute it to fome imaginary and unknown Being, of whofe Exiftence, Nature, Actions, and Manner of Operation, we have not the leaft Knowledge or Affurance; we are indeed fenfible that the Caufes of many Functions in the human Body are merely mechanical; and we alfo know in general, that Life, Health, and all the Actions of the human Body, proceed from the conjunct Action of innumerable phyfical Caufes, affembled in fuch a manner into one united Body and Mind, as to be capable of continuing and reftoring the feveral Offices of the human Machine; nor does it require any more than one original Caufe to put it in motion; like a Clock, which when once put

in

in motion, will continue the same, and perform its several Actions during the whole Space of Time for which the Wheels and Works are adapted.

6 The Chemists have generally made use of Similies, taken from their own Operations, in order to explain the Separation of the fluid and nutritious Juices from the excrementitious and useless Part of the Aliment; *e. g.* If an Ounce of Silver be dissolved in *Aqua fortis*, the Liquor appears uniform, limpid, and bitter to the Senses ; but if Spirit of Salt be poured into that Solution, there arises a Commotion, and the Silver precipitates to the bottom, reduc'd to the Form of what they term a *Calx.*

7 Much in the same manner *Verheyn* imagined the Food was dissolved in the Stomach by an acid *Menstruum*, which upon mixing with alcaline Bile, occasioned a Fermentation, at which time the most subtil and fluid Part, which had acquired a volatile saline Nature, was impelled into the Veins, while the more gross, useless, and heavy Parts were converted into Fæces, *&c.* But all this Scheme falls to nothing, upon demonstrating that no such Effervescence happens in the human Body.

8 A Parcel of lazy Philosophers, who explain'd every thing, as well as Physic, by the mere Sophistry of the Schools, improperly accounted for Digestion by unknown Faculties, as the attractive, retentive, digestive, expulsive, and assimilating Faculties ; but they are not much less excusable than the Chemists, who had Experiments to alledge for the improper Deductions or Explanations made from them; whereas the Peripatetics neither made false Propositions, nor alledg'd Experiments, but entertain'd us with mere Words; which Words may be admitted, if we do not take up with them

for

for an Explanation of the Appearances, of which they are Names only.

8* A Ferment was defined by the ancient Chemiſts to be a Subſtance, which being mixed with another, converted it into its own Nature. Thus a Grain of Wheat becomes augmented in a proper Soil to a hundred, each of which are capable of producing a hundred more; ſo that the ſecond Produce of the firſt will be a thouſand Grains of Wheat, all of the ſame mealy and nutritious Nature: but the ſame Soil will alſo nouriſh very ſtrong Plants, ſuch as *Spurge*, *Euphorbium*, and *Muſtard*; there muſt therefore be ſomething in the Wheat which converts the common nutritious Juice of the Earth into its own particular Subſtance; which would have been quite different in other Plants: but how ſmall is that ſeminal Particle, the whole Grain of Wheat does not exceed the Weight of a phyſical Grain; and if you again ſeparate the Seed-Leaves, or *Placenta*, with the Integuments, mealy Cells, and Radicle, there will then remain a Particle ſo ſmall, as not to exceed a little Grain of Sand; and yet in that Particle, no bigger than a ſmall Grain of Sand, lies conceal'd the Power by which the Juice of the Earth is converted into ten thouſand Plants; a Juice, which in its own Nature is quite different from the Subſtance which it forms: and this Power of Tranſmutation has been denominated by the Chemiſts a *Ferment*. They were indeed excuſable, as being ignorant of the mechanical Structure of the human Body, whereby all Sorts of Aliments are converted into animal Fluids and Solids, and render'd capable of re-producing our Species: but who would believe that a Man may be form'd of Flour and Water, yet we ſee that Children are nouriſh'd and grow therewith: and from the ſame Sub-

ſtance,

ftance, by the Power of the human Body, may be
formed *Semen Mafculinum*, which being received
into the *Uterus*, re-produces our Species : And in
this Senfe the Term may be excufed, being otherwife but little agreeable to the Idea which it ex-
preffes ; but if by the Word *Ferment* we underftand
with the modern Chemifts, a Subftance capable of
exciting an inteftine Motion in Bodies, whereby an
Alteration or Change is made in their Nature ; or if
we underftand by it a Conflict of oppofite Salts,
the Word is then fpurious, may be the caufe of
Error, and ought to be rejected.

9 If thefe imaginary Hypothefes reach'd no farther than the Profeffor's Chair who ftarted them,
it would be Matter of little confequence to avoid
them, and they would do no great Damage ; but
they even advance into the Practice of Phyfic, and
are often fatal to the Health and Lives of Patients.
Thus the Patrons of an acid Ferment being the chief
Caufe of Digeftion in the Stomach, deriving Fevers alfo from a Redundancy of the fame Acid, attempted their Cure by volatile, oily, lixivious, and
alcaline Salts ; which for a while became almoft an
univerfal Practice, and may ferve as an Inftance
how the elegant Notions of a Profeffor may be
propagated by his Pupils, to the great Prejudice
of the Healths and Lives of the Sick.

10 By which Motion the Aliment is preffed backward, forward, and into the lacteal Veffels ; otherwife the Aliment would find a fpeedy Paffage thro'
the Inteftines out of the Body ; but it is fo retained in their Cells by the periftaltic Motion, that
only the groffer Parts are propelled into the large
Inteftines, and the more fluid retained in the fmall
ones by a furprifing Artifice, not to be parallel'd
by any other Contrivance.

11 If the Heart of a ftrong Man fhould ftop but
one Moment, he falls down, grows cold, appears
dead,

dead, his Limbs become ſtiff, and all the ſolid
Parts of the Body come nearer into contact with
each other, the Fluids being propell'd from all the
ſmall Branches of the conical Veſſels from their
Extremities, towards the Heart. In like manner
alſo the Chyle may continue to be propell'd thro'
the Lacteals and thoracic Duct into the ſubclavian
Vein, by the Force of the periſtaltic Motion, yet
remaining; But the Heart is no ſooner irritated by
this new Supply, or by any other Means, than it
returns to its former Action; and if the Machine
is entire, the Man may by that means be revived.
In a common *Syncope* we find that the Functions
are reſtored by the Aſperſion of cold Water; and
there have been ſeveral Inſtances of People who
have been given out for dead in a Plague, that
have recovered their Life and Senſes upon being
expoſed to the Cold, various Agitations, and the
ringing of Bells. *Pyerus* having therefore taken
the Hint from Nature, produced the like Effect
in his anatomical Diſſections, recalling the Heart
to its proper Motion by inflating the Veins.

Concerning the Nature and Expulſion of the Fæces.

WE come now to a naſty, but neceſſary Buſineſs, the Expulſion of the Fæces, being
one of the Neceſſaries of Life, without which we
cannot long ſubſiſt. When the Great *Alexander*
was upon his Succeſſes congratulated by his Flat-
terers with the Name of a God, he frankly con-
feſſed that his Subjection to Sleep and Women
proved him but a Man; he might alſo have added;

ded, that, like other Men, he was necessitated to this Office of going to stool.

§. 108. The *grosser Parts* [1] of the Aliment, which are so compact and solid, that they cannot be sufficiently attenuated to enter the Lacteals, by the Action of Mastication and Chylification in the Stomach and *Duodenum*; are yet more perfectly drained of their succulent and dissolved Parts in the two other small Intestines; which are for that End furnish'd with a vermicular Contraction, numerous Valves, and various Convolutions, to the Length of about 37 Hands Breadth, being also lubricated internally by the *oily Mucus* [2] of their Glands: In the Capacity of these small Intestines, the courser Parts of the Aliment are therefore gradually propell'd forward, compressed, further divided, diluted, macerated, and their fluid Parts inbibed or drawn off by the Lacteals; while the *Remainder* [3] being deprived of almost all its Juices and more soluble Parts, is in that State *protruded* [4] thro' the End of the *Ileum*, which usually opens almost perpendicularly into the left Part of the large Cavity in the *Cæcum* [5], by a narrow and oblong Aperture, furnished with a sort of Valves or folding Lips, and a Set of muscular Fibres, that close the Aperture, and prevent a Return of the Fæces, which are by that Valve directed into the ample Cavity of the *Intestinum Cæcum*.

[1] Such as cannot be sufficiently attenuated and dissolved into Particles small enough to enter the

Orifices

Orifices of the Lacteals, but are caft out of the Body, after having endured the Action of the digeftive Organs for fome time, in the fame manner as the hard Integuments and furfuracious Parts of farinaceous Seeds, which being depriv'd of their mealy and juicy Parts, remain ligneous and ufelefs in Emulfions.

² Through the whole Tract of the fmall Inteftines there are a Number of fmall Glands, fituated in Clufters, firft obferved by *Pyerus*, ferving to feparate a gelatinous *Mucus*, partly oily, and partly aqueous, which is referved in Cells, from whence it is expreffed very plentifully to the Fæces in their Paffage. When this lubricating *Mucus* is wanting in lean and hypochondriac People, it occafions cholicky Pains and Piles; to remedy which nothing is more ferviceable than oily Glyfters; but there have been alfo Obfervations of the Fæces being fo concreted and indurated in large Lumps, that they have entirely obftructed the Cavity of the Inteftine adhering to its Sides, and intercepting the Courfe of the Fæces.

³ Thefe Fæces are the *Refiduum* of all the Aliment feparated from its moft fluid and milky Part, and from its alimental Juice, which is ftill more fubtle than Milk itfelf, and is that Fluid with which the *Fœtus* is nourifhed in the Womb of the Mother; for there is a confiderable Quantity of Fæces found in the large Inteftines of the *Fœtus*, and in their *Appendicula Vermiformis*, which at the time of Birth are found full of Fæces, reprefenting the Juice of Poppies, ufually called *Meconium*. But thefe Parts of the Aliment which have been drained of their Juices in the fmall Inteftines, become altogether ufelefs as foon as arrived into the larger Inteftines; for the *Inteftina Craffa* are not furnifhed with a villous Coat, like the *Tenuia*, nor with exhaling Arteries, difcharging a diluting Lymph; alfo the

Fæces

Fæces of a human Body are so light, as to swim upon Water when discharg'd out of the Body.

⁴ It seems no easy Matter to explain by what Means the Fæces are propell'd thro' so long a Tube as the Intestines, and to overcome so many Resistances from the Valves, when the peristaltic Motion moves them upwards as well as downwards ; for it is certain when the peristaltic Motion of the lower Intestines is retrograde, all their Contents are drove back, insomuch that Glysters have been seen to return into the Stomach. It may perhaps be answered, that the Intestines act more strongly, as they are full, as their Action is weakest when they are empty ; to which may be added, that the Fæces are collected not suddenly, and at once, but by degrees.

⁵ Following the Antients, we call that Part of the *Colon* the *Cæcum* ; which is large and globular at its end or beginning, and so capacious, as at some times to equal two Spans ; and in this the Fæces are collected as they slip thro' the *Ilium*. We cannot agree with the modern Anatomist *Vesalius*, and others, that the *Appendicula Vermiformis* should be called *Cæcum*, since that cannot be reckoned one of the large Intestines ; but the *Intestinum Cæcum* is the Seat of flatulent Disorders in hypocondriac People and pregnant Women, occasioned from the Air distending the Sides of the Intestine ; which Air is set at liberty by Putrifaction of the Matter, and exerts a considerable Force ; this Air passing thro' the whole *Colon*, occasions intolerable Pain, which is frequently attributed to the Spleen and Stomach, when they are not the least in Fault. I have even seen an Instance among Men who led sedentary Lives, where the hard Fæces have been gradually accumulated to so large a Quantity in this Intestine, as to occasion the Death of a considerable

Person,

Person, whose *Cæcum* was found distended with hard Fæces to such a degree, that upon opening him it appeared not lesser than a Man's Head. For it is to be observed, that all the more fluid Parts of the Aliment are absorbed in the small Intestines, and the remaining dry Fæces adhere sometimes like Glue to the Valve of the *Colon*, insomuch that I have frequently perceived it by the Touch in Women big with Child ; and from this Quarter proceeds many of the Disorders of Artists and Men of Letters, whose Fæces are obstructed from the inflected Posture of sitting still after Meals.

§. 109. The Reservoir or *Diverticulum* of the large *Cæcum*, is furnish'd with a small vermicular Appendix, or little *Intestine* ¹, and a *Valve* ², described by *Tulpius*, together with Ligaments which close the same, and prevent a Return of the Fæces into the *Ilium*; this Intestine ascending *perpendicularly* into the *Colon*, renders it impossible for the Fæces to return into the *Ilium*; but they stagnate, and are retained some time here, and are strongly compressed, not only by their own Weight, but also by the Contraction of the Intestine and circumjacent Parts ; by which means they are deprived of all their more fluid and aqueous Parts, which being absorb'd by the *Lymphatics* 4, are convey'd to the *Receptaculum Chyli* and *Thoracic* Duct, till at length the Fæces are form'd into hard, dry, figur'd, putrid, and fœtid Excrement, different from the Contents of *any* 5 of the other Intestines. The *Colon* is next, furnish'd with numerous and large *Valves* 6, disposed in three Ranks, formed and

supported

supported by the Action of three muscular Ligaments which contract the Capacity of the Inteftine, and detach muscular Fibres, to ftrengthen its thin and membranous Structure, which would be otherwife too weak to caufe a perpendicular Afcent of the Fæces; and being variously *inflected* 7, of a large Diameter, and about eight Hands Breadth long, is well adapted to collect, retain, and retard the Fæces, drain off their aqueous Parts, and *putrify* 8 the reft. The ftrong Fibres of its mufcular and membranous Coat being then irritated to *Contraction* 9 by the hard Fæces (which wou'd not pafs if the Tube was not diftractile, and their Surfaces lubricated with an oily *Mucus* from the *Glands* 10) they are by that means protruded into the *Rectum*, in which the Fæces are gradually collected without our Knowledge, but are difcharged indeed not without our Knowledge and Influence of the Mind, tho' they cannot be well retain'd by the Mind, when it is requifite they fhould be difcharged, without exciting a *convulfive Motion* 11, and very uneafy Senfation, which is a Circumftance much conducing to the Well-being of the Animal.

¹ This is a fmall flender Procefs of the *Cæcum*, arifing ufually from its bottom or fide, at fome diftance from the *Colon* in that Part which is oppofite to the Infertion of the *Ilium*; this Procefs, or fmall membranous Bag, is furnifh'd with glandular Cells, which difcharge a *Mucus* to the Fæces. This Appendix is larger in the *Fœtus*, which ferves to increafe the Space deftin'd for the Reception of its

Meconium,

Meconium, or Fæces, which at that that time fills all the large Inteſtines; but the ſmall Inteſtines admit no Part of the Excrement: but when the Fæces are accumulated in thoſe Parts to ſuch a degree that they cannot be eaſily contain'd, by diſtending and irritating the Inteſtine, it occaſions Pain, and cauſes the Infant to ſtruggle, whereby the natural Birth is promoted.

- ² This Valve has been deſcribed by *Varolius* and *Bauhine*, but moſt exactly by *Tulpius*, it being formed by an Inſertion of the *Ilium* ſome way into the *Colon*, in the ſame manner as the *Duodenum* is inſerted within the *Pylorus*: the *Ilium* and *Colon* at their Juncture do not make a right Angle in the human Body, as they do in Brutes; but the *Ilium* hangs pendulous a little way within the *Colon*, and being as it were divided in the middle, forms the Valve of the *Colon*, the Aperture of which is ſtrengthened by an annular Series of muſcular Fibres. The Uſe of this Valve is, to admit the groſs and fœcal Parts of the Aliment out of the *Ilium* into the *Colon*, and to prevent their Return again by any Cauſe from the *Colon* into the *Ilium*; the Valve being folded together in ſuch a manner, and contracted by its muſcular Fibres, that nothing can paſs out of the large into the ſmall Inteſtines; as readily appears from the Laws of Hydraulics and the Structure of the Part. Sometimes this Valve is lacerated, and becomes paralytic and relaxed, by ſome Violence or convulſive Motion; in which Caſe the Fæces of the large Inteſtines are regurgitated even by the Mouth, which filthy and terrible Diſorder, is from its own Nature called *Miſerere mei*. Below the Inſertion of this Valve is ſituated the large Cavity of the *Inteſtinum cœcum*, in which the Fæces are convey'd and accumulated.

This

³ This perpendicular Afcent of the *Colon*, and Incurvation thereof at the Liver, it being more inflected by the fedentary Pofture of the Studious, occafions the Fæces to ftagnate, and be retained longer ; and during the Putrifaction of the Fæces in this Cavity, they difcharge a confiderable Quantity of elaftic Air, whence flatulent Diforders, and the Symptoms familiar to hypochondriacal and ftudious Perfons.

⁴ *Malpighius* has obferved thefe Lymphatics in the Cells or Appendices of the *Inteftina Craffa* in an Afs, which he faw open into their Cavity, for the abforbing a turbid or dirty Lymph ; they are not indeed fo eafily perceived in the human Body, but that they are there, is apparent from the Inftances we have of Men kept alive a confiderable time barely by nourifhing Glyfters ; alfo from the Ufe of Glyfters made of Honey, Nitre and Water, in inflammatory Difeafes ; which would hardly be of any Service, if there was not a Paffage from the large Inteftines into the Blood, no Part of the Liquor in the Glyfter being difcharged again ; which evidently demonftrates an Abforption of the fame made by the Lymphatics : this Lymph is not indeed putrid, but is in a State tending to Putrifaction, and is of fome Ufe to the Blood when it arrives there.

⁵ The Fæces of the Inteftines are not fœtid when in the *Ilium*, notwithftanding they are pretty dry and exhaufted ; but as foon as they have paffed thro' the Valve of the *Colon*, they acquire a putrid and fœcal Stench, from ftagnating fo long in that Part, and from the fermenting Contents already in the Inteftine, with which they are mixed ; fo that from their natural Tendence to Putrifaction, and become alcalious in a warm and moift Place, they muft neceffarily put on the fore-mentioned

Y   Appear-

Appearance. This Change being quickly made in the Fæces, occafioned *Helmont* to imagine that it arofe from a Ferment refiding in the *Appendicula Vermiformis*, which converted the ufelefs Parts of the Food by its Acrimony into Dung ; but the fore-mentioned Caufes feem altogether fufficient, without any particular Ferment in this Part, which ufually contains nothing but a *Mucus*, difcharged by many fimple Glands ; nor do the Fæces become putrid and fœtid all at once, for they are more fo in the *Rectum* than in the *Colon*, and ftill more fo as they arrive nearer the *Anus*.

⁶ There are three ftrong Ligaments detach'd from the *Appendicula Vermiformis* on each fide, thro' the whole Length of the *Colon*, which contract that Inteftine like fo many Mufcles, and terminate in the *Rectum* ; thefe Ligaments are at leaft fix times fhorter than the *Colon* itfelf, fo that upon feparating them from that Inteftine, it becomes much elongated, thinner and narrower, its thicknefs being entirely owing to thefe Ligaments : the Ufe of thefe Ligaments is to elevate the *Rectum*, and contract the Length of the *Colon*, or approximate one end towards the other, by that means to contract it in length, and form it into Wrinkles or Cells, which do not confift in a Corrugation of the villous Coat, which is not to be found in the large Inteftines, but of the nervous Coat ; which being feparated from its Ligaments, the *Colon* becomes four times as long as before: this is a furprifing Contrivance, to render the Inteftines capable of retarding the Fæces, without being of any great Length or large Diameter ; for if the Paffage of the Fæces had been direct and open, the Animal would have been continually difturbed with the difagreeable, but neceffary Evacuation of this Part ; the *Colon* is therefore formed of a middle

Capacity,

Capacity, and replenifhed with moveable Valves, fo that it can dilate and make way for the larger Fæces, and contract itfelf to the fmaller. Thefe Valves are very large in the Colons of Rabbits, Hares, Birds, and Horfes, in order to divide and give the Fæces a globular Figure; but there are not any to be found in the *Rectum.* Another Ufe of thefe Valves is, to fuftain the Weight of the Fæces, and to facilitate their Afcent in the *Colon.*

⁷ The various Inflections of the *Colon* in the human Body, accurately defcribed by *Vefalius,* is very different from that in Brutes; for the *Colon* firft afcends from its Origin at the right *Ilium* up to the Liver and *Duodenum,* where it is inflected acrofs at right Angles under the Stomach towards the Spleen; where being again inflected, it forms a Dilatation, which receives the *Flatus* in hypochondriacal People and the Fæces of Women with Child; from thence it defcends in a right Angle down to the left *Ilium,* where afcending a little obliquely towards the right Side, it makes its laft Inflection, and forms the *Rectum* defcending upon the *Os facrum.* Hence we obferve, that the Fæces are twice obliged to afcend perpendicularly, paffing over the Refiftance of four Angles, two right, and two acute. In that Curvature of the *Colon,* form'd by its tranfverfe Progrefs from the Right to the Left Side, and defcending near the Spleen, is the Seat of thofe Pains in the Studious and Sedentary; which are often improperly attributed to the Spleen, fince they proceed from the confin'd *Flatus* diftending the Inteftine, which is in the Angle obftructed by the indurated and accumulated Fæces: which fame Diforder alfo occurs in Women with Child, when the diftended *Uterus* occupies almoft the whole Capacity of the *Abdomen.* That the Spleen is not the Seat of thefe

Complaints,

Complaints, appears from their Removal by a laxative Medicine, which cannot be suppofed capable of extending its Effects to that *Vifcus*.

⁸ All the recent Parts of Animals and Vegetables, when confined in a clofe and warm Place, putrify and degenerate into a ftinking Excrement. and as this is the Cafe in the Inteftines, we find they undergo the like Changes there; the more readily, as the Excrements are charged with animal Humours, efpecially the Bile, which is of an alcalefcent Nature, and tends greatly to Putrifaction; therefore human Excrements afford a volatile alcaline Salt by Diftillation, even tho' the Perfon was fed only upon acid Food. It is alfo obfervable the inteftinal Fæces afford *Phofphorus* in the greateft Plenty.

⁹ This Motion of the large Inteftines is different from the periftaltic Motion of the fmall Inteftines, by which the latter are kept in conftant and fucceffive Agitations or Contractions; for the Contraction of the large Inteftines is mufcular, and perform'd only when the Fæces are prefent, ftimulating by their Quantity and Acrimony, and ceafing again when the Inteftines are not irritated by their Fæces.

¹⁰ Thefe are large folitary Glands, which difcharge their *Mucus* by large Ducts into the Cavity of the Inteftines.

¹¹ There are Nerves extremely fenfible diftributed to the laft of the large Inteftines, which renders the Preffure and Retention of the hard Fæces fo intolerable, as to occafion that uneafy Senfation or Motion to Stool, which is not properly a Pain, but a fort of Convulfion of all the Mufcles confpiring to expel the offending Matter with fo much Impetuofity, that the Fæces are frequently incapable of being retain'd behind the *Rectum*, notwithftanding

withstanding all the Influence of the Mind to prevent their Exclusion. Related to this Motion, is
the Throws of the Mother in Labour, who is no
sooner seized by her Labour Pains, than a violent
Tenesmus follows, with a Protrusion of the Head of
the Infant to the Mouth of the *Uterus*, in such
manner, that the Mother is rather tortured with an
intolerable *Conatus* than real Pains. A like *Conatus* or *Tenesmus* is also observed amongst the Inhabitants of the *Indies*, who are fatigued with such
an uneasy Sensation from a Vellication of the Nerves
in the *Rectum*[1] and *Anus* by sharp Humours, as to
oblige them to be constantly going to Stool, without Effect, where-ever they are going, till they at
last perish in great Misery with a Convulsion of all
the Extremities.

§. 110. The Fæces are then forced into the
Rectum[1], which descends almost perpendicularly thro' the *Pelvis*, and being well lubricated on its internal Surface, without any Valves,
and without any muscular Ligament, by that
means the Fæces meet with a more easy De-
scent, whilst they irritate its muscular Fibres
to contract by their Weight and Acrimony, or
both. The muscular Coat of this Intestine consists of strong *longitudinal* Fibres, arising from
an Expansion of the Ligaments of the *Colon*
meeting together, invest all the whole external Part of the *Rectum*, and joining the Extremity of the *Colon* and *Rectum* to each other,
they also contract the Length and Diameter of
the latter ; to do which they are also assisted
by *spiral*[2] or circular Fibres, whereby the Fæces are driven down even to the *Sphincter*, stop-

ping

ping at the flefhy Columns and *Valves* 3 at the End of this laft Inteftine.

1 When the three Ligaments of the *Colon* have reached the *Rectum*, they become expanded, and diftribute their Fibres equally over that Inteftine, without contracting it into Valves: Thefe elevate and fuftain the *Rectum* fo ftrongly, that if it ever fuffers a *Prolapfus*, it is always by way of Inverfion.

2 Thefe longitudinal and fpiral Fibres affift each other in their Action; the longitudinal Fibres draw the Inteftine backward over the Fæcus, and elevate it after they are difcharged, to prevent a *Prolapfus Ani*, while the fpiral Fibres do by this Contraction protrude the Fæces forward. It is alfo obfervable, that this Motion of expelling the Fæces, is never retrograde or reverted, as that of the fmall Inteftines frequently is.

3 Thefe fimple and compound Valves at the Extremity of the *Anus*, have been accurately defcribed by *Morgagni* in his *Adverfaria Anatomica* III. *Fig.* I.

§. 111. Then the large, thick, flefhy, and orbicular or oval *fphincter* 1 Mufcle of the *Anus*, embracing the End of the *Rectum*, being relaxed 2, the elevating Mufcles are next contracted, whofe Fibres are inferted under the former, arife from the infide of the *Os Pubis*, *Ifchium* and *Sacrum*, confifting of many ftrong converging Fibres, which being inferted under the *Sphincter*, are extended to the very End of the *Anus*, which they dilate and elevate; by which means the Fæces are more expofed to the

the Preſſure of the *Peritonæum* and circumjacent Parts above the *Pelvis*; then the *Pelvis*
being ſtrictly compreſſed by the Air inſpired,
retained, and rarefied in the *Thorax*, together
with the Contraction of the *Diaphragm* and abdominal Muſcles, the Fæces meet with a ready
Deſcent thro' the *Rectum*, whoſe Sides are
plentifully lubricated with a ſoft *Mucus* 3, preffed out from its numerous Cells and ſmall Glands
by the Fæces; which being now excluded, all
the preceding are relaxed, and the *Sphincter*
Muſcle alone is ſtrongly contracted. The large
Quantity of *Fat* 4 which inveſts this Inteſtine
on every Side, with the ample circumambient
Space fill'd with nothing but ſoft Fat, render it
very well adapted to receive and retain the Fæces
to be expell'd.

¹ It has been controverted amongſt Anatomiſts,
how it cou'd be poſſible that the *Sphincter* ſhou'd
retain the Fæces, ſince *Bernoulli* has demonſtrated
that an annular or circular Muſcle cannot be contracted above one third Part of its Diameter; but
the *Sphincter*-Muſcle of the *Anus* is not a Line without Breadth; but being contracted, it forms its
large internal Membrane into *Rugæ*, which protruding into the Cavity of the Inteſtine, fills up
its Space, and prevents any thing from eſcaping.
Anatomiſts are uſed to deſcribe the *Elevatories Ani*,
as ariſing from each Side of the *Anus*, and terminating in the Margin or Extremity of the *Rectum*;
which is falſe, for they ariſe befo e from the *Os
Pubis*, and behind from the *Os Sacrum*; alſo on each
Side from the *Oſſa Ilia*; from whence deſcending,
their muſcular Fibres inveſt the whole Surface of the

Rectum; so that they not only elevate, but also strongly dilate the same; which has justly been observed by *Bidlow*, *Cowper*, and *Santorini*.

₂ The *Sphincter*-Muscle of the *Anus* is not relaxed by the Will: I even much doubt whether the Mind has a confiderable Influence upon any of the *Sphincters*; it is relaxed or opened, by becoming Paralytic, from the Preffure of the *Faeces*; so that being deprived of its Influx of the nervous Fluid, it cannot exert its wonted Refiftance, especially as the *Diaphragm* preffes down all the *Viscera* of the *Abdomen* with a confiderable Force, which at laft terminates or acts only upon the *Sphincter*. The Force of the retained Air in Infpiration ought alfo to be allowed a Share, with the forcible Depreffure of the *Diaphragm*, in expelling the Faeces, which always ceafe to be difcharged upon Expiration; so that as the *Fœtus* does not refpire, it alfo does not difcharge its Faeces by the *Anus*, whilft inclofed in the *Uterus*; and if it difcharge any Faeces thro' the *Uterus* in the Birth, we may be certain it has breathed, and that if it be not inftantly delivered, it will not long furvive; in this Action therefore the Air, which is taken in with a ftrong and deep Infpiration, is retained and rarefied in the Lungs; the *Glottis* being clofed, and its Expiration prevented, whilft it acts upon the defcending *Diaphragm*, which preffed down the Stomach, Liver, and all the Inteftines upon the *Pelvis*, which being furnifhed with no antagonifing Mufcles, receives the Force of all the other Parts of the *Abdomen*, whereby the Urine and Faeces are expelled with a confiderable Force.

₃ There are in this Part abundance of very large mucous Ducts, or *Lacunae*, into which a *Fiftula* of the *Anus* often infinuates, and becomes very obftinate, confuming all the Fat of this Inteftine, infomuch

much that its Sides become inflamed and ulcerated,
by·rubbing againſt each other, withŏut any Lubrication; but the *Sphincter* itſelf is ſeldom corroded,
except in the. Venereal Diſeaſe. If this *Mucus* is
wanting, as it frequently is in Infants, the Child is
in danger of periſhing, if an oily Glyſter be not
injected, to lubricate the Excrement, which is then
indurated and dried like Chalk. Alſo in the blind ›
Piles the acute Pain may be prevented by injecting
half an Ounce of Oil before going to Stool, which
Experiment has never miſcarried in all the Patients
who have had the ſame adminiſtred by my Advice.

⁴ The *Inteſtinum Rectum* is very fat, infomŭch
that it is vulgarly called by Butchers the fat Gut,
which is even ſo in emaciated Subjects; beſides
which it is alſo furniſhed with numerous mucous
Glánds, whoſe Contents are preſſed out by the Contraction of the longitudinal Fibres, which ſhorten
the Inteſtine.

§. 112. From hence appears what Materials
compóſe the Fæces ; and whether they do not
conſiſt in Part of the uſeleſs Superfluities of the
*Bile*¹, *Blood*², *Mucus*, *Saliva*, Lymph, and
pancreatic Juice; the *Cauſe*³ of their Formation into Excrement ; and whether it be from
a Stercoracious *Ferment*⁴, or Part of the Fæces before retained; why the Inteſtines are
more copiouſly repleniſh'd with ſmall *Glands*⁵
and *Mucus*, as they are nearer their Extremity; of what Uſe is the *Appendiculæ Adipoſæ*⁶
of the *Colon* and *Rectum*; why ſtrong People
are *coſtive*⁷, and their Fæces few, light, and
indurated; and why ſuch are frequently ſubject

ject to the *Piles*[8]; why expelling the Fæces also difcharges the *Urine*[9]; why thofe who have a *Stone*[10] in their Bladder are troubled with a *Tenefmus*; why People who have Dyfenteries are fo frequently troubled with the *Strangury*[11]; and why a Strangury is often accompanied with a *Tenefmus*[12]; and laftly, why the *Rectum* is fufpended *freely*[13], without being connected to any Bone or Mufcle in a large Cavity, filled only with Fat.

[1] *Helmont* ftrenuoufly denies that any Part of the Bile is difcharged with the Fæces, or tinges them; but their yellow Colour is a fufficient Proof of the Bile being prefent, as it is a common Obfervation, that the ftronger the Bile, the deeper yellow is the Fæces; and the weaker the Bile, the paler are the Fæces; fo that in the Jaundice they are often whitifh, or Afh-colour'd.

[2] There are many Arguments to prove that the Blood itfelf difcharges its excrementitious Parts by the Inteftines. As, (1) The lax Structure of the mefenterick Veffels, tranfmitting the ceraceous Injection into the Cavity of the Inteftines. (2.) Their frequent Inofculations with each other; fo that by injecting one Trunk, all the reft are diftended. (3.) The *Meconium* in the *Fœtus*, which feems to be rather formed from the Blood than the Liquor of the *Amnios*, which has been attenuated by the Action of fo many Veffels, and is much more fubtil than the Blood itfelf; tho' the *Meconium* abounds fo as to fill all the large Inteftines, and is fo feculent as to refemble *Opium*. Alfo, (4.) The Depuration of the Blood by the Inteftines, which is fo ftrongly promoted by the Exhibition of brifk Purges, which excite frequent and copious Difcharges.

charges. There are alfo other Reafons to prove
that the Liver, Spleen, and whole Mafs of Blood,
may be freed from their noxious Parts by the Inteftines; which was the Opinion of the Antients.
We are alfo furnifh'd with another Argument from
fad Experience; for fince the Invention of the triangular Dagger, called a Bayonet, there have been
frequent Inftances of Wounds dividing the Inteftines; in the Cure of which, nothing was more
neceffary than fupplying the Patient with Aliment
affording little or no Fæces, till within the Space
of fourteen Days the Inteftines were again united;
this was performed by feeding the Patients with
Broth only, by which means there were no Fæces
difcharged for the Space of 14 or 21 Days; at the
end of which time, when the Excrements were
voided, they appeared like *Meconium*, proceeding
chiefly from the animal Humours difcharged into
the Inteftines.

³ By draining the Aliment of all fuch Parts as
are aceffent and nutritious, the Remainder being
conftantly fupplied with animal Juices, tending to
Putrifraction with the addition of Heat and Reft;
whence it follows, from their own Nature and
fpontaneous Changes, that they become putrid and
excrementitious.

⁴ According to the conftant Obfervation of *Helmont*, who could never find fœtid Excrement in the
Ilium, nor any Contents of the *Colon* which were
not fœtid; he therefore fought for the Caufe of this
Change in the Confines of the *Ilium* and *Colon*;
and as he was previoufly biafs'd with the Notion
of Fermentation, he fuppofed a yellow Ferment in
the *Cæcum* which putrified the Fæces; and returning to the Kidneys, tinged the Urine of a yellow
Colour; which, he fays, *Galen* wrongly attributes
to the Bile. But that Gentleman feems either ne-

ver

ver to have read the Writings of *Harvey*, or elfe he perufed them when he was too old to change his Opinion; but he might have known that all Vegetables, even the moft acid, putrify only by ftagnating in a clofe, warm, and moift Place.

⁵ Becaufe the Fæces are drier, harder, and more acrimonious, as they approach nearer to the Extremity of the Inteftines.

⁶ The cellular Coat is more confpicuous in the large than fmall Inteftines, and is more plentifully fupplied with Oil between their external and mufcular Coat; but the *Omentum* is wanting to thefe Inteftines, and their mufcular Fibres require more Lubrication; without which their nervous Coat would be injur'd by the Attrition of the hard Fæces, not without danger of Inflammation or Excoriation; we therefore meet with a Portion of Fat about the *Anus* near an Inch thick, which being diffolved by Heat, tranfudes into the Cavity of the Inteftine, to lubricate its internal Surface with the Fæces, that their Attrition might not produce Pain, Inflammation, or Ulcer; and accordingly we obferve that fat People are feldom troubled with the Piles, but lean Perfons very often.

⁷ It is a commonly receiv'd Opinion, that it is more healthy to be loofe than coftive; and many being prejudiced with that Notion, are continually irritating their Bowels with cathartic and laxative Medicines, by which means they become infenfible and fluggifh to the natural and weaker *Stimulus* of the Bile; but it is certain, contrary to this Opinion, that the digeftive Organs are always ftronger, in proportion as the Fæces are harder, lighter, and more figur'd; for that is a certain Token that all their ufeful Juices have been abforbed by the Lacteals. Nor is there any room to fufpect Danger from a Conftipation of the Bowels

els for the Space of fix, or even twelve Days, if
the *Abdomen* appears foft, and not tumified, and
the Appetite ftrong in the mean time; whereas a
fluid State of the Fæces denotes, and is a Caufe of
Weaknefs; it fignifies that the Aliment has been
acted upon by a Force too weak in the digeftive
Organs, whence a great Part of the Chyle is loft,
and difcharged with the Fæces; but the hard and
dry Fæces are lighter than foft and fluid, becaufe
the Bread, *&c.* of which they are compofed, are
lighter than Water; but the Fæces of People in a
Dyfentery fink to the bottom of Water; dry Fæces, without a Tumour of the *Abdomen*, are therefore healthy, and fignify that the Aliment is perfectly digefted or attenuated, affording a large
Quantity of Chyle to fupply the Blood and all the
other Juices, affording very few Fæces. To this
Place belongs the Obfervation of *Sanctorius*, that
Perfpiration being increafed, the other Excretions
are diminifhed; and the contrary.

⁸ This Propofition, notwithftanding its Truth,
feems to be a Paradox. We find that Women
have a falutary Difcharge of Blood from their
Uterus every Month, which frees them from a
Plethora, and prevents many confequent Diforders;
in like manner there is no reafon why a fimilar
Difcharge of fuperfluous Blood in Men fhould not
be equally ferviceable. The *Italians*, *Spaniards*,
and *Dutch*, congratulate their Friends upon the
Acceffion of a large hæmorrhoidal Flux in Diforders; and when the hæmorrhoidal Difcharge is
either diminifhed, or wholly fupreffed, violent
Head-achs, and many other Diforders follow. Alfo
if bleeding at the Nofe is ufeful to a plethoric
young Man, why may not the like Difcharge in
the Piles prove of the fame Ufe? Our next Bufinefs is to explain why healthy and ftrong People,
who

who are ufually coftive, are more fubject to the
Piles than others; in them the hard and globular
figur'd Fæces filling the whole Cavity of the Inteftine, cannot be difcharg'd without violent ftrain-
ing; fo that by the ftrong Preffure of the Diaphragm and abdominal Mufcles upon the *Rectum*
to difcharge its Fæces, the Veins diftributed upon
the Surface of that Inteftine are ftrongly compreffed, and their Blood ftopt in its Paffage; fo that
being ftill drove forward by their Artery into them,
they are more diftended with Blood; and being
almoft deftitute of Elafticity, they remain dilated
even after the Preffure ceafes, which occafions varicofe Tumours or Knots, continuing diftended
with thick Blood; which upon a Repetition of the
former Preffure burft, and difcharge a Quantity
of thick and dark-colour'd Blood, which is called
the open Piles; but while the varicofe Tumours
remain entire, they are called the dry or blind Piles.
If the Coats of the Veins were thick and ftrong,
the Piles remain blind, or dry, with great Pain;
but if they were thin and weak, they break eafily.
Men of Letters are frequently fubject to this Diforder from a Conftipation of their Bowels; whence
arifes Pain and many bad Symptoms, in thofe Perfons whofe Nerves are eafily diforder'd from the
fmalleft Caufes of any other kind; thefe will find
the moft Benefit by injecting an Ounce of Oil into
the *Anus* before they go to ftool, ordering them to
abftain from warm, dry, and aftringent Food, and
to eat frrequently of Garden Fruits. Women are
feldom diforder'd with the Piles, except when they
are near Lying-in, when the *Uterus*, which is then
greatly diftended, compreffes the hæmorrhoidal
Veins.

⁹ Becaufe the fame Force of the *Diaphragm* and
abdominal Mufcles which difcharge the Fæces,

will

will alfo comprefs the Bladder ; but the fame Force which difcharges the Urine, will not alfo expel the Fæces ; becaufe the Bladder may be emptied by a lefs Preffure than what is required to overcome the Refiftance of the *Sphincter Ani.* It is alfo obfervable, that fome of the Fibres of the *Elevatores Ani* inveft part of the *Urethra,* and proftrate ; whence it frequently happens, that the *Mucus* of thofe Parts is frequently preffed out at the fame time when the Fæces are difcharged ; which is a Cafe occurring in the moft healthy Men, without any Caufe of a *Gonorrhæa,* which is frequently fufpected by Phyficians.

¹⁰ Becaufe the Neck of the Bladder is incumbent upon the *Rectum,* by which means the Refiftance of a Stone ftimulates the *Rectum,* the fame as hard Fæces.

¹¹ From a fharp Matter lodg'd in the Interftices of the *Anus,* which corroding the *Rectum,* puts it into a convulfive Motion, which by Continuity of Parts is communicated to the Bladder, whence a Strangury is frequently met with in Dyfenteries ; but a Strangury is alfo fometimes occafioned by hard Fæces ftopping in the *Rectum,* and preffing upon the Neck of the Bladder, which irritates it in the fame manner as a Stone.

¹² The Bladder contracting itfelf with a great Force to difcharge its Contents, is formed into a globular Figure ; and being incumbent upon the *Anus,* gives the Senfation of hard Fæces ; befides which the Bladder is alfo irritated and follicited to difcharge its Contents by the Acrimony of the Urine, as we have fometimes obferv'd from drinking new Ale ; which Irritation is communicated by a Confent of Parts to the *Rectum,* which is nearly attach'd to the Neck of the *Bladder* and *Urethra.*

¹³ The

¹³ The generality of the fofter Parts of the human Body are conftantly attach'd or fix'd to fome Bone, only the *Uterus* and *Rectum* are at liberty on every fide; which was neceffary, that they might be equally and largely dilated. When a Perfon has been conftipated for the Space of above fix Days, the hard Fæces are fometimes fo compacted together in the *Rectum*, that they dilate it like a Ball, and prevent the Paffage of any Glyfter; in which Cafe the hard Fæces are to be taken out with an Inftrument, and afterwards a Glyfter injected.

Concerning the Action of the Mefentery on the Chyle.

§. 113. THE Chyle (§. 105.) being impelled into the open Mouths of the *Lacteals* ¹ (§. 103.) by the periftaltic Motion (§. 103, 104.) is by the fame Motion and Preffure of the abdominal Mufcles and *Diaprhagm* impelled forward towards its Receptacle. But fince we are taught by many Experiments, that the Lacteals open *obliquely* ² into the Cavity of the Inteftines, their Mouths being extremely fmall, we are affured that only the more white and *fluid* ³ Part of the Chyle, feparated from the more grofs, *ramous* ⁴, fibrous, and yellow or afh-coloured Part, enters by their Orifices, which pafs immediately thro' the mufcular Coat of the Inteftines, and terminating in

larger ⁵

larger 5 Veſſels under the external Coat of the Inteſtines, proceed towards the *Meſentery* 6.

1 As ſoon as a Particle of the Chyle has enter'd an Orifice of the Lacteals, it meets with a Valve which ſeparates it from the Inteſtine, and prevents it from returning back; the Chyle is alſo drawn in by means of theſe Valves, as if it were in a ſort of *Vacuum*.

2 That the Lacteals have an oblique Inſertion into the Inteſtines, is evident ; becauſe neither Water nor Wind can be forc'd out of the Inteſtines into them; and becauſe their Orifices and firſt Progreſs cannot be ſeen even with a Microſcope. From this Obliquity of their Inſertion it happens, that the Inteſtines being diſtended, tranſmit nothing into the lacteal Veſſels ; but when the Inteſtines are contracted and render'd ſhorter, that Part of the Chyle intercepted by the *Rugæ* of their villous Coat, is compreſſed; and at the ſame time the muſcular Fibres being contracted, the Chyle is retained in the *Villi* of their internal Coat; in the next Inſtant, when the muſcular Fibres are relaxed, the Chyle in the Lacteals which paſs thro' the muſcular Coat, runs toward their cellular Coat ; and thus by the ſucceſſive Contraction and Preſſure of the muſcular Coat of the Inteſtines upon the Origin of the Lacteals, one Part of the Chyle drives the other forward towards the Meſentery.

3 A great Part of the Food with which we are nouriſhed being converted into Chyle, is form'd into Globules, which are yet much leſs than thoſe of the Blood; theſe Globules have been obſerved by *Lewenhoeck* in Wine, Ale, and Dough: ſpherical Particles can more eaſily enter the cylindrical Orifices of the Lacteals, as they are of a leſs Diameter, and more compacted by the Power of the

digeſtive

digeſtive Organs, the Parts of the Chyle becoming leſs porous or more denſe by Attenuation; and their white Colour, joined with their ſmooth Surface, is a Mark of Denſity.

4 Thus it is manifeſt, that a Feather or Piece of Wool ſwimming in a Fluid, will never paſs thro' a narrow Aperture; but only ſuch Subſtances as are more denſe, or contained under a leſs Surface, will make their way into and through ſmall Orifices.

5 Immediately above the Inteſtines, and ſometimes even in their cellular Coat, there are Lacteals viſible to the naked Eye, and large enough to admit a Probe, as *Ruyſch* informs us, and *Nuck* has delineated.

6. It is not every Anatomiſt that gives us a true Idea of the Structure of the Meſentery. The *Peritonæum* inveſting all the *Viſcera* of the *Abdomen*, alſo covers the *Aorta*, *Vena Cava*, and Nerves. When the Veſſels ſtrike off from the Loins, they do not perforate, but are intercepted in a Reduplication of the *Peritonæum*; theſe Veſſels are the ſuperior and inferior meſenteric Arteries, with the Receptacle of the Chyle, and correſponding Veins leading to the *Cava*. This Reduplication of the *Peritonæum* alſo intercepts and ſuſtains the lacteal Veſſels and Branches of the *Vena Porta*.

§. 114. Hence it appears, why a great variety of acrimonious, hard, and ſharp Subſtances, which are ſwallowed, prove *inoffenſive* 1 to human Bodies, and no ways detrimental to their Health; and if we compare the *Structure* 2 of the *Oeſophagus*, Stomach, and Inteſtines, with that of the other *Viſcera*, they will appear very different: As for inſtance, the Largeneſs

nefs or Difproportion of the Cavity of the Inteftines with the *narrow*3 Orifices of the Lacteals which thence arife; to which we may
add the Aptnefs of the fmall *Sphincters* 4 at the
Mouths of the Lacteals, to be contracted by
acrimonious Particles, which guards them
from a too eafy Admiffion of fuch Humours.

1 Thus we feed on almoft all Sorts of Subftances; but were many of them to enter the Blood,
they would become Poifons; fome Parts of the
Chyle are acrimonious, hard and vifcid, others oily,
and rancid, and yet we receive no Injury from either.

2 Their Compofition being of tough and ftrong
Membranes, which ftrongly refift the Action and
Injuries of other Bodies, infomuch that boiling the
Inteftines for the Space of ten Hours does not diffolve them; nor are they digefted after they have
undergone the Actions of the Teeth and Stomach
of a voracious Dog. The internal Coat of the Inteftines of Sheep, &c. remain tough and whole,
after they have been boiled long enough to render
the minc'd Meat within them foft and tender; as
in *Bolognia* Puddings, Sauffages, &c. There is a
great difference between the tough Confiftence of
the Inteftines when formed into Cat-gut or elaftic
Fiddle-ftrings, and the foft Subftance of the Liver, which crumbles between one's Fingers.

3 Which only tranfmit fuch Parts of the Aliment
as have before been form'd into Globules, of a determinate Size, by the digeftive Organs; all Particles of any other Figure, coming obliquely upon
the Mouths of the Lacteals, being excluded; and
if they are acrimonious, they ftimulate their membranous Mouths or Sphincters to Contraction.

4 There

There are a vast Number of Nerves, and those extremely sensible, distributed to the Intestines, which are easily vellicated by any thing acrimonious; these contract the whole Capacity of the Intestines, as well as the small Orifices of the Lacteals, whereby they refuse Admittance to acrimonious and injurious Substances; which Office is by *Helmont* attributed to his *Archæus*. By the same Contraction they also press out a Lymph from the ultimate Branches of the mesenteric Arteries, to mollify and dilute the acrimonious Food. If a Grain of Salt slips into the Lungs, it occasions incessant coughing; if any thing alike acrimonious should penetrate to the Brain, it will there occasion surprising Commotions. We see that Wine affects the Tongue with a pleasant Acidity, but if a little of it falls into the Eyes, it produces great Irritation till it is wash'd out by the Flux of Tears. The whole Surface of the Skin is also corrugated or contracted into numerous small Tubercles by the Action of injurious Cold, whereby the Orifices or Sphincters of the Pores are contracted, the Air excluded, and their contained Fluids, which would have been discharged in a warm Air, are thus retained. So it is also in the Intestines, Poisons do not enter the lacteal Vessels; but being mix'd with the Chyle, are excluded by their Sphincters, being afterwards discharged by the convulsive Irritation which they excite.

§. 115. The several Causes which impel the Chyle into the Lacteals (§. 113.) still continue to *protrude*[1] fresh Chyle, and press forward what was before received, by which means the Chyle is forced thro' the Lacteals, seated in the cellular Substance of *Ruyfch*, between the *Du-*

plicature

plicatue ² of the *Mefentery*, where it is detained from flowing back again by femilunar Valves
fix'd by *Pairs* ³ in the Lacteals, and its Courfe
determined towards the Loins.

¹ The lacteal Veffels pafs through the mufcular
Coat of the Inteftines, and creep along the cellular
Coat, without perforating the external; fo that
having reach'd the cellular Subftance of the Mefentery, they are by that defended and lubricated
in their Courfe.

² The Force which firft impell'd the Chyle into
the Lacteals, feems to ceafe. where thofe Veffels
perforate the mufcular Coat of the Inteftines, where
it is protruded forward by fucceffive Supplies of
fucceeding new Chyle, whilft its Return is prevented by their Valves.

³ Thefe Valves fuftain the Weight of the Chyle
in its Afcent, and prevent it from returning back
the way it came; they appear to be fo numerous
and ftrong, that *Mercury* being injected by the
Lacteals, could never break thro' their Refiftance,
fo as to pafs into the Cavity of the Inteftines; nor
can Air be forced thro' thofe Veffels into the Inteftines by inflating the thoracic Duct and Lacteals,
&c. Thefe Valves alfo prevent the preceding
Chyle from obftructing the Progrefs of that which
follows; fo that the Chyle meets with lefs Refiftance in its Progrefs, proportionable to the Number
of Valves; and the Space between the two preceding Valves being emptied, makes a fort of *Vacuum*,
into which the fucceeding Chyle flows without any
Refiftance; and in this Refpect they feem not to
differ from thofe in the Lymphatics which were demonftrated by *Ruyfch* in his younger Days; notwithftanding his Antagonift *Bilfius*, who being not

skill'd in Physic, 'tho' well versed in living Diffe-ctions, maintain'd that the lacteal Vessels had no Valves, and that *Flatus* might be easily drove thro' them into the Intestines from the Receptacle; but *Rusch* ty'd a lacteal Vessel of a Horse lately kill'd in two places, and inserted a small Steel Tube, made by our Countryman *Musschenbroeck*, and in-flating it with Air, dry'd and inverted it, and de-monstrated double Valves.

§. 116. The Lacteals in a human Mesente-ry being extremely minute at their Origin, unite and meet together in acute Angles, form-ing *larger* [1] Vessels; which Vessels afterwards recede from each other, and forming a Sort of Islands, they meet together again, and uniting in their Progress, they form still larger Vessels; all which are furnished with many distinct Valves. In these Vessels, call'd Lacteals of the first Order, the Chyle is more perfectly mixed, *attenuated* [2], and rendered more fluid.

[1] Hence the intimate Mixture, Uniformity, and Attenuation of the Chyle in these Vessels; for if different Juices, conveyed by separate Canals, at last return into one Vessel, they will undergo an intimate Mixture: but this Communication of the lacteal Vessels with each other is often repeated, by which means their Mixture is render'd still more uniform; which it would not be if the Vessels ran parallel, or had but one Communication with each other: thus if two Vessels, conveying different Fluids, communicate with each other but in one part only, the Liquors will flow out of their con-taining Tubes distinct in their Direction and Co-
lours,

lours, the Red by itfelf, and alfo the Blue; or they will be but half mixed, half of the blüe Liquor flowing thro' the red Veffel, and half of the red thro' the blue: but if the Tubes frequently unite, feparate, and again communicate, the Liquor will be of one Colour in both of them. In the fame manner the Chyle, which comes feculent from the large Inteftines, meets and mixes with the more mild and fubtil Chyle of the fmall Inteftines, fo as to form one fimilar milky Fluid.

² If a Liquor be moved with a very great Velocity, its Parts will not be divided. or attenuated without the Refiftance of fome Solids, upon which the Parts of the Liquor may impinge, and be divided from each other; and this is admirably well effected by the Angles of the Veffels: for if one Veffel be divided into two Branches, its contained Liquor will ftrike upon the Angle of its Divifion, and be thereby attenuated; and thus the Chyle is prevented from congealing or running into Grumes by its flow motion thro' the Lacteals: by increafing the Contact of Particles, they attract and adhere to each other more ftrongly, and thence lofe their Motion; but if their Contact be perpetually changed, and the Particles feparated, they will not concrete together.

§. 117. The Lacteals being thus diftributed through the Mefentery, fome in right Lines, others in oblique ones, varioufly interfecting and inofculating with each other, proceed to the very foft and fcattered *Glands* ¹ difperfed thro' the middle of the Mefentery; and meeting together in thefe Glands, which they *penetrate* ² and *inveft* ³, they pafs out again from them in larger and lefs numerous Branches,

Z 4 diftended

distended with the Chyle, now render'd more fluid and diluted. These Lacteals, which convey the Chyle to the Receptacle at the Loins, are also furnish'd with many distinct Valves, and are denominated Lacteals of the second Order.

' *Eustachius* was the first that described these Glands, which he did so well, that *Ruysch* with his Injection, and the other minute Anatomists, could make but little Improvement therein ; they are usually distributed in the human Mesentery, without observing any constant or regular Order, only they usually adhere to the Sides of the Blood Vessels at their Ramifications, as *Eustachius* has accurately expressed in his Figure of them. These Glands gradually shrink and disappear in old People, insomuch that I and my Friend *Ruysch* could scarce perceive any Remains of them in the Mesentery of an old Woman which he injected. And the same has been also observed by *Ruysch*, not only in the Glands of the Mesentery, but also in the Glands of the Breasts, *Thymus*, &c. but without any evident Cause. The Glands of the Mesentery are so soft, that they may be squeez'd to pieces by the Fingers. In the generality of Brutes these Glands are not dispersed thro' the Mesentery as in the human Body, but collected into one large Gland, which being fixed in the Center of the Mesentery, adheres to the Loins, and was by *Asellius* called *Pancreas*, from its Similitude to that Gland ; and other succeeding Anatomists also adding the Name of its first Describer, have called it *Pancreas Asellii*. So that Brutes have but one Order of Lacteals, the Structure of the other Parts of their Mesentery being different from that of the human.

This

² This is demonstrated by the remarkable Observation of *Nuck*, made in the Body of a Clown, who being kill'd at a public Feasting, was publicly opened by Order of the Magistrates, to discover the nature of his Wound. In this Subject the *Mercury* which was injected into the Lacteals of the first Order, penetrated the mesenteric Glands, and fill'd several of their Vessels, passing afterwards into the Lacteals of the second Order, beyond them. We do not know of any Anatomist that has described this Structure before *Nuck*, which has been universally received by his Successors.

³ All the Lacteals enter some Gland or other of the Mesentery, but in their Passage they ride over and invest some Glands without entring them; and other Glands they pass under in the same manner; but at those Glands which they penetrate into, they are not lost, but come out again at the opposite side of the Gland which they enter'd.

§. 118. From hence it appears, that nothing is separated from the Chyle by the mesenteric Glands; but that the Chyle is by them *diluted* ¹ with Lymph, and rendered more fluid in its Passage.

¹ It has been the Opinion of some considerable Anatomists, that the most subtil Part of the Chyle was absorbed by the mesenteric Glands, the Remainder passing on thro' the Lacteals of the second Order; but if any thing was separated from the Chyle in those Glands, it must either be of a thinner or thicker Consistence than the Chyle itself; if it was thinner, the Remainder of the Chyle would be more inspissated, which is contrary to Experience, by which we find that the Chyle in the

Lacteals

Lacteals of the second Order is more dilute; if it was thicker, it would then require Veffels to convey it much larger than are thofe of the Lymphatics, and confequently they would be fubject to our Obfervation or Infpection.

§. 119. That the Chyle is thus diluted in the mefenteric Glands, will more evidently appear, if we confider, that thefe *hollow* [1] Glands are every where fupplied with Arteries, diftributed up and down in a particular manner, and not wound up in a Bundle; that they are alfo fupplied with many Nerves, and receive the Lymphatics, with their Lymph, from many *Vifcera* of the *Abdomen*; which mixing with the Chyle in thefe Glands, dilutes it, and renders it more fluid; the Chyle may alfo be diluted in thefe Glands by a thin Humour, feparated from the Extremities of the Arteries, diftributed in their Cavities; which feems probable, from the Experiment of *Cowper*, who tells us, that *Mercury* injected by the mefenteric Arteries entered the Lacteals.

[1] The Structure of thefe Glands has been much controverted by Anatomifts. *Nuck* will have them to be of a reticular Texture, bound up in a common Integument. *Malpighius* fuppofes Follicles or Cells interfperfed between the reticular Texture of Fibres, which arife from the common external and ftrong Membrane which inveft thefe Glands, which Cells he tells us are cover'd with the fmall Arteries diftributed upon their Membranes; he fuppofes thefe Cells receive and retain a Liquor, which is difcharged by the excretory Ducts in thefe Glands

into

into the Lacteals of the fecond Order. *Ruyfch* informs us in his later Obfervations, that many fmall Arteries enter the mefenteric Glands, and being diftributed into exceeding fmall Branches, terminate at their ultimate Divifion in fmall fpherical Bodies like Grapes, which he alfo takes to be fmall Veffels. The Opinion of *Malpighius* and *Ruyfch* appear not to be repugnant to each other; but there feems to be fomething concealed in their Structure, which we have never yet been able to difcover; however, it is more than probable that the mefenteric Arteries difcharge a Liquor at their Extremities, which mixes with the Chyle, or elfe there would be no neceffity for fuch a Number of them to be diftributed to fo fmall Glands; which is alfo fupported by *Cowper*'s Experiment; by which it appears that there is a free Paffage thro' the mefenteric Arteries into the Lacteals. But there has been alfo particular Veins lately difcovered by *Ruyfch*, and defcribed in his excellent anatomical Collections, delineated in a Copper Plate, which he added in a Letter to myfelf; thefe Veins pafs under the mefenteric Glands, and feem to carry back the fuperfluous Part of the nutritious Blood.

§. 120. The Chyle is therefore not only retarded, *mixed together* [1], and diluted in thefe Glands; but it is alfo probable, that it is further attenuated by the addition of a Fluid difcharged from the *Nerves* [2].

[1] It is fhook together and mixed by the Contraction of the external fibrous Coat, by the Vibrations of the Arteries and external Preffure; which *Nuck* fuppofes to be the principal, if not the only Office of the mefenteric Glands.

[2] It

2 It is obfervable that there are many Nerves diftributed in the Mefentery, but they cannot be for Senfation, for that Part has hardly the common Senfe of feeling; nor can they be for mufcular Motion, which has no place here, but are all wove into a large *Plexus*, the moft confiderable in the *Abdomen*, well defcribed by *Winflow*, feated in the middle of the Mefentery, and largely expanded throughout the fame: Therefore as thefe Nerves do not appear to be fubfervient to the fore-mention'd Ufes, there is room to fufpect that they difcharge a Fluid into the Glands by their ultimate Branches, which mixing with the Chyle, renders it more Fluid, and fit for Nutrition.

§. 121. The larger lacteal Veffels *uniting* [1] again beyond the mefenteric Glands, proceed towards the *Receptacle* [2] of the Chyle at the Loins, opening into the fame by a triple Orifice; by which is alfo difcharg'd a large Quantity of *Lymph* [3] convey'd by the lymphatic Veffels from almoft all the Parts below the *Diaphragm*, as into a common Channel.

[1] Notwithftanding thefe are larger, or lefs ramified, they are rather more plentifully fupplied with Valves than thofe of the firft Order; which was neceffary, to diminifh the Refiftance of the Chyle, as the propelling Force of the Inteftines becomes lefs.

[2] This Receptacle is formed by the Union of three or four of the laft or largeft Lacteals, as *Cant* demonftrates, who firft gave a good Defcription of this Part; tho' it is fometimes formed of but one or two Lacteals, varying according to the Number of larger Veffels proceeding to the Receptacle,

tacle, which are fometimes more, and fometimes lefs ; but the fmall Glands of *Bartholin* are Collections or Convolutions of innumerable lymphatic Veffels.

3 The Lymph of almoft all the *Vifcera* of the *Abdomen* and inferior Limbs, which makes no inconfiderable Quantity ; for if two Ounces of Blood are expell'd by the Heart at each Contraction, and but one 16th Part of the whole Mafs be taken as Lymph, it will eafily appear, that as 7200 Ounces of Blood pafs thro' the Heart in an Hour, the Quantity of Lymph in that time will be 4 or 500 Ounces, or above 37 Pounds ; but that Quantity of Lymph much exceeds the Chyle difcharg'd into this Receptacle, whence it is greatly diluted, and more eafily affimilated. Thefe lymphatic Veffels have been chiefly defcrib'd by *Nuck,* whofe Tables have been wrong efteem'd fpurious, for I have a hundred times feen all the Lymphatics fpread upon a Table ; to do which, that expert Anatomift inferts a fmall fharp pointed Tube of Steel into one of the leaft Lymphatics, by which he injects Mercury amalgamed with Lead or Tin, fo as to congeal when in the Veffels ; by this means he compofed a complete Hiftory of all the lymphatic Veffels, a fair Specimen of which laborious Performance he has given us in his *Adenographia* where he has accurately defcribed the lymphatic Veffels, as the Blood-Veffels are ufually by other Anatomifts ; but Death too foon deprived us of that excellent Anatomift, to the great Damage of the Science.

§. 122. And that this is the conftant Courfe of the Chyle and Lymph, is apparent from the *Valves* 1 in the Lacteals, and Experiments

made

made with *Ligatures* 2, as well as from various *Diseases* 3, of the Lymphatics.

1 Which prevent the Passage of the Chyle, Water, or Mercury, from the Receptacle downwards towards the Intestines, but easily admit those Fluids from the Intestines towards the Receptacle; so that the *Receptaculum Chyli* is a sort of Heart or Foutain-head of all the Lymph of the *Abdomen.*

2 Which being made upon the Lymphatics, cause them to swell between the Ligature and their Extremities, or Parts from whence they arise, but to become flaccid in that Part between the Ligature and Receptacle. If the Abdomen of a living Animal be expeditiously open'd, and a Ligature made about the *Pancreas Asellii,* if warm Water be then injected into the *Abdomen,* the lymphatic Vessels will be very turgid and conspicuous; but if the Ligature be removed, they quickly become flaccid, and disappear. In like manner, to demonstrate the Lymphatics of the Head, a Ligature is made about the jugular Veins, as it was about the Receptacle of the Chyle, in order to demonstrate the Lymphatics of the *Abdomen.* To this we may add, that if a Mastiff Dog be strangled, so as not to be quite dead, by opening the left Cavity of his *Thorax,* and pressing with the Finger upon the thoracic Duct, when discover'd, it swells below the Finger, so as to be near bursting, and many of the lymphatic Vessels are by that means render'd conspicuous; but in this Operation the Anatomist should be provided with several Sponges, some dipt in Water, others in Spirit of Vitriol, to wash out the extravasated Blood, and prevent a fresh Afflux. Add to this, that if a small Tube be inserted into a lymphatic Vessel, and Air be inflated thereby, or some Liquor

quor injected; it will pass into the *Cava* and Heart, and describe the Course of the Blood ; but if the Air and Liquor be injected towards the smaller Branches of the Lymphatic, it will find no Passage, by meeting with a Resistance from the Valves.

³ In the *Morbus Regius*, which is a kind of Jaundice, almost all the Glands in the Body are obstructed and tumified, attended with a slow Consumption. Upon opening Bodies diseased with this Disorder, the mesenteric Glands are usually found schirrous, which obstructing the Course of the Chyle, cause a Consumption ; and by denying a Passage to the Lymph, occasions a Distention or Rupture of its Vessels, whence proceeds one of the worse Kinds of Dropsy, termed *Ascites.*

§. 123. This lymphatic Juice, or Lymph, consists of the purest, most aqueous, and spirituous or subtle Parts of the arterial Blood, and is impregnated with the most volatile of its Salts ; as appears from the Nature of its secretory and excretory Organs, and from its sensible Qualities.

The Action of the thoracic Duct upon the Chyle.

§. 124. WHEN the Chyle has been diluted with the Lymph discharged into the Receptacle, and separated from all the Parts below the *Diaphragm*, it is then, by the foremention'd Causes (§. 113.) and especially

cially by the Contraction of the *Diaphragm* 1
and Pulsation of the *Aorta* 2, pressed into and
thro' the thoracic *Duct* 3 of *Pecquet*; which
being full of Valves, ascends a little above its
Insertion, and then dips down into the *right* 4
or left subclavian Vein (usually the last) opening in the 'Space between the external and internal Jugulars, and discharges the Chyle and
Lymph, into the venal Blood of the *Subclavian* and *Cava*, by two semilunar *Valves* 5;
which meeting together, form an oblong Aperture or Slit, admitting the Chyle by a small
Stream into the Vein, but preventing any Return of the venal Blood in the Thoracic Duct,
into which is also discharged all the *Lymph* 6
from all Parts of the *Thorax*, whether *Viscus*,
Membrane, or Muscle; as all the Lymph of
the *Abdomen* was discharged into the Receptacle.

1 As the Receptacle of the Chyle is lodg'd upon
the *Vertebræ* of the Loins, between the muscular
Crura of the *Diaphragm*, it must necessarily be
compressed, and its Contents discharged at every
Contraction of that Muscle in Respiration; but as
the Chyle cannot pass downward by that Pressure,
being prevented by the Valves, the Pressure of the
Diaphragm will exert all its Force in propelling
the Chyle upward into and thro' the thoracic Duct,
which will be still promoted by the 2 *Diastole* of the
Aorta, by the side of which the thoracic Duct is
connected, and ascends.

3 The thoracic Duct was first described by *Eustachius* in a Horse; after him it was first discover'd
by *Pecquet* in a Dog, who by compressing the Mesentery,

fentery, perceived the Chyle pafs through a fmall
Channel in the *Thorax*, and from thence into the
Vein which in the Dog anfwers to the fubclavian
in Men; but as that Animal is deftitute of Clavicles, the Veins are only denominated axillary.
The fame Duct was alfo delineated by him as it
appeared in Dogs; but *Vanhorne* and *Bartholin*
were the firft that defcribed it in a human Body;
and fince *Cantius* has lately delineated it by large
and neat Figures.

⁴ The Defcriptions of Anatomifts vary with regard to the Infertion of the thoracic Duct, Nature
herfelf not always obferving the fame Rules therein; for the thoracic Duct has been obferved to
open into either of the fubclavian Veins; it generally divides itfelf in the upper Part of the *Thorax*,
and uniting again at the fecond *Vertebra*, it afcends
a little above its Infertion, and is then inflected
downward to its Opening in the fubclavian Vein,
into which it is inferted by a double Valve, like
the *Inteftinum Illium*, into the *Colon*; and not with
a fingle Valve, as it has been figur'd by *Lower*
from Brutes. Provident Nature has taken care to
place this Duct in a Part of the *Thorax* where it is
in no danger of being compreffed or wounded by
external Injuries, which would foon put a Period
to Life; as we learn from the Experiment of
Lower, who lacerating the thoracic Duct in a Dog,
obferved that the Animal perifhed in a few Days,
notwithftanding he was fupplied with the beft
Food; and, upon opening him, his *Thorax* was
found replete with Chyle.

⁵ The Aperture of the Valve at the Infertion of
the thoracic Duct is difpofed in a different manner
from the reft of the Valves in the Veins, being in
the Figure of a half Moon, fo as to entirely clofe
up the Mouth of the thoracic Duct; and being

A a   preffed

preffed together by the Blood in its Paffage to the Heart thro the fubclavian Vein, it will not admit any Part thereof into the Duct; but being a little way opened by the Chyle preffed thro' the thoracic Duct by the fore-mention'd Forces, it admits that Fluid, with the Lymph that accompanies it, into the Blood.

[6] The whole Mafs of Lymph, which is feparated from the *Vifcera*, and other Parts of the *Thorax*, is all difcharg'd into this Duct; upon tying which all the lymphatic Veffels of the *Thorax* become turgid and diftended with Lymph; it being deny'd a Paffage into the Duct. There muft certainly be fome material Reafon why the Creator fhould rather caufe all the Chyle in Quadrupeds to afcend into the Blood by one large Duct, rather than let it be abforbed by the numerous fmall Veins of the Mefentery; and the moft probable Reafon for this Mechanifm feems to be, that the Chyle fhould receive a large Quantity of Lymph before it enters the Blood, in order to dilute and attenuate it; otherwife it might be apt to produce Obftructions in the fmall Veffels of the Lungs, and occafion a *Peripneumony*, or Inflammation of that *Vifcus*.

§. 125. Thus we are acquainted with the Means by which fo large Quantities of Chyle and Lymph are eafily convey'd thro' this *narrow* [1], crooked, and perpendicular Duct (which in part is, and may with eafe be totally *compreffed* [2]) into the Blood, and that even when a Man is in an erect Pofture. Thefe Means will fufficiently appear, if we confider, 1. The contractile Power of the Inteftines, together with the Means (§. 103, 104, 86.) which affift the Expulfion of the Chyle out of them into the Lacteals.

&teals. 2. The *Valves* 3 in the Lacteals, Receptacle, and thoracic Duct, which are admirably adapted to take off the perpendicular Weight, and *expedite* 4 the Paſſage of the Chyle thro' them. 3. The Impulſe of the meſenteric Arteries, which either interſect or run parallel with the Lacteals in the Meſentery. 4. The ſtrong and alternate Preſſure of the abdominal Muſcles being returned by the *Peritonæum* 5 upon the ſoft, *thin* 6, and lax Membranes of the Meſentery, inveſting the Lacteals; together with, 5. The like Preſſure of the *Diaphragm* upon the Receptacle. 6. The ſtrong and conſtant contractile *Niſus* of the Membranes, conſtituting the thoracic Duct itſelf, which appears to be *conſiderable* 7 by its Contraction, even after Death. 7. The ſtrong and inceſſant Pulſation of the *Aorta* 8, which aſcends by the Side of the thoracic Duct, and laſtly, 8. The Action of the Lungs and *Thorax* in Reſpiration.

¹ Small, if compar'd with the Quantity of Chyle and Lymph paſſing thro' it; which would be too large for this Duct, if it was not preſſed forward with a conſiderable Force and Velocity.

² The thoracic Duct is preſſed by the whole Weight of the Atmoſphere dilating the Lungs, which is ſufficient to ſuſtain a Column of Water in a Tube 32 Foot high, and a perpendicular Column of Mercury to the height of about 30 Inches; but the *Thorax* is fulleſt at the time of Inſpiration, when there is no Space left between the Lungs and the Ribs, and therefore the thoracic Duct muſt of neceſſity be compreſſed by the Lungs expanded

with

with Air in Infpiration; and even when the weight
of the Air is nothing in Expiration, it is preffed
by the Pulfation of the *Aorta*, &c.

³ Which Valves fuftain the Weight of the Chyle,
that it might not be thereby forc'd downward lower than the next fubjacent Valve, which will by its
Elafticity re-act, and return the Force from the
perpendicular Preffure upon the Chyle again ;
which, with the external Preffure, will caufe it to
afcend.   It is an Affertion of *Bilfius*, that the Chyle
is diftributed from the thoracic Duct, as from a
Fountain, to the Breafts, and all Parts of the Body ; but he afterwards refutes his own Notions in
his Commentary on the Valves.

⁴ The Velocity with which the Air rufhes into
a *Vacuum*, has been formerly demonftrated by
Pappin ; its Force has been alfo by me demonftrated to be twice equal to the fwifteft Wind, which
according to *Marriotte* runs 22 Feet in a Second ;
the Chyle will therefore run with a great Celerity
in the thoracic Duct, fince that Tube is divided
into fo many void Interftices as it hath intercepting Valves; therefore if one Interftice be empty'd,
the Chyle will flow into it from the fecond with a
great Velocity ; and fo from the third into the fecond, &c. fucceffively ; which fwift Motion was
neceffary, to prevent the Chyle from running into
Concretions before it had arrived into the fmall
Veffels of the Lungs.

⁵ The Mefentery is not ftretch'd down pendulous by the Weight of the Inteftines, nor the Cavity of the *Abdomen* empty, as fome have falfely
imagin'd; but the whole lower *Venter* is quite full,
and all its *Vifcera* compreffed.   If one inferts their
Finger at a Wound of the *Abdomen*, which has
been by Accident inflicted upon a healthy Perfon,
the Finger will be compreffed with a greater Force
than

than one would imagine. In Infpiration the *Dia-phragm* preffes down all the *Vifcera* with a confide-rable Force towards the *Pelvis,* and there again preffed upward by the abdominal Mufcles in Expi-ration, and therefore the Lacteals will be compref-fed by both ; and thus the Chyle will be propell'd thro' them, partly by the Contraction of the In-teftines themfelves, and partly by the Preffure of the circumjacent Parts.

⁶ Which, if it be not over-diftended with Fat, communicates the whole Preffure which it receives to the fubjacent Lacteals.

⁷ Its conftituent Membranes are thin, but ela-ftic ; for in a Body which has been not long froze to death, the thoracic Duct, which a little before appeared diftended with Chyle, becomes the next Moment contracted, pellucid, and entirely empti-ed, fo as to difappear from the Eyes of the Spe-ctators.

⁸ Which is by fome eftimated to be more than equal to 100 Weight ; to this we may add, that we have feen a Juggler at a Fair, who lying upon his Back, laid a heavy Anvil of Iron upon his Breaft, which might be fenfibly perceiv'd to afcend at every Contraction of his Heart.

§. 126. The Effects therefore which the Chyle fuffers in its Paffage from the Inteftines into the venal Blood, will appear reducible to the four following Heads, to which they may be referr'd, as

1. The Slownefs of its Motion thro' the Inte-ftines, Lacteals, and mefenteric Glands; which is demonftrable from the great Length of the firft, when ftript from the Mefentery, and

from the Number and Minutes of the two laſt: The Effects of all which muſt be a Digeſtion and *Depuration* [1] of the Chyle from its groſſer Parts.

2. The Motion and Preſſure communicated externally to the Veſſels, and by the Veſſels to their contained Fluids; the Effects of which are, a Protruſion, Attenuation, and Mixture of the Chyle, with a Preſervation of its Fluidity. Here we ſhou'd conſider, (1.) The Poſition of the Lacteals, which gradually increaſe in Size, are all furniſhed with Valves, and frequently open into each other; then recede, and preſently after unite again *(per* §. 116.) (2.) The ſtrong Preſſure of the *Diaphragm* and Muſcles of the *Abdomen*, with its compreſſed *Viſcera*, being returned upon the Lacteal Veſſels, which run almoſt on the outſide of the Meſentery, with hardly any Covering (§. 86.) (3.) The degree of *Heat* [2] and Moiſture adminiſter'd to the Chyle, moſt apt to promote Digeſtion, and produce Effects well known and obſerved by the Chemiſts. And (4.) The conſtant Pulſation of the *Aorta* on the thoracic Duct, and of the meſenteric Arteries upon the Lacteals, moſt of the laſt running cloſe by each other; ſo as to receive a vibratory Motion.

3. The Dilution of the Chyle, by mixing with, (1.) all the *Lymph* [3] of almoſt the whole Body; (2.) with the moiſt Dew or *Vapours* [4] in the *Abdomen*, which is chiefly abſorbed by the Lymphatics leading to the Receptacle; and we may add, (3.) that the Juice of the *Nerves* [5], mixing

mixing with the Lymph in all its conglobate Glands, contributes much to dilute and attenuate the Chyle.

4. The *Affimilation* [6] of the Chyle, to render it fit to circulate thro' all Parts of the Body, before it enters the venal Blood; which is done by meeting and mixing with various Humours, in its Paffage from the Mouth to the fubclavian Vein. (1.) It is gradually and fucceffively fupplied and digefted with Juices, which have been before elaborated in, and often circulated thro' all the Veffels diftributed throughout the *Body* [7]; as the *Saliva* and *Mucus* of the Mouth, Lymph and *Mucus* of the *Oefophagus,* Stomach, Inteftines, pancreatic Juice, cyftic and hepatic Bile, the Lymph from all Parts of the Body; and probably the Juice from the fmall Nerves in the lymphatic Glands of all Parts. (2.) And laftly, it is accurately mix'd and attenuated by the united Force of the whole chylopoietic Machine, which contributes to thofe Effects by the Figure, Difpofition, and Motion of its feveral Parts and Veffels.

[1] By the great Length of the Inteftines, the folid and excrementitious Part of the Chyle is retained and feparated, by their numerous Turnings, from the more fluid and uniform Part. The Chyle is found by Experience to be 24 or 30 Hours in its Paffage thro' the Inteftines, whereas it is not above 10 or 12 in paffing the Lacteals; for upon opening an Animal eight Hours after a Meal, the Lacteals are found diftended with Chyle; but the

next day after they will appear to contain nothing but an excrementitious Lymph. The longer the Food is retained in the Inteſtines, the more Chyle is drawn off from it by the Lacteals ; and that its Stay there is ſometimes very conſiderable, may appear from a healthy Man living at *Delph*, who did not go to ſtool oftner than once in 16 Days.

² Nature often produces Effects by a ſmall Force, which cannot be produc'd by more violent Means ; thus all Animals are bred and brought to Perfection in a Heat of 94 Degrees; and it is not probable that there are any Animals whoſe Heat exceeds that of the human Body, ſince a human Heart bears a greater Proportion to the reſt of the Body than the Heart of an Ox, &c. All Vegetables are nouriſh'd and brought to Perfection by a Heat ſtill leſs than the fore-mentioned Degree ; it being the Property of a Heat like that of the human Body, to attenuate all animal and vegetable Juices, and diſſolve them into exceeding ſmall Particles, ſo as to form a ſubtil Liquor ; which Heat has uſually a greater Effect, in proportion as the Juices are retained in a more cloſe Place. We ſee by a Heat of 94 Degrees, the thick White of an Egg is in the Space of 22 Days ſufficiently attenuated to enter into and form the ſubtil Humours of the Chick.

³ All the Lymph of the *Abdomen* is convey'd to the Receptacle of the Chyle, as that of the *Thorax* is into the thoracic Duct, while the Lymph which comes from the Head and Neck, is alſo diſcharg'd either into the thoracic Duct, or into the adjacent jugular Veins. This Lymph is eaſily diſtinguiſhable from the Chyle by its external Appearance and reddiſh Hue ; and being much thinner than the Chyle, it dilutes the ſame, and renders it more eaſily convertible into animal Juices. This Lymph which is mix'd with the Chyle, is compos'd both

of

of that Lymph which is feparated from the lymphatic Arteries, and of all thofe Juices in the human Body, which are of a more fubtil Confiftence
than the Lymph itfelf. Some indeed deny the Exiftence of thefe lymphatic Arteries, becaufe their
Eyes will not convince them ; even the Microfcope will but juft exhibit the fmalleft of the red
or fanguiferous Arteries, which being much larger,
and conveying a colour'd Liquor, are more confpicuous ; whereas the lymphatic Arteries, which are
fo much fmaller, and convey a pellucid Liquor,
whofe Globules are 6 times fmaller than thofe of the
Blood, cannot be render'd vifible to the Eye, tho'
armed with that Inftrument. The other Part of the
Lymph, compofed of thofe Juices in the Body,
which are thinner than the Blood, will alfo appear
to be confiderable ; for all the animal Juices feparated from the Blood, return again into the Circulation, except what is difcharged by the Kidneys
and Skin ; all the other Juices return again from
their Sources by the reductory Veins : And if there
are any other Veins befides thofe which convey
Blood, they muft be the valvular Lymphatics ;
the return'd Juices are therefore convey'd by the
Lymphatics to, and mix'd with the Chyle.

⁴ *Hippocrates* diftinguifh'd the folid Parts of the
human Body into Cavities and Veffels ; the Cavities in a healthy Body, he fays, are full of Vapours,
but in a difeafed Body full of fharp Humours, or
Ichor. And it is certain that all the Cavities and
Interftices in the human Body are fupplied with a
warm and moift Vapour, which renders the Membranes and mufcular Fibres pliable and fit for motion, and prevents them from adhering to each
other. But this Vapour is never difcharg'd in fuch
Quantities as to turn into Liquor, and prove offenfive ; for upon opening the *Thorax* or *Abdomen*

of

of a living Brute, nothing but a Vapour exhales, without any Water remaining ; this Vapour muft therefore return again into the Blood, which it can do by no other Veffels that we are yet acquainted with, than the lymphatic Veins. Dogs have a communicating Paffage from their Teſticles into the Cavity of their *Abdomen* ; which is not found in Men. *Nuck* therefore wounded the *Scrotum* of a Dog, and injected a Pound of Water thereby into the Cavity of the *Abdomen*, fewing up the Wound after the Operation ; the Dog afterwards voided all the Water by Urine within the Space of three Days, fo that no Part thereof was found remaining in the *Abdomen* ; there muſt therefore be an open and continued Paffage from the Cavity of the *Abdomen* to the Receptacle of the Chyle. The warm and fubtil Vapour which is natural to the Body, will be therefore much more eafily admitted by the fame Veffels, tho' its Quantity be not inconfiderable ; which is argued by the Largenefs of the Cavities which are moiften'd therewith, as thofe of the *Pelvis, Scrotum, Abdomen, Thorax, Pericardium, Cranium,* Ventricles of the Brain, Cavity of the Lungs, Stomach, Inteftines, &c. The fame is alfo argued from the fudden Increafe of a Dropfy, where the Veffels are not affected, but only the Abforption of this Vapour obftructed. As this Vapour therefore appears to be fo copious, it muſt have no fmall Share with the other Part of the Lymph in affimilating the Chyle, and rendring it more eafily convertible into Blood and other Juices proper to the human Body.

    ⁵ The nervous Juice, which we fuppofe to be mixed with the Lymph, muſt be very much fubtiliz'd by paffing thro' the many Series of the fmalleſt Veffels before it enters the fmaller Cavities of the Nerves ; but we do not propofe this as certain,

                       but

but probable, as we are not led thereto by the full
Evidence of our Senses and Experiments, but
barely by Reason and Analogy.

‘ The human Body would never continue in that
State in which it appears, if it was not to be constantly repair'd and renew'd ; which is perform'd
by Assimilation, or the Conversion of the crude
and foreign Parts of the Chyle into animal Solids
and Fluids of our own Nature. To facilitate this
Change or Conversion of the Aliment, provident
Nature has cautiously supplied the Chyle with a
large Quantity of a Fluid, partaking of all the
Juices in the Body, except the Blood; that it might
not be pour'd crude into the Veins: thus the Chyle
contains a Quantity of Bile capable of being again
separated under the Form of that Juice; a Quantity of *Saliva*, which will again return by the salival
Glands ; and so of the Lymph, &c. insomuch that
the crude Part of the Chyle will be little or nothing
comparatively, and almost lost in the large Quantity of Juices which are already proper to the
Animal ; as a little Vinegar loses its Strength in a
large Quantity of Honey.

‘ We need not wonder that a Pound of vegetable Juices should be converted from their own Nature into animal Substance, if we consider that it
mixes with above 24 Pounds of animal Juices,
with which it is intimately mixed and digested in
its Passage from the Mouth before it reaches the
venal Blood. Were the nutritious Juices of our
Food to be conveyed into the Blood without this
Mixture, they would be destructive rather than
preservative to the Animal ; as may appear from
the Diseases which are so frequent and epidemical
in these Parts soon after the yearly Charity of di-
stributing Food to the Poor. But the Principal of
these animal Juices is the Bile, a kind of liquid

Soap,

Soap, fo acrimonious, that Nature could not prepare it in any of the Veſſels, but digeſts it in a diſtinct Cell, the Gall-bladder, where it becomes
thicker and ſtronger by its Stay and Heat of the
Party ; nor do I believe there is any ſincere Bile
contained in any of the other Veſſels in the whole
human Body.

127. If we now examine the Subſtance of
the Chyle when arriv'd thus far, we ſhall find
it conſiſt of all thoſe Principles which compoſe
Blood ; as *Water* [1], Spirit, Oil and Salts, intimately mix'd and united together.

[1] All theſe Principles are alſo contained in the
Food itſelf, of which the Chyle is formed. In this
Place it ſeems of Importance to take notice of
Lewenhoeck's Obſervations, that all the nutritious
Juices, upon which we live, are compoſed of ſmall
Globules, which are uſually larger than thoſe of the
Blood, but of a laxer Texture, and more eaſily di-
viſible. When theſe Juices of our Food have been
converted into Chyle, there then appears to be but
few of the larger Globules, but a great Number of
the ſmaller, into which the larger ſeem to have been
diſſolved ; theſe by their greater Tenuity are more
eaſily abſorbed by the Veſſels, and paſs more freely
thro' them ; it then remains that theſe ſmaller Globules be united into larger and more compact ones,
like thoſe of the Blood, after the Chyle has arriv'd
into the ſecond Paſſages, or Blood-Veſſels. The
uniform Nature of the Chyle is apparent from its
ſenſible Qualities, its ſmooth or even Taſte and
Fluidity, the ſpherical Figure of its Particles, it
being inodorous, &c.

§. 128. Nor

§. 128. Nor is it furprifing that *Diforders* ᵗ fo feldom happen in the Mefentery, notwith-ftanding it feems to be greatly fubjected to ob-ftruction, and its Confequences, from its Veffels being the firft that receive the crude Chyle; to prevent which, Nature has every where ufed the ftricteft Precaution.

ᵗ Even in old Men of 90 Years of Age the Me-fentery generally appears found and entire, except that its Glands are ufually fhrunk or contracted. And the Chyle itfelf is a fubtil Liquor, that has un-dergone many Depurations, is abforbed by the fmall-eft Veffels, and does not ftagnate, but is conftant-ly protruded with a confiderable Force and Velo-city thro' the Lacteals, by the Action of the *Dia-phragm* and *Aorta*, its Paffage being ftill promo-ted by the numerous Valves in the Lacteals; not to mention the Efficacy of the Vapours, in which the Mefentery is fufpended in the *Abdomen*, to prevent and diffipate Obftructions. But notwith-ftanding all this Provifion of Nature, Obftructions are often formed in the Mefentery, either from a Coagulation of the Chyle, or Concretion of thofe Parts in the fmalleft Veffels, which had been dif-folved in the Inteftines, promoted by a weak Ha-bit and inactive Life; by which means the Chyle, not being propelled forward with a proper Force, ftagnates, concretes together, and while its more fluid Part is drained off, the Remainder has been fometimes obferved to put on a ftony Confift-ence; whence ftrumous Glands of the Mefentery and Pancreas, which frequently occur in thofe who are fubject to Strumofity of the Glands in the Throat; but ftrumous Glands of the Neck are not to be efteemed either the Caufe or Effect of

ftrumous

ftrumous Glands in the Mefentery, tho' they are
ufual Companions, and proceed from the fame latent Caufe.

§. 129. We are from hence alfo informed,
that the thoracic Duct ferves not only to convey the Chyle, but alfo the *Lymph* [1] into the
Blood, and perhaps a Part of the nervous Juice;
upon which account I frequently call the thoracic Duct the *Vena Cava* [2] of the Lymph,
from its fimilitude to that Veffel; for as the
one returns all the Blood mixed together towards the Heart, fo, this returns the Chyle,
Lymph, and all the more fubtil Juices; hence
in dead Subjects, after fafting, this Duct re-
fembles a large Lymphatic fill'd with a pellucid
Liquor.

[1] The Lacteals convey Chyle to the Quantity of
a Pound or two, only during the time of Digeftion; at other times they are pellucid, not differing
from the Lymphatics, as they then only return the
Saliva, Juices of the Stomach and Inteftines, with
the thin hepatic Bile and infipid Juice of the *Pancreas*. In long fafting, the Lacteals and their
Orifices are kept open, and from clofing, by the
Return of thefe Juices, and the great Quantity
of Lymph which is that way conftantly returned
into the Blood; which was the more neceffary, as
empty Veffels in the human Body quickly collapfe
and grow together.

[2] As being the common reductory Channel of
all the Juices in the human Body, which are thinner than the Blood itfelf. This Duct is much fmaller
than the fanguiferous *Vena Cava*, becaufe it was
neceffary

neceſſary that the Chyle ſhould paſs thro' it with a greater Velocity than the Blood thro' the former.

§. 130. Having thus traced the Paſſage of Chyle into the Veins; in order to underſtand its further Progreſs and Changes, it will be neceſſary to conſider the Circulation of the Blood, with which it now mixes, and the Conſequences thereof; which we ſhall therefore make the Subject of our next Diſcourſe.

The Chyle now pours itſelf into the purple Ocean of the Blood, and never after appears ſeparately under any other Form or Name but that of Milk, which is found circulating in the Veins of live Animals about three or four Hours after a Meal, retaining its white Colour diſtinct, according to the Obſervation of *Lower.*

F I N I S.

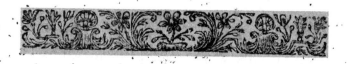

BOOKS printed for WILLIAM INNYS, in Pater-Noster-Row.

1. **B**Oerhaave's Aphorisms concerning the Knowledge and Cure of Diseases, translated from the last Edition, printed in Latin at Leyden, 1728. with useful Observations and Explanations. By J. Delacoste, M. D. 8vo.

2. Herman Boerhaave's Materia Medica: Or, a Series of Prescriptions adapted to the Sections of his practical Aphorisms concerning the Knowledge and Cure of Diseases; translated from the Latin Original of the last genuine Edition of the Author, 8vo. 1741.

3. Pharmacopœia Edinburgensis: Or, the Dispensatory of the Royal College of Physicians in Edinburgh; translated and improved from the fourth Edition of the Latin, and illustrated with Notes. By Peter Shaw, M. D. The fifth Edition, with Additions, 1746.

4. Pharmacopœia Bateana: Or, Bates's Dispensatory; translated from the last Edition of the Latin Copy, published by Mr. James Shipton; containing his choice and select Recipe's, their Names, Compositions, Preparations, Virtues, Uses and Doses, as they are applicable to the whole Practice of Physic and Chirurgery; the Arcana Goddardiana, and their Recipe's, interspersed in their proper Places, which are almost all wanting in the Latin Copy; compleated with above 600 chymical Processes, and their Explications at large, various Observations thereon, and a Rationale upon each Process. To which are added, the fam'd Dr. Goddard's Drops, Ruffel's Powder, Rabell's styptic Powder, Tinctura de Sulphure Metallorum, and the Emplastrum Febrifugium. The fifth Edition. By William Salmon, M. D. 1720.

5. Pharmacopœia Extemporanea: Or, a Body of Medicines, containing a thousand select Precepts, answering most Intentions of Cure; to which are added useful Scholia, a Catalogue of Remedies, and a copious Index for the Assistance of young Physicians The third Edition with Additions, by the Author Tho. Fuller, M. D. 8vo. 1740.

6. Pharmacopœia Domestica: Or, the Family Dispensatory, with Remarks on the Composition, and an Explanation of their Virtues, designed for the Use of Physicians in the Country. By the late Tho. Fuller, M. D. in 8vo.

9 781014 428936